The doctrine of fluxions, founded on Sir Isaac Newton's method, published by himself in his tract upon the quadrature of curves. By James Hodgson, ...

James Hodgson

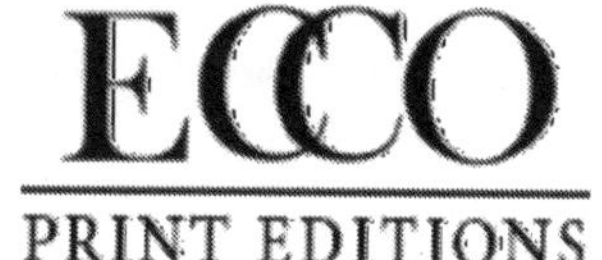

The doctrine of fluxions, founded on Sir Isaac Newton's method, published by himself in his tract upon the quadrature of curves. By James Hodgson, ...
Hodgson, James
ESTCID: T111669
Reproduction from British Library
With an index.
London : printed by T. Wood, for the author: sold by W. Mount and T. Page: W. Innys and R. Manby: B. Motte and C. Bathurst: J. Clarke, and J. Stagg, 1736.
xvi,452,[12]p. : ill. ; 4°

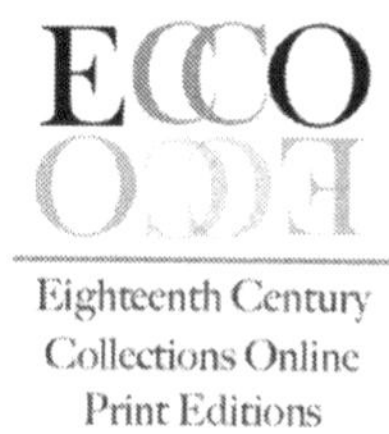

Gale ECCO Print Editions

Relive history with *Eighteenth Century Collections Online*, now available in print for the independent historian and collector. This series includes the most significant English-language and foreign-language works printed in Great Britain during the eighteenth century, and is organized in seven different subject areas including literature and language; medicine, science, and technology; and religion and philosophy. The collection also includes thousands of important works from the Americas.

The eighteenth century has been called "The Age of Enlightenment." It was a period of rapid advance in print culture and publishing, in world exploration, and in the rapid growth of science and technology – all of which had a profound impact on the political and cultural landscape. At the end of the century the American Revolution, French Revolution and Industrial Revolution, perhaps three of the most significant events in modern history, set in motion developments that eventually dominated world political, economic, and social life.

In a groundbreaking effort, Gale initiated a revolution of its own: digitization of epic proportions to preserve these invaluable works in the largest online archive of its kind. Contributions from major world libraries constitute over 175,000 original printed works. Scanned images of the actual pages, rather than transcriptions, recreate the works ***as they first appeared.***

Now for the first time, these high-quality digital scans of original works are available via print-on-demand, making them readily accessible to libraries, students, independent scholars, and readers of all ages.

For our initial release we have created seven robust collections to form one the world's most comprehensive catalogs of 18th century works.

Initial Gale ECCO Print Editions collections include:

> ***History and Geography***
> Rich in titles on English life and social history, this collection spans the world as it was known to eighteenth-century historians and explorers. Titles include a wealth of travel accounts and diaries, histories of nations from throughout the world, and maps and charts of a world that was still being discovered. Students of the War of American Independence will find fascinating accounts from the British side of conflict.

Social Science

Delve into what it was like to live during the eighteenth century by reading the first-hand accounts of everyday people, including city dwellers and farmers, businessmen and bankers, artisans and merchants, artists and their patrons, politicians and their constituents. Original texts make the American, French, and Industrial revolutions vividly contemporary.

Medicine, Science and Technology

Medical theory and practice of the 1700s developed rapidly, as is evidenced by the extensive collection, which includes descriptions of diseases, their conditions, and treatments. Books on science and technology, agriculture, military technology, natural philosophy, even cookbooks, are all contained here.

Literature and Language

Western literary study flows out of eighteenth-century works by Alexander Pope, Daniel Defoe, Henry Fielding, Frances Burney, Denis Diderot, Johann Gottfried Herder, Johann Wolfgang von Goethe, and others. Experience the birth of the modern novel, or compare the development of language using dictionaries and grammar discourses.

Religion and Philosophy

The Age of Enlightenment profoundly enriched religious and philosophical understanding and continues to influence present-day thinking. Works collected here include masterpieces by David Hume, Immanuel Kant, and Jean-Jacques Rousseau, as well as religious sermons and moral debates on the issues of the day, such as the slave trade. The Age of Reason saw conflict between Protestantism and Catholicism transformed into one between faith and logic -- a debate that continues in the twenty-first century.

Law and Reference

This collection reveals the history of English common law and Empire law in a vastly changing world of British expansion. Dominating the legal field is the *Commentaries of the Law of England* by Sir William Blackstone, which first appeared in 1765. Reference works such as almanacs and catalogues continue to educate us by revealing the day-to-day workings of society.

Fine Arts

The eighteenth-century fascination with Greek and Roman antiquity followed the systematic excavation of the ruins at Pompeii and Herculaneum in southern Italy; and after 1750 a neoclassical style dominated all artistic fields. The titles here trace developments in mostly English-language works on painting, sculpture, architecture, music, theater, and other disciplines. Instructional works on musical instruments, catalogs of art objects, comic operas, and more are also included.

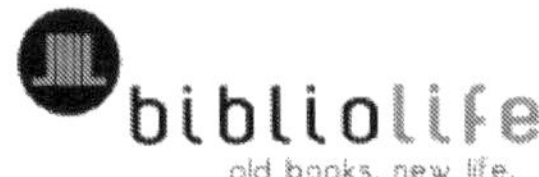
bibliolife
old books. new life.

THE DOCTRINE OF FLUXIONS,

FOUNDED ON

Sir ISAAC NEWTON's Method,

Published by HIMSELF in his TRACT

UPON THE

QUADRATURE of CURVES.

By *JAMES HODGSON*, F. R. S.
And Master of the Royal Mathematical-School in
CHRIST-HOSPITAL.

Etiamsi omnia à Veteribus inventa sunt · hoc semper Novum *erit, Usus, & Inventorum ab aliis Scientia & dispositio.*
SENEC. Epist. 64.

LONDON

Printed by T. WOOD, for the AUTHOR

Sold by W. MOUNT and T. PAGE on *Tower-hill* W. INNYS and R. MANBY in *Ludgate street* B. MOTTE and C. BATHURST at the *Middle Temple-Gate, Fleet-street* J. CLARKE under the *Royal Exchange*, and J. STAGG in *Westminster-Hall.*

MDCCXXXVI.

TO THE

ROYAL SOCIETY

Of *LONDON*,

FOUNDED BY

King CHARLES II.

For the Improvement of

NATURAL KNOWLEDGE,

And now Flourishing under the Influence
and Encouragement

Of His Sacred MAJESTY

King GEORGE II.

PATRON,

This TREATISE upon the

DOCTRINE of FLUXIONS,

Is most Humbly Dedicated, by

Their most Obedient Servant,

JAMES HODGSON.

THE

INTRODUCTION.

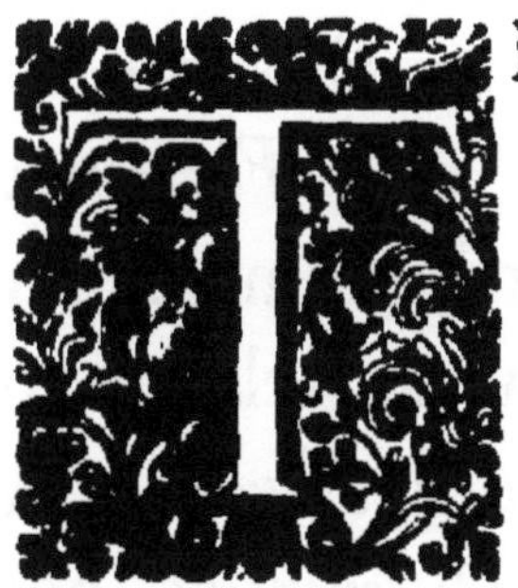

HE Deſign of publiſhing the following Treatiſe, is to introduce the true Method of *Fluxions*, moſt of the Books that have hitherto appeared upon that Subject having in them little more than the Name, the Principles upon which they have proceeded being the ſame with the *Differential Calculus*; ſo that by calling a *Differential* a *Fluxion*, and a ſecond *Differential* a ſecond *Fluxion*, *&c.* they have ſo confuſedly jumbled the Methods together, that People, who have not been throughly acquainted with them, have been led into many Miſtakes: For although the way of Inveſtigation in each be the ſame, and both center in the ſame Concluſions, yet whoever will compare the Principles, upon which the Methods are founded, will find that they are very different. The *Differential* Method teaches us to conſider Magnitudes as made up of an infinite Number of very ſmall conſtituent Parts put together; whereas the *Fluxionary* Method teaches us to conſider Magnitudes as generated by Motion. A Line is deſcribed, and in deſcribing is generated, not by an Appoſition of Points, or *Differentials*, but by the Motion, or Flux, of a Point; and that Velocity with which the generating Point moves, when the Line begins to ariſe, or in the firſt Moment of its Generation, or Formation, is called its *Fluxion*; ſo that to call a *Differential* a *Fluxion*, or a *Fluxion* a *Differential*, is an Abuſe of Terms, and an Impoſition upon the Reader; for a *Fluxion* has no Relation to a *Differential*, nor a *Differential* to a *Fluxion*; a *Fluxion* cannot be compared with a *Differential*, nor a *Differential* with a *Fluxion*, becauſe they are of a different Nature The *Fluxion* ſhews us the Law and Manner of Flowing, by which we are taught how to determine the Proportion of Magnitudes one to another, from the Celerities of the Motions by which they are generated, which is a pure and abſtracted way of Reaſoning, and agreeable to the Method made uſe of by the ancient Geometers, whereas the *Differential* being but an infinitely ſmall Part of the Magnitude itſelf, in the forming of Magnitudes after this way, we are to conceive them as made up of an infinite Number of theſe ſmall conſtituent Parts, diſpoſed of

in

in ſuch a manner, as to produce a Magnitude of a given Form; and that theſe ſmall conſtituent Parts are to each other as the Magnitudes of which they are *Differentials*, and conſequently, that one infinitely ſmall Part, or *Differential*, muſt be infinitely great, with reſpect to another infinitely ſmall Part, or *Differential*, which muſt happen when we conſider Magnitudes formed after the *Differential* Method. Theſe things being well conſider'd, it muſt be confeſs'd that the Way of conſidering the different Degrees of Magnitudes, as ariſing from an increaſing Series of Mutations of Velocity neceſſary to the Generation of the Quantities to be formed, is much more ſimple, and leſs perplexed than the other, and conſequently, all the Operations that are founded upon the Method of *Fluxions* muſt be much more clear, accurate and convincing than thoſe that are founded upon the *Differential Calculus*. In the former Method Quantities are rejected, becauſe they really vaniſh; in the latter they are rejected, becauſe they are infinitely ſmall; which cannot but leave the Mind in ſome Ambiguity or Confuſion. And therefore to treat of *Fluxions* upon *Differential* Principles, is leading the Reader quite wrong, and giving him ſuch falſe Conceptions of things, which he will, if ever, with great Difficulty get clear of; for People having been long accuſtomed to one way of conſidering things, it is not very eaſy to get over the Prepoſſeſſions, and to bring themſelves into a quite different Way.

WHAT I have here ſaid relating to the *Differential* Method, will, I hope, be no ways conſtrued as if I intended to leſſen, or depreciate that Method; far be it from me: On the contrary, I highly value and eſteem it, and always made uſe of it, 'till I became acquainted with the *Fluxionary* Method: but what I mention it here for, is to compare the two Methods together, that the Excellency of the *Fluxionary* Method above the *Differential*, may the more evidently appear; and thence to ſhew, how wrong it is to make uſe promiſcuouſly of two Methods, ſo very different in Principles, as if they were one and the ſame Method.

NOW as the Principles upon which the *Fluxionary* Method is founded are every way as ſimple as thoſe upon which the *Differential* is founded, and as eaſy to be underſtood by young Beginners, it is but Juſtice to ſet them out right at firſt, that they may not, after they have ſpent ſome Time, and made ſome Progreſs in the Science, be forced to unlearn what they have taken Pains to attain; which will always be the Caſe of thoſe who begin with the *Differential* Method, in order to learn *Fluxions*.

In the firſt *Section* you have the Arithmetick of *Exponents*; wherein, from the Nature of *Powers*, and the Manner of their Generation, I have deduced, and demonſtrated the Rules made uſe of.

In the next *Section* you have the Doctrine of *Infinite Series*; wherein is ſhewn how to extract *Roots* out of given *Powers*. And in order to prove the Truth of the Inveſtigations, it has been ſhewn how the *Roots* themſelves may be involved, ſo as to reſtore the Original *Powers*; by which Means the Learner will not only be inſtructed how to raiſe any *Multinomial* to any given *Power*, or to extract any *Root* out of the ſame, but be of himſelf able to perform what is requiſite in the Doctrine of *Series*, without having recourſe to *Series* formed or contrived for that Purpoſe.

But becauſe in raiſing *Multinomials* to high *Powers*, or extracting *Roots* of the ſame, the Operation by the former Manner is tedious, I have proceeded to ſhew how the *Binomial*, *Trinomial*, *Quadrinomial* and *Infinite Multinomial Series* may be found; and at the ſame time have ſhewn their Uſes in raiſing *Powers*, and extracting of *Roots*, whereby the Coincidences of the different Ways are ſhewn in the Production of the ſame Quantities

In the third *Section* you are told the Meaning of a *Fluxion*, and the Manner how *Mathematical Quantities* are generated; from whence the Nature of *Fluxions* in general is very amply explained: By which it will easily be perceived, that a first *Fluxion* is not *Incomprehensible*, and that it is not so difficult to form a just Idea of it in the Mind, as some have imagined.

In the fourth *Section* you have the *Notation* of *Fluxions*, or the Manner how the several Orders of *Fluxions* are distinguished one from the other. And in the next *Section* you have the *Algorithm* of first *Fluxions*, wherein the Rules are demonstrated, and illustrated with Variety of Examples

In the sixth *Section* you are taught how to find second, third, &c. *Fluxions*: wherein I have endeavoured, in a more particular Manner, to shew what is meant by second, third, &c. *Fluxions*: whence it will manifestly appear, that there is nothing *obscure* or *mysterious* in them, but that they may be as easily conceived, and as fully comprehended, as first *Fluxions*.

In the seventh *Section* are demonstrated the Rules for finding the *Fluxions* of *Exponential Quantities*: And in the eighth *Section* you have Methods for finding the *Fluents* from given *Fluxions*. After which follows their Uses in drawing *Tangents* to *Curves*; in the Soluti-

on

on of Problems *de Maximis & Minimis*; in the Invention of *Points* of *Inflection* and *Retrogression*; in the finding the *Evoluta* of a given *Curve*; in finding the *Caustick Curves* by *Reflection* and *Refraction*; in the *Rectification* of *Curves*; in finding the *Areas* of *Curvilinear Spaces*, in finding the *Values* of the *Surfaces* of *Solids*, as alſo their *Contents*; and in finding their *Centers* of *Gravity*, *Percuſſion* and *Oſcillation*; wherein I have endeavoured to render the Inveſtigations plain and eaſy And in explaining the Nature of *Fluxions*; in demonſtrating the *Fundamental Rules*, and indeed throughout the whole Work, my principal Aim has been ſtrictly to adhere to the *Method* publiſhed by the *Inventor* Himſelf, in his Introduction to his Tract on the *Quadrature* of *Curves*. For whatever may have induced ſome People to imagine that Sir *Iſaac Newton*, after having revolved in his Mind the Doctrine of *Fluxions* for forty Years, has not delivered himſelf ſo clearly as he might have done, and have therefore endeavoured to explain it better; for my part, I muſt confeſs, I cannot ſee the leaſt Shadow of Reaſon for ſuch an Objection, and Attempt. Nor can I think there is any more Difficulty in conceiving or forming an adequate Notion of a naſcent or evaneſcent Quantity, than there is of a Mathematical Point, which, though it be void of Magnitude, is the Foundation, or

Root, from whence all kinds of Magnitudes take their Riſe For whoever conſiders how a Line is generated, cannot but eaſily conceive, that the generating Point in moving according to ſome Direction, and therefore deſcribing a flowing Line, muſt, in a very ſmall Part of Time, deſcribe a very ſmall Part of the generated Line, which is what is meant by an *Increment*; and as at the Inſtant of Time that the generating Point ſets out, or begins to move, at that very Inſtant an *Increment* begins to be generated, or exiſt, this ariſing *Increment*, or this ariſing *Quantity*, is called a naſcent *Increment*, or a naſcent *Quantity*; and, on the contrary, after a Line has been generated, if we imagine the generating Point to return back, and move towards the Place it firſt ſet out from, in this Caſe the Line will conſtantly decreaſe, and the very ſmall Part of it run over in a very ſmall Part of Time, is called a *Decrement.* And as the generating Point, in returning back to its firſt Situation, muſt of Neceſſity, by this contrary Motion, continually diminiſh the Line, ſo when it arrives at the Place from whence it firſt ſet out, the Line will, by this means, be totally deſtroyed or annihilated, and that *Decrement* with which it vaniſhed, or ceaſed to exiſt, is what is meant by an *Evaneſcent Decrement*, or an *Evaneſcent Quantity:* And as *Increments*, generated after this Manner, become greater or

leſs,

leſs, in Proportion to the Velocity which the generating Point begins to move with, ſo the different Degrees of Velocity with which ſuch *Increments* do ſo ariſe, are called their reſpective *Fluxions*; where all Conſiderations of Time, and Acceleration of Motion are totally and abſolutely excluded, and muſt therefore be in the firſt *Ratio* of the *Increments*, as ariſing, or in the laſt *Ratio* of the *Decrements*, as vaniſhing.

As the main or fundamental Point in the Method of *Fluxions*, upon which all the future Operations depend, is to find the *Fluxion* of the *Rectangle*, or Product of two indeterminate or flowing *Quantities*; and as ſome Difficulty has ariſen, and may ſtill ariſe, about rejecting the little *Rectangle* DdFH, expreſſed by $y\,x\,o\,o$, in the Product ariſing from the Multiplication of x by y, conſidered as flowing Quantities, I believe it will be eaſy, from the Principles here laid down, to account for it in a clear and ſatisfactory Manner And to this end, let x and y repreſent two flowing or indeterminate *Quantities*, z the Product ariſing from the Multiplication of the one by the other, then will $z = xy$: Let o be a very ſmall *Quantity*. Now if we ſuppoſe the *Quantities* x and y in a flowing State, it is manifeſt, that while x flows into, or becomes $x + \dot{x}\,o$, y flows into or becomes $y + y\,o$· Multiplying therefore theſe two *Quantities* the one into the other, we ſhall have

$x'\,y$

$xy + yxo + xyo + xyoo = z + zo$; for while xy, by flowing, becomes $xy + yxo + xyo + xyoo$, z, by flowing, becomes $z + zo$. Taking away then xy from one Side of the Equation, and z, its equal, from the other Side, we ſhall have $yxo + xyo + yxoo = zo$.

Make AB $= y$, AC $= x$, and ſuppoſe the Lines AB, AC in a flowing State; then while AB flows into, or becomes A b, y will flow into, or become $y + yo$; and in the ſame Time AC will become AE, and x will become $x + xo$; whence we ſhall have $xy = z$ for the Value of the *Rectangular Space* ABDC, xyo for the Value of the incremental Space B b d D, yxo for the Value of the incremental Space CDHE, and $yxoo$ for the Value of the *Incremental Space* D d F H. Let us now imagine the Lines b F and E F to return back, and to move according to the Direction b A and E A; that is, that the Point b moves according to the Direction b B, the Point E according to the Direction EC, while the Point F, common to the Lines F b and FE, muſt move according to the Direction F D; it is manifeſt, that the

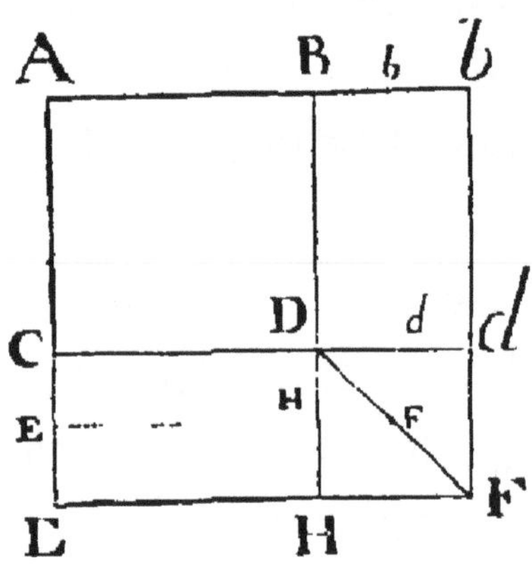

nearer

nearer the Lines *b* F and F E approach to the Lines BD and DC, the nearer will the Line *b* F approach to an Equality with the Line BD, and the nearer will the Space B*b*F D approach to an Equality with the Space B*bd*D, alſo the nearer will the Line E F approach to an Equality with the Line CD, and the nearer will the Space EFDC approach to an Equality with the Space EHDC, and the leſſer will be the *Rectangular Space* D*d*F H: For when the Lines *b*F and EF are got into the Situation *b*F and EF, the Space D*d*F H is become D*d*FH, the Difference between the Spaces *b*FDB and *bd*DB is expreſs'd by the little Triangle D*d*F; alſo between the Spaces EFDC and EHDC by the little Triangle HDF, 'till at laſt, when the Lines *b* F and E F arrive at, or coincide with the Lines B D and C D, they will become equal, and the Space *b*F D B, in its evaneſcent State, will become equal to the Space B*bd*D, and at the ſame time the Space EFDC, in its evaneſcent State, will become equal to the Space EHDC, and at that Inſtant the *Rectangular Space* D*d*FH, expreſſed by $xyoo$, will vaniſh, and we ſhall have $xyo+yxo=zo$. Now if each Side of the Equation be divided by o, the Quotient will give $xy+yx=z$, for the *Fluxion* of the Product xy, or of the *Rectangle* ABDC; inaſmuch as *Fluxions* are in the laſt *Ratio* of their evaneſcent *Decrements*, that is, in the *Ratio* with which they vaniſh.

WHENCE,

WHENCE, and from what is contain'd in the following *Sheets* (I presume) it may be justly inferr'd, that the *Doctrine of Fluxions*, as deliver'd by Sir *Isaac Newton*, may be clearly *Conceiv'd*, and distinctly *Comprehended*; that the Principles upon which it is founded are *True*; that the Demonstrations of the fundamental Rules are *Conclusive*; that it requires no *Explanation*, nor need it fear any *Opposition*.

IT is now some Years since the greatest Part of this Book was prepared for the *Press*; but being employ'd in publishing the *Posthumous Works* of Mr. *Flamsteed*, and after they were finish'd, meeting with unexpected Hindrances, I for some time laid aside all Thoughts of compleating it: but as something of this Nature seem'd greatly to be wanted, and not knowing or hearing of any Persons being engag'd in a Work of this Kind, I resolved to put the last Hand to it, and to send it into the World, in hopes it might be useful to young Beginners, for whom it was principally intended. For by giving them a clear and adequate Notion of the *Nature* and *Grounds* of *Fluxions*, they would be able to penetrate farther into the Depths of this admirable *Science*, and become Masters of the more sublime *Discoveries* that have been made by this incomparable Method of Reasoning.

FLUXI-

FLUXIONS.

PART I.

Containing an Account of the Nature of FLUXIONS:

Together with a Demonſtration of the FUNDAMENTAL RULES.

In EIGHT SECTIONS.

SECT. I.

Contains an Account of the Nature and Properties of Powers, and their Exponents, with a Demonstration of the Rules made use of in Exponential Arithmetick.

SECT. II.

Treats of Infinite Series.

SECT III.

Contains an Account of the Nature of Fluxions, and the Generation of Mathematical Quantities.

SECT. IV.

Contains the Notation of Fluxions.

SECT. V.

Contains the Algorithm of Fluxions

SECT. VI.

Contains the Operations in Second, Third, Fourth, &c. *Fluxions.*

SECT VII.

Treats of the Fluxions of Exponential Quantities, that is, of such Quantities, or Powers, whose Exponents themselves are Variable or Flowing Quantities.

SECT. VIII.

Contains the Inverse Method of Fluxions, or Rules for finding the Fluents from given Fluxions

FLUX-

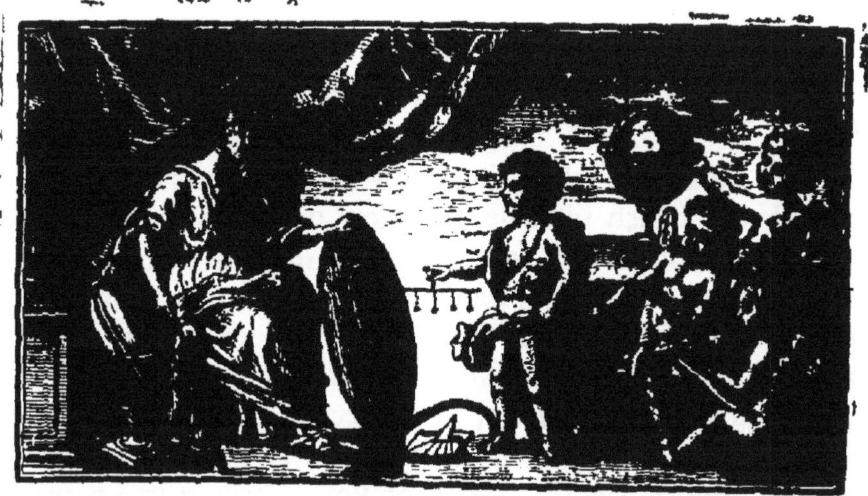

FLUXIONS.

SECT. I.

Of the Nature and Generation of Powers, *and their Exponents.*

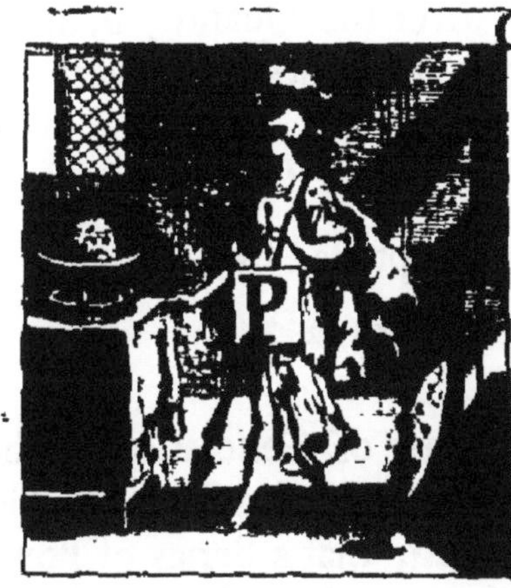

POWERS are the Reſult of, or ariſe from, the Multiplication of the ſame Quantity, a certain Number of times into itſelf; where Unity being the firſt Multiplicand, the Products produced are called the firſt, ſecond, third, fourth, *&c.* Powers For Example, If Unity be multiplied by the Quantity *a*, the Product *a* is called the firſt Power of *a*, and if this Power be multiplied again by *a*, the Product *a a* thence reſulting, is called the ſecond Power of *a*; and if this Power be multiplied again by the ſame Quantity *a*, the Product *a a a* is called the third Power of *a*, this again being multiplied by *a*, the Product *a a a a* is the fourth Power of *a*, *&c.*

THE Numbers, which ſhew how many Letters the Powers conſiſt of, which likewiſe ſhew how many times the Quantity has been involved, to produce the reſpective Powers, are very properly called their Indices, or Exponents, inaſmuch as they indicate, or ſhew, the Rank, or Place, that every Power obtains in the Order of Powers, ſo that the Index of the Simple, or firſt Power of a is 1, of the ſecond Power of a or $a\,a$ is 2, of the third Power of a or $a\,a\,a$ is 3, *&c.* and, conſequently, the Indices of a Series of Powers ariſing in a natural and orderly Progreſſion from Unity, will be a Series of Numbers, beginning in a natural Order, *viz.* 1, 2, 3, 4, 5, *&c.*

AND inaſmuch as theſe Indices expound the Number of times that any Quantity has been involved, to produce the given Power, the Products, or Powers themſelves, are very neatly, and elegantly expreſſed, by placing the Index over the Root, or Simple Power, thus the fourth Power of a, or $a\,a\,a\,a$, is very properly expreſs'd by placing the Index 4 over the Quantity a, after this manner a^4, as is the fifth Power of a, or $a\,a\,a\,a\,a$, by placing the Index 5 over the Quantity a, in the ſame manner a^5, and conſequently the Series of Powers

$$a,\ a\,a,\ a\,a\,a,\ a\,a\,a\,a,\ a\,a\,a\,a\,a,\ a\,a\,a\,a\,a\,a,$$

are very ſignificantly expreſſed by

$$a^1,\ a^2,\ a^3,\ a^4,\ a^5,\ a^6,\ \&c.$$

FROM a Conſideration of the Law of Generation of theſe Powers, with the Manner of Formation of a Series of Geometrical Proportionals, it is manifeſt, that a Series of Powers is no other than a Series of Numbers, or Quantities, in a Geometrical Proportion continued, as are their Indices a Series of Numbers, or Quantities, in Arithmetical Proportion continued, for as the Series of Powers are in a conſtant Ratio of 1 to a (for a to $a\,a$, is as 1 to a), So the Indices themſelves are in an Arithmetical Proportion, inaſmuch as they increaſe by equal Differences, for the Difference between 1 and 2, is the ſame with the Difference between 2 and 3, *&c.*

AND

AND hence it is, that if the first Term of the Geometrical Series be 1, the first Term of the Arithmetical Series will be 0; for as 1, *a*, *aa*, are in continual Proportion Geometrically, and 0, 1, 2, in a continual Proportion Arithmetically, inasmuch as 1 and 2 are the respective Indices of *a* and *aa*, it follows, that 0, the first Term in the Arithmetical Series, must be the respective Index of 1, the first Term in the Geometrical Series, and, consequently, the Series of Powers, 1, *a*, *aa*, *aaa*, *aaaa*, *aaaaa*, *aaaaaa*, &c will have, for their respective Indices, a Series of Numbers, beginning from 0, and increasing in a natural Order, as

0, 1, 2, 3, 4, 5, 6, &c.

AGAIN, as a^2 and a^1 are the Powers corresponding to the Indices 2 and 1, in the Arithmetical Series, the Power a^0 must correspond with the Term 0 in the same Series For as a^2 is the Result of two Multiplications, of the Multiplier *a*, and a^1, or $a \times 1$, the Result of one such Multiplication, so a^0 is the Result of no Multiplication at all, and, consequently, since from the Nature of Geometrical Proportionals, 1 will be the next Term below *a*, and since from the Nature of Powers, a^0 is the next Term below *a*, in the Series of Powers, it is manifest that these two Expressions are the same And hence we are let into the Reason of the practical Operations in Powers, and their Indices, or Exponents, and why. First,

THAT the Sum of any two or more Indices, or Exponents of Powers, will be the Index of a Power resulting from the Multiplication of the several Powers into each other, that is, why $a^2 \times a^4 = a^{2+4} = a^6$, or why $a^2 \times a^4 \times a^6 = a^{2+4+6} = a^{12}$

FORASMUCH as a Series of Powers is a Series of Numbers in Geometrical Proportion continued, and that their respective Indices form a Series of Numbers in an Arithmetical Progression, and that from the known Laws of Proportion the Sum of any two, or more Terms, in the Arithmetical Series, will produce a Number, which shall be a Term in the Arithmetical Series corresponding to a Term in the Geometrical Series, resulting from

from the continual Multiplication of the correſpondent Terms in the Geometrical Series, it follows, that the Sum of two or more Indices will give a Number, that ſhall be the Index of a Power produced from the continual Multiplication of the Powers one into the other, and, ſecondly, why the Difference of any two Indices will produce the Index of a Power reſulting from the Diviſion of the two reſpective Powers the one by the other; that is, why

$$\frac{a^6}{a^2} = a^{6-2} = a^4, \text{ or why } \frac{a^{12}}{a^8} = a^{12-8} = a^4.$$

FORASMUCH as the Difference of any two Terms in an Arithmetical Series, is equal to a Term in the ſame Series, ariſing from the Diviſion of the two correſpondent Geometrical Terms, it follows, that the Index of any Power to be divided, leſſen'd by the Index of the Power by which it is to be divided, will give the Index of a Power reſulting from the Diviſion of the two given Powers

HENCE we are taught, how from the Index of any Power to find the Index of the Square, Cube, Biquadrate, *&c* or the Index of the Square, Cubic Root *&c.* of the ſame Power, or, which is the ſame thing, a ready and expeditious way of raiſing any Power, conſider'd as a Root, to any given Power, or for extracting any Root out of the ſame.

FOR ſince to raiſe any Power, is to multiply the ſuppoſed Root a certain Number of times into itſelf If the Index of the given Root be multiplied by the Index of the Power, it will give a Number expreſſing the Index of the Power to be found Thus the Index of the Square of a^3 will be a^{3+3}, or $a^{2\times3}$, or a^6, the Index of the Cube of a^3 will be a^{3+3+3}, or $a^{3\times3} = a^9$, the Biquadrate of the ſame $a^{3+3+3+3}$, or $a^{3\times4} = a^{12}$, *&c* and the ſame Law will obtain for any Power conſider'd as a Root

AND again, inaſmuch as to extract the Root out of any Power, is to find a Root, which, being multiplied as often into itſelf as there are Involutions in the given Power, will reſtore

the

the Power again If the Index of any Power be divided by the Number expressing the Number of Involutions, the Quotient will give the Index of the Power to be found, considered as a Root. Thus the Index of the square Root of a^{12} is $a^{\frac{12}{2}} = a^6$, the Cube Root of the same Power a^{12} will be $a^{\frac{12}{3}}$, or a^4, the Biquadrate Root of the same $a^{\frac{12}{4}}$, or a^3, the Cube Root of the Square Root, or the sixth Power of the same, will be $a^{\frac{12}{6}}$ or a^2, *&c.*

As every Number may be considered as the Infinite Power of the *Momentum* of that Number, and a certain Power of the *Momentum* of the same Number, and as the same Number may be consider'd as the *Momentum* of the Power of some other Number, so every Number may be considered as any Power of some Number considered as a Root, or as any Root of some certain Number considered as a Power.

And hence it is, that the Series of Powers, a^1, a^2, a^3, a^4, a^5, a^6. *&c.* may be continued downwards, or backwards, from Unity, in a reciprocal Order, *ad Infinitum*, and is therefore called the reciprocal Series, wherein the same Ratio of the Terms to each other will be constantly observed, for the Terms,

$$\&c.\ \frac{1}{a^6},\ \frac{1}{a^5},\ \frac{1}{a^4},\ \frac{1}{a^3},\ \frac{1}{a^2},\ \frac{1}{a},\ a,\ a^2,\ a^3,\ a^4,\ a^5,\ a^6,\ \&c$$

having the same Ratio throughout the whole, are a Series of Geometrical Proportionals, or Powers, infinite in Number, arising from the *Momentum* of the Quantity represented by a, and as the Indices of the Powers on the Right Hand of Unity are represented by a Series of Numbers in an Arithmetical Progression, *ad Infinitum*, being each of them Affirmative, so the Indices of the several Powers on the Left Hand of Unity, and decreasing from Unity in the same manner as the Series on the Right Hand increases, will have for their Indices, or Exponents, a Series of Numbers, increasing, in the same Order, from Unity towards the Left Hand, as the Indices of Powers on the Right Side of Unity increased

to

towards the Right Hand, but will be all of them Negative, or leſs than nothing

For as the Index of a^2 is $+ 2$, the Index of $\frac{1}{a^2}$ muſt be $- 2$; inaſmuch as to leſſen the Index, and divide by a given Power, is the ſame thing, as has been already ſhewn Moreover, ſince $a \times \frac{1}{a}$ produces $\frac{a^2}{a^2}$ or 1, ſo the Sum of their reſpective Indices muſt produce 0, the Index of Unity, and to take away the Poſitive Index 2, we muſt ſubjoin a Negative Index of the ſame Value, and, conſequently, the Index of $\frac{1}{a^2}$ muſt be $- 2$.

So that as a^{+2}, the ſecond Power removed from Unity towards the Right Hand in the Order of Powers, has $+ 2$ for its Index, ſo $\frac{1}{a^2}$, the ſecond Power from Unity, in the the Order of Powers towards the Left Hand, and decreaſing in the ſame Proportion from Unity as the Power a^2 increaſed, will have $- 2$ for its Index, and the ſame Law will hold good in all Powers whatſoever that are removed at equal Diſtances from the Place of Unity

And that this may the more evidently appear, let the Indices of the reciprocal Series be repreſented by the Letters b, c, d, e, *&c.* and let the Quantities a^b, a^c, a^d, *&c* be ſuppoſed to diminiſh in the ſame Ratio as the Quantities a^1, a^2, a^3, increaſe, or, which is the ſame thing, let the Quantities a^b, a^c, a^d, *&c* be reſpectively equal to $\frac{1}{a}$, $\frac{1}{a^2}$, $\frac{1}{a^3}$, *&c* then will the former Series be expreſſed thus,

$$\&c\ a^m,\ a^n,\ a^e,\ a^d,\ a^c,\ a^b,\ a^0,\ a^1,\ a^2,\ a^3,\ a^4,\ a^5,\ a^6,\ \&c.$$

Now, becauſe from the Nature of Powers, and their Exponents, or Indices, $2 + b = 1 + 0 = 1$, therefore $b = 1 - 2$, that is $b = -1$ In like manner, becauſe $3 + c = 1 + 0 = 1$, there-

therefore $c = 1 - 3$, and, consequently, $c = -2$ Again, because $4 + d = 1 + 0$, therefore $d = 1 - 4$, and $d = -3$

AND after the same manner e will be found equal to -4, $n = -5$, $m = -6$, &c *ad Infinitum*, whence the former Series $\frac{1}{a^6}, \frac{1}{a^5}, \frac{1}{a^4}, \frac{1}{a^3}, \frac{1}{a^2}, \frac{1}{a^1}$, is much more elegantly and significantly expressed thus, a^{-6}, a^{-5}, a^{-4}, a^{-3}, a^{-2}, a^{-1}

IN extracting the Roots of Powers, if the Index of the Root to be extracted, or the Number of Involutions supposed to be contained in the given Power (for every Number, whose Root is required, is supposed to be made up of the same Number of Involutions, tho' the Quantity, through a Defect in our way of Notation, cannot be exactly expres'd) be not an Aliquot Part of the Index of the given Power, then such Root will be expres'd by a Fractional Number, as if it were required to extract the Cube Root out of the fifth Power of a, inasmuch as the Number 3, the Number of Involutions, of which a in this Case is supposed to be compounded of, is not an Aliquot Part of, or contained an even Number of Times in the Number 5, the given Index of the Power of a, the Index of the Power after such Extraction will be expres'd by a Fractional Number after this manner $a^{\frac{5}{3}}$, and signifies, that by this Expression is meant the Cube Root of the fifth Power of a, whatsoever be the Quantity represented by the Letter a, and after the same manner is any given Root, out of any given Power of any Quantity, when the Indices are not multiple the one of the other expres'd

AND the same Law holds good when the Indices are negative, for $a^{-\frac{3}{2}}$ expresses the Square Root of a Number, which being multiplied into itself three times, will produce the Quantity a as $a^{\frac{3}{2}}$, expressed the Square Root of a Number arising from the Multiplication of the Quantity a three times into itself, and the same will hold good in extracting any Root out of any Power, whether the Power have a negative or positive Index.

AND hence ariſes the Uſe of the Knowledge of Fractions in the Compoſition and Diſſolution of Powers, and the manner of compounding negative and poſitive Quantities, according to any Compoſition whatſoever.

THE Laws hitherto delivered relating to Powers, when the Indices, or Exponents, are expreſs'd by Numbers, will take Place when the ſame Indices are expreſſed more generally by Letters of the Alphabet ſuch as m, n, p, q, *&c.* Thus if the Power a^n were to be ſquared, the Power then ariſing would be a^{n+n}, or a^{2n}. If the ſame Power were to be cubed, the Reſult would be a^{n+n+n}, or a^{3n}, and univerſally, if the Power a^n were to be raiſed to any given Power t, the Power to be produced will be a^{tn}. Again, if the Square Root of the Power a^n were to be extracted, the Anſwer would be $a^{\frac{1}{2}n}$, or $a^{\frac{n}{2}}$ If the Cube Root were to be found, the Quantity thence ariſing would be $a^{\frac{1}{3}n}$, or $a^{\frac{n}{3}}$ And, laſtly, if the $\frac{1}{m}$ Root of the ſame Power were to be extracted, the Reſult would be $a^{\frac{1}{m}n}$, or $a^{\frac{n}{m}}$.

AGAIN, if the Power a^n were to be multiplied by the Power a^m, the Product would be the Power a^{n+m}; and if the ſame Power a^n were to be divided by the ſame Power a^m, the Quotient would be the Power a^{n-m}. In like manner, if the Power a^n were to be multiplied by the Power x^m, the Product will be $a^n x^m$, and if the ſame Power a^n were to be divided by the Power x^m, the Quotient will be $\frac{a^n}{x^m}$.

HENCE we are fully inſtructed in the Reaſon of the Practical Operations in Exponential Arithmetick; and

I THAT the Addition of the Indices is equivalent to the Multiplication of the Powers, as $a^2 \times a^4 = a^{2+4} = a^6$, and $a^n \times a^m = a^{n+m}$

II THAT

II. THAT the Subſtraction of Indices produces the ſame Effect as the Diviſion of Powers, thus $\frac{a^6}{a^2} = a^{6-2} = a^4$, and $\frac{a^{n+m}}{a^m} = a^{n+m-m} = a^n$.

III THAT the Multiplication of Indices is equivalent to the Involution of Powers. For the Index of the Cube of a^n will be $a^{n+n+n} = a^{3n}$

IV. THAT the Diviſion of Indices is equivalent to Evolution, or the extracting of Roots, as the Cube Root of a^3 will be $a^{\frac{3}{3}} = a^1$, and the Cube Root of $a^{\frac{n3}{3}} = a^n$; and the ſame Laws will extend to any other Powers how complicate ſoever.

SECT. II.

Of Infinite Series.

AS in Ordinary Arithmetick, when the Diviſor is not an Aliquot Part of the Dividend, or any Number, conſidered as a Power, is a Surd or Irrational Number, the Quotient, or Root, may be found infinitely near the Truth by different Fractional Approximations, according to the Pleaſure of the Artiſt. So in Specious Arithmetick, when the Dividend is not an exact Multiple of the Diviſor, or the Quantity, conſidered as a Power, has not an exact Root, the Quotient, or Root, in this Caſe, may be found, by different ſucceſſive Series of Terms, continually decreaſing; 'till at laſt the Difference between the true Quotient, or Root, and the Sum of the ſeveral Approximating Terms, thus produced, will be infinitely ſmall, and, at laſt, vaniſh and the Reſults in this Caſe are called Infinite Series, or Approximations.

For Example, Suppoſe $y + yx = v$, then $y = \frac{v}{1+x}$.

And dividing v by $1 + x$, according to the common Rules for Diviſion of Algebra, as in the following Operation

$$1 + x)\, v\, (v - vx + vxx - vx^3 + vx^4, \text{ \&c.}$$
$$v + vx$$
$$\overline{\qquad - vx \qquad}$$
$$- vx - vxx$$
$$\overline{\qquad + vxx \qquad}$$
$$+ vxx + vx^3$$
$$\overline{\qquad - vx^3 \qquad}$$
$$- vx^3 - vx^4$$
$$\overline{\qquad + vx^4, \text{ \&c.} \qquad}$$

Or,

Or by dividing v by $x+1$, in the same manner as in the following Example

$$x+1)\,v\,\left(\frac{v}{x}-\frac{v}{xx}+\frac{v}{x^3}-\frac{v}{x^4},\ \&c.\right.$$

$$v+\frac{v}{x}$$

$$-\frac{v}{x}$$

$$-\frac{v}{x}-\frac{v}{xx}$$

$$+\frac{v}{xx}$$

$$+\frac{v}{xx}+\frac{v}{x^3}$$

$$-\frac{v}{x^3},\ \&c.$$ we shall

have $y=\begin{cases} v-vx+vxx-vx^3+vx^4-vx^5+vx^6,\ \&c. \\ \frac{v}{x}-\frac{v}{xx}+\frac{v}{x^3}-\frac{v}{x^4}+\frac{v}{x^5}-\frac{v}{x^6},\ \&c. \end{cases}$

or $y=v\times\begin{cases} 1-x+xx-x^3+x^4-x^5+x^6,\ \&c. \\ \frac{1}{x}-\frac{1}{x^2}+\frac{1}{x^3}-\frac{1}{x^4}+\frac{1}{x^5}-\frac{1}{x^6},\ \&c. \end{cases}$

AGAIN, by the same way of Investigation, if $yb\mp yx=aa$, we shall find $y=\frac{aa}{b\mp x}=\frac{a^2}{b}\pm\frac{a^2x}{b^2}+\frac{a^2x^2}{b^3}\pm\frac{a^2x^3}{b^4}+\frac{a^2x^4}{b^5}$, &c.

AGAIN, if $ſ-\frac{1}{2}ſa^2+\frac{1}{24}ſa^4-\frac{1}{720}ſa^6$, &c. $=r^2$;

then will $ſ=r^2+\frac{1}{2}r^2a^2+\frac{5}{24}r^2a^4+\frac{61}{720}r^2a^6$, &c.

For $s = r^2 \frac{1}{1 - \frac{1}{2}a^2 + \frac{1}{24}a^4 - \frac{1}{720}a^6}$, &c and dividing 1 by $1 - \frac{1}{2}a^2 + \frac{1}{24}a^4$, as in the following Operation:

$$1 - \frac{1}{2}a^2 + \frac{1}{24}a^4 - \frac{1}{720}a^6, \&c \,)\, 1 \quad (1 + \frac{1}{2}a^2 + \frac{5}{24}a^4 + \frac{61}{720}a^6, \&c$$

$$1 - \frac{1}{2}a^2 + \frac{1}{24}a^4 - \frac{1}{720}a^6, \&c.$$

$$+ \frac{1}{2}a^2 - \frac{1}{24}a^4 + \frac{1}{720}a^6, \&c.$$

$$+ \frac{1}{2}a^2 - \frac{1}{4}a^4 + \frac{1}{48}a^6, \&c$$

$$+ \frac{5}{24}a^4 - \frac{14}{720}a^6, \&c.$$

$$+ \frac{5}{24}a^4 - \frac{5}{48}a^6, \&c$$

$$+ \frac{61}{720}a^6, \&c.$$

we shall have $s = r^2 \times 1 + \frac{1}{2}a^2 + \frac{5}{24}a^4 + \frac{61}{720}a^6$, &c

AND by the same way of Investigation,

if $t = \frac{r\,r}{a + \frac{1}{3}a^3 + \frac{2}{15}a^5 + \frac{17}{315}a^7}$, &c.

Then $t = r^2 \times \frac{1}{a} - \frac{1}{3}a - \frac{1}{45}a^3 - \frac{2}{945}a^5$, &c $=$

$= \frac{r^2}{a} - \frac{r^2 a}{3} - \frac{r^2 a^3}{45} - \frac{2 r^2 a^5}{945}$, &c. Again, if $t\,a - \frac{1}{6}t\,a^3 + \frac{1}{120}t\,a^5$, &c. be divided by $1 - \frac{1}{2}a^2 + \frac{1}{24}a^4 - \frac{1}{720}a^6$, &c.

Then $t = a + \frac{1}{3}a^3 + \frac{2}{15}a^5 + \frac{17}{315}a^7$, &c.

For

For $t = \frac{a - \frac{1}{6}a^3 + \frac{1}{120}a^5 - \frac{1}{5040}a^7, \ \&c.}{1 - \frac{1}{2}a^2 + \frac{1}{24}a^4 - \frac{1}{720}a^6, \ \&c}$, and dividing $a - \frac{1}{6}a^3 + \frac{1}{120}a^4, \&c.$ by $1 - \frac{1}{2}a^2 + \frac{1}{24}a^4, \&c.$ according to the common Rules of Specious Arithmetick, in the manner following.

$$1 - \frac{1}{2}aa + \frac{1}{24}a^4 - \frac{1}{720}a^6, \&c \ \Big) \ a - \frac{1}{6}a^3 + \frac{1}{120}a^5 - \frac{1}{5040}a^7, \&c$$

$$a - \frac{1}{2}a^3 + \frac{1}{24}a^5 - \frac{1}{720}a^7, \&c.$$

$$\frac{1}{3}a^3 - \frac{1}{30}a^5 + \frac{1}{840}a^7, \&c.$$

$$\frac{1}{3}a^3 - \frac{1}{6}a^5 + \frac{1}{720}a^7, \&c.$$

$$\frac{2}{15}a^5 - \frac{4}{315}a^7, \&c.$$

$$\frac{2}{15}a^5 - \frac{2}{30}a^7, \&c$$

$$+\frac{17}{315}a^7, \&c$$

we ſhall have $a + \frac{1}{3}a^3 + \frac{2}{15}a^5 + \frac{17}{315}a^7, \&c. = t$ for the Quotient.

And after the ſame way,

if $y = \left\{ \frac{1 - \frac{1}{2}ax^2 - \frac{1}{8}a^2x^4 - \frac{1}{16}a^3x^6 - \frac{5}{128}a^4x^8, \&c}{1 - \frac{1}{2}bx^2 - \frac{1}{8}b^2x^4 - \frac{1}{16}b^3x^6 - \frac{5}{128}b^4x^8, \&c.} \right.$ we ſhall

find

find $y = 1 + \frac{1}{2}bx^2 + \frac{3}{8}b^2x^4 + \frac{5}{16}b^3x^6 + \frac{35}{128}b^4x^8$, &c

$$- \frac{1}{2}ax^2 + \frac{1}{4}abx^4 + \frac{3}{16}ab^2x^6 + \frac{5}{32}ab^3x^8, \&c.$$

$$- \frac{1}{8}a^2x^4 - \frac{1}{16}a^2bx^6 - \frac{3}{64}a^2b^2x^8, \&c.$$

$$+ \frac{1}{16}a^3x^6 + \frac{1}{32}a^3bx^8, \&c.$$

$$- \frac{5}{128}a^4x^8, \&c.$$

Let us now suppose $yy = 1 - xx$, then by extracting the Root on each side of the Equation according to the common Rules, we shall have $y = 1 - \frac{1}{2}x^2 - \frac{1}{8}x^4 - \frac{1}{16}x^6 - \frac{5}{128}x^8 - \frac{7}{256}x^{10}$, &c. as will appear by the following Investigation

$$1 - xx\left(1 - \frac{1}{2}x^2 - \frac{1}{8}x^4 - \frac{1}{16}x^6 - \frac{5}{128}x^8 - \frac{7}{256}x^{10}, \&c.\right.$$

$$\overline{1}$$

$$2 - \frac{1}{2}x^2\Big) \; - xx$$

$$- xx + \frac{1}{4}x^4$$

$$2 - xx - \frac{1}{8}x^4\Big) - \frac{1}{4}x^4$$

$$- \frac{1}{4}x^4 + \frac{1}{8}x^6 + \frac{1}{64}x^8$$

$$2 - xx - \frac{1}{\cdot}x^4 \; \&c\Big) - \frac{1}{8}x^6 - \frac{1}{64}x^8, \; \&c$$

$$- \frac{1}{8}x^6 + \frac{1}{16}x^8 + \frac{1}{64}x^{10}, \; \&c$$

$$- \frac{5}{64}x^8 - \frac{1}{64}x^{10}, \; \&c.$$

$$- \frac{5}{64}x^8 + \frac{5}{128}x^{10}, \; \&c$$

$$- \frac{7}{128}x^{10}, \; \&c$$

After

After the same manner of Investigation, the Root of $\sqrt{aa \pm xx}$, or $\overline{aa \pm xx}|^{\frac{1}{2}}$, will be found to be

$$a \pm \frac{x^2}{2a} - \frac{x^4}{8a^3} \pm \frac{x^6}{16a^5} - \frac{5x^8}{128a^7} \pm \frac{7x^{10}}{256a^9}, \&c$$

Of $\frac{1}{x}\sqrt{x - xx}$, or $\frac{1}{x} \times \overline{x - xx}|^{\frac{1}{2}}$, will be

$$x^{-\frac{1}{2}} - \frac{1}{2}x^{\frac{1}{2}} - \frac{1}{8}x^{\frac{3}{2}} - \frac{1}{16}x^{\frac{5}{2}} - \frac{5}{128}x^{\frac{7}{2}}, \&c$$

Of $\sqrt{dx - xx}$, or $\overline{dx - xx}|^{\frac{1}{2}}$, will be

$$d^{\frac{1}{2}}x^{\frac{1}{2}} - \frac{x^{\frac{3}{2}}}{2d^{\frac{1}{2}}} - \frac{x^{\frac{5}{2}}}{8d^{\frac{3}{2}}} - \frac{x^{\frac{7}{2}}}{16d^{\frac{5}{2}}} - \frac{5x^{\frac{9}{2}}}{128d^{\frac{7}{2}}}, \&c$$

Again, suppose it were required to find the Cube Root of the same Quantity $1 - xx$, or, which is the same thing, suppose $y^3 = 1 - xx$, and it were required to find the Value of y

By extracting the Cube Root on each Side of the Equation by the common Methods, after the manner following, we shall have

$$y = 1 - \frac{1}{3}x^2 - \frac{1}{9}x^4 - \frac{5}{81}x^6 - \frac{10}{243}x^8 - \frac{22}{729}x^{10}, \&c.$$

For $\overline{1 - xx}|^{\frac{1}{3}}\left(1 - \frac{1}{3}xx - \frac{1}{9}x^4 - \frac{5}{81}x^6 - \frac{10}{243}x^8 - \frac{22}{729}x^{10}\right.$

$$1$$

$3\ \big)\ -xx$

$$-xx + \frac{1}{3}x^4 - \frac{1}{27}x^6$$

$3 - 2x^2\ \big)\ -\frac{1}{3}x^4 + \frac{1}{27}x^6$

$$-\frac{1}{3}x^4 + \frac{2}{9}x^6 - \frac{1}{27}x^8$$

$$+\frac{1}{27}x^8 - \frac{1}{81}x^{10}, \&c$$

$$3 - 2x^2 + \frac{1}{3}x^4, \&c \Big) - \frac{5}{27}x^6 \qquad + \frac{1}{81}x^{10}, \&c.$$

$$- \frac{5}{27}x^6 + \frac{10}{81}x^8 + \frac{5}{243}x^{10}, \&c$$

$$- \frac{10}{81}x^8 - \frac{2}{243}x^{10}, \&c$$

$$- \frac{10}{81}x^8 + \frac{20}{243}x^{10}, \&c.$$

$$- \frac{22}{243}x^{10}, \&c$$

AGAIN, if the Biquadrate Root of the same Quantity were required, the Operation will be as follows.

$$1 - xx \Big(1 - \frac{1}{4}x^2 - \frac{3}{32}x^4 - \frac{7}{128}x^6 - \frac{77}{2048}x^8, \&c$$

$$1$$

$$- xx$$

$$- xx + \frac{3}{8}x^4 - \frac{1}{16}x^6 + \frac{1}{256}x^8, \&c$$

$$- \frac{3}{8}x^4 + \frac{1}{16}x^6 - \frac{1}{256}x^8, \&c$$

$$- \frac{3}{8}x^4 + \frac{9}{32}x^6 - \frac{9}{128}x^8, \&c$$

$$+ \frac{27}{512}x^8, \&c.$$

$$- \frac{7}{32}x^6 + \frac{7}{512}x^8, \&c$$

$$- \frac{7}{32}x^6 + \frac{21}{128}x^8, \&c.$$

$$- \frac{77}{512}x^8, \&c.$$

SUP-

SUPPOSE it were required to find the $\frac{1}{5}$ Power of the same Quantity $1 - xx$, we shall have

$$1 - \frac{1}{5}x^2 - \frac{2}{25}x^4 - \frac{6}{125}x^6 - \frac{21}{625}x^8, \text{ \&c for the Root}$$

For $\overline{1 - xx}|^{\frac{1}{5}} = 1 - \frac{1}{5}x^2 - \frac{2}{25}x^4 - \frac{6}{125}x^6 - \frac{21}{625}x^8$, &c

$$\begin{array}{l}
1 \\
\underline{\quad} \\
-xx \\
-xx + \frac{2}{5}x^4 - \frac{2}{25}x^6 + \frac{1}{125}x^8, \text{ \&c.} \\
\hline
5 - 4x^2, \text{\&c}\Big) - \frac{2}{5}x^4 + \frac{2}{25}x^6 - \frac{1}{125}x^8, \text{ \&c.} \\
\qquad - \frac{2}{5}x^4 + \frac{8}{25}x^6 - \frac{12}{125}x^8, \text{ \&c} \\
\qquad\qquad + \frac{8}{125}x^8, \text{ \&c} \\
\hline
\qquad - \frac{6}{25}x^6 + \frac{3}{125}x^8, \text{ \&c} \\
\qquad - \frac{6}{25}x^6 + \frac{24}{125}x^8, \text{ \&c} \\
\hline
\qquad\qquad - \frac{21}{125}x^8, \text{ \&c.}
\end{array}$$

AND after the same manner may any other Root of the Quantity given be found, and the same Rules will serve in Trinomials, Quadrinomials, &c

FOR Example, Suppose it were required to find the Square Root of the infinite Multinomial $\overline{1 - \frac{1}{2}x^2 - \frac{1}{8}x^4 - \frac{1}{16}x^6 - \frac{5}{128}x^8 - \frac{7}{256}x^{10}, \text{ \&c}}|^{\frac{1}{2}}$ By proceeding after the same

Method

Method as in the Binominal, we shall have $1 - \frac{1}{4}x^2 - \frac{3}{32}x^4 - \frac{7}{128}x^6$, &c for the Square Root, as in the following Operation.

$$1 - \frac{1}{2}x^2 - \frac{1}{8}x^4 - \frac{1}{16}x^6 - \frac{5}{128}x^8 - \frac{7}{256}x^{10}, \text{ \&c.}$$

$$1$$

$$2 - \frac{1}{4}x^2 \Big) - \frac{1}{2}x^2 - \frac{1}{8}x^4$$

$$- \frac{1}{2}x^2 + \frac{1}{16}x^4$$

$$2 - \frac{1}{2}x^2 - \frac{3}{32}x^4 \Big) - \frac{3}{16}x^4 - \frac{1}{16}x^6 - \frac{5}{128}x^8$$

$$- \frac{3}{16}x^4 + \frac{3}{64}x^6 + \frac{9}{1024}x^8$$

$$2 - \frac{1}{2}x^2 - \frac{3}{16}x^4, \text{ \&c} \Big) - \frac{7}{64}x^6 - \frac{49}{1024}x^8 - \frac{7}{256}x^{10}, \text{ \&c}$$

$$- \frac{7}{64}x^6 + \frac{7}{256}x^8 + \frac{21}{2048}x^{10}, \text{ \&c.}$$

$$- \frac{77}{1024}x^8 - \frac{77}{2048}x^{10}, \text{ \&c.}$$

$$- \frac{77}{1024}x^8 + \frac{77}{4096}x^{10}, \text{ \&c}$$

$$- \frac{231}{4096}x^{10}, \text{ \&c}$$

$1 - \frac{1}{4}x^2 - \frac{3}{32}x^4 - \frac{7}{128}x^6 - \frac{77}{2048}x^8 - \frac{231}{8192}x^{10}$, &c. the same with the Biquadrate Root of $1 - xx$ in Page 18.

AGAIN,

AGAIN, Suppose it were required to find the Cube Root of the same Infinite Multinomial, the Operation will be as follows

$$1 - \frac{1}{2}x^2 - \frac{1}{8}x^4 - \frac{1}{16}x^6, \text{ \&c.} \left(1 - \frac{1}{6}x^2 - \frac{5}{72}x^4 - \frac{55}{1296}x^6 \text{ \&c.} \right.$$

$$1$$

$$\overline{\qquad\qquad\qquad\qquad\qquad\qquad}$$

$$-\frac{1}{2}x^2 - \frac{1}{8}x^4 - \frac{1}{16}x^6, \text{ \&c.}$$

$$-\frac{1}{2}x^2 + \frac{1}{12}x^4 - \frac{1}{216}x^6, \text{ \&c.}$$

$$\overline{\qquad\qquad\qquad\qquad\qquad\qquad}$$

$$-\frac{5}{24}x^4 - \frac{25}{432}x^6, \text{ \&c}$$

$$-\frac{5}{24}x^4 + \frac{5}{72}x^6, \text{ \&c}$$

$$\overline{\qquad\qquad\qquad\qquad\qquad\qquad}$$

$$-\frac{55}{432}x^6, \text{ \&c.}$$

AND by proceeding after the same manner as in the former Examples, may the $\frac{1}{4}$, $\frac{1}{5}$, $\frac{1}{6}$, &c Root of the Infinite Multinomial be investigated.

AND that these are the true Roots of the given Powers, will be evident by restoring the Powers themselves from the Roots by the common Rules of Multiplication, as in the following Example.

1 —

$$1 - \frac{1}{6}x^2 - \frac{5}{72}x^4 - \frac{55}{1296}x^6, \&c.$$

$$1 - \frac{1}{6}x^2 - \frac{5}{72}x^4 - \frac{55}{1296}x^6, \&c.$$

$$1 - \frac{1}{6}x^2 - \frac{5}{72}x^4 - \frac{55}{1296}x^6, \&c.$$

$$- \frac{1}{6}x^2 + \frac{1}{36}x^4 + \frac{5}{432}x^6, \&c$$

$$- \frac{5}{72}x^4 + \frac{5}{432}x^6, \&c.$$

$$- \frac{55}{1296}x^6, \&c$$

$$1 - \frac{1}{3}x^2 - \frac{1}{9}x^4 - \frac{5}{81}x^6, \&c.$$

$$1 - \frac{1}{6}x^2 - \frac{5}{72}x^4 - \frac{55}{1296}x^6, \&c.$$

$$1 - \frac{1}{3}x^2 - \frac{1}{9}x^4 - \frac{5}{81}x^6, \&c$$

$$- \frac{1}{6}x^2 + \frac{1}{18}x^4 + \frac{1}{54}x^6, \&c.$$

$$- \frac{5}{72}x^4 + \frac{5}{216}x^6, \&c.$$

$$- \frac{55}{1296}x^6, \&c.$$

$$1 - \frac{1}{2}x^2 - \frac{1}{8}x^4 - \frac{1}{16}x^6, \&c.$$

AGAIN,

AGAIN, by multiplying $1 - \frac{1}{2}x^2 - \frac{1}{8}x^4 - \frac{1}{16}x^6$, &c by itself, we shall have $1 - xx$, as in the following Example

$$\begin{array}{rrrrrrl}
1 & -\frac{1}{2}x^2 & -\frac{1}{8}x^4 & -\frac{1}{16}x^6 & -\frac{5}{128}x^8 & -\frac{7}{256}x^{10}, & \&c \\
1 & -\frac{1}{2}x^2 & -\frac{1}{8}x^4 & -\frac{1}{16}x^6 & -\frac{5}{128}x^8 & -\frac{7}{256}x^{10}, & \&c \\
\hline
1 & -\frac{1}{2}x^2 & -\frac{1}{8}x^4 & -\frac{1}{16}x^6 & -\frac{5}{128}x^8 & -\frac{7}{256}x^{10}, & \&c \\
 & -\frac{1}{2}x^2 & +\frac{1}{4}x^4 & +\frac{1}{16}x^6 & +\frac{1}{32}x^8 & +\frac{5}{256}x^{10}, & \&c. \\
 & & -\frac{1}{8}x^4 & +\frac{1}{16}x^6 & +\frac{1}{64}x^8 & +\frac{1}{128}x^{10}, & \&c \\
 & & & -\frac{1}{16}x^6 & +\frac{1}{32}x^8 & +\frac{1}{128}x^{10}, & \&c. \\
 & & & & -\frac{5}{128}x^8 & +\frac{5}{256}x^{10}, & \&c \\
 & & & & & -\frac{7}{256}x^{10}, & \&c \\
\hline
1 & -xx & .\ 0 & 0 & .\ 0 & 0 & \\
\hline
\end{array}$$

And after this manner may any Power of any Root be found.

AGAIN, by multiplying the Quotient by the Divisor, as in ordinary Arithmetick, the Dividend will be restored, thus in the Example of Division in Page 15.

Multi-

Multiplying $a + \frac{1}{3}a^3 + \frac{2}{15}a^5 + \frac{17}{315}a^7$, &c the Quotient

by $1 - \frac{1}{2}a^2 + \frac{1}{24}a^4 - \frac{1}{720}a^6$, &c the Divisor

$$a + \frac{1}{3}a^3 + \frac{2}{15}a^5 + \frac{17}{315}a^7, \text{ \&c.}$$

$$- \frac{1}{2}a^3 - \frac{1}{6}a^5 - \frac{1}{15}a^7, \text{ \&c}$$

$$+ \frac{1}{24}a^5 + \frac{1}{72}a^7, \text{ \&c.}$$

$$- \frac{1}{720}a^7, \text{ \&c.}$$

The Product $= a - \frac{1}{6}a^3 + \frac{1}{120}a^5 - \frac{1}{5040}a^7$, &c Dividend.

And after the same manner may any Product be found.

Let us now suppose n to represent the Index of any Power, whether whole Number or Fraction, Positive or Negative, and $\overline{p+px}$ the Quantity proposed, whose Power is to be raised, or Root to be extracted, then will $\overline{p+px}^n = p^n + np^nx + \frac{n}{1} \times \frac{n-1}{2}p^nx^2 + \frac{n}{1} \times \frac{n-1}{2} \times \frac{n-2}{3}p^nx^3 + \frac{n}{1} \times \frac{n-1}{2} \times \frac{n-2}{3} \times \frac{n-3}{4}p^nx^4$, &c and putting $p^n = A$, $np^nx = B$, $\frac{n}{1} \times \frac{n-1}{2}p^nx^2 = C$, $\frac{n}{1} \times \frac{n-1}{2} \times \frac{n-2}{3}p^nx^3 = D$, &c.

$$\overline{p+px}^n = p^n + nAx + \frac{n-1}{2}Bx + \frac{n-2}{3}Cx + \frac{n-3}{4}Dx + \frac{n-4}{5}Ex, \text{ \&c.}$$

For

FOR assume $\overline{1+x}^{n} = 1 + Ax + Bxx + Cx^3 + Dx^4 + Ex^5 + Fx^6$, &c.

Then $n \times \overline{1+x}^{n-1}\,\dot{x} = A\dot{x} + 2Bx\dot{x} + 3Cx^2\dot{x} + 4Dx^3x + 5Ex^4x + 6Fx^5x$, &c.

And $n \times \overline{1+x}^{n-1} = A + 2Bx + 3Cx^2 + 4Dx^3 + 5Ex^4 + 6Fx^5$, &c. Whence

$$\frac{n \times \overline{1+x}^{n-1}}{\overline{1+x}^{n}} = \frac{A + 2Bx + 3Cx^2 + 4Dx^3 + 5Ex^4 + 6Fx^5, \text{ \&c.}}{1 + Ax + Bx^2 + Cx^3 + Dx^4 + Ex^5 + Fx^6, \text{ \&c}}$$

And $n + nAx + nBx^2 + nCx^3 + nDx^4 + nEx^5 + nFx^6$
$= A + 2Bx + 3Cx^2 + 4Dx^3 + 5Ex^4 + 6Fx^5$, &c.
$+ Ax + 2Bx^2 + 3Cx^3 + 4Dx^4 + 5Ex^5$, &c

Whence, by comparing the respective Terms on each Side of the Equation together, we shall have $n = A$, also
$nA = 2B + A$ & $nB = 3C + 2B$ & $nC = 4D + 3C$ & $nD = 5E + 4D$
$nA - A = 2B$ $nB - 2B = 3C$ $nC - 3C = 4D$ $nD - 4D = 5E$
$\frac{n-1}{2} \times A = B$ $\frac{n-2}{3} \times B = C$ $\frac{n-3}{4}\,C = D$ $\frac{n-4}{5}\,D = E$

Whence $\overline{1+x}^{n} = 1 + nx + n \times \frac{n-1}{2}x^2 + n \times \frac{n-1}{2} \times \frac{n-2}{3}x^3 + n \times \frac{n-1}{2} \times \frac{n-2}{3} \times \frac{n-3}{4}x^4 + n \times \frac{n-1}{2} \times \frac{n-2}{3} \times \frac{n-3}{4} \times \frac{n-4}{5}x^5 + n \times \frac{n-1}{2} \times \frac{n-2}{3} \times \frac{n-3}{4} \times \frac{n-4}{5} \times \frac{n-5}{6}x^6$, &c. and multiplying each Side of the Equation by p^n we shall have $\overline{p+px}^{n} = p^n + np^nx + n \times \frac{n-1}{2}p^nx^2 + n \times \frac{n-1}{2} + \frac{n-2}{3}p^nx^3 + n \times \frac{n-1}{2} \times \frac{n-2}{3} \times \frac{n-3}{4}p^nx^4 + \frac{n}{1} \times \frac{n-1}{2} \times \frac{n-2}{3} \times \frac{n-3}{4} \times \frac{n-4}{5}p^nx^5 + n \times \frac{n-1}{2} \times \frac{n-2}{3} \times \frac{n-3}{4} \times \frac{n-4}{5} \times \frac{n-5}{6}p^nx^6$, &c.

&c. and putting $p^n = A \cdot n p^n x = B$ $n \times \frac{n-1}{2} p^n x^2 = C$. $n \times \frac{n-1}{2} \times \frac{n-2}{3} p^n x^3 = D$. $n \times \frac{n-1}{2} \times \frac{n-2}{3} \times \frac{n-3}{4}$ $p^n x^4 = E$ $\frac{n}{1} \times \frac{n-1}{2} \times \frac{n-2}{3} \times \frac{n-3}{4} \times \frac{n-4}{5} p^n x^5 = F$, we shall have $\overline{p+px}^n = p^n + nAx + \frac{n-1}{2} Bx + \frac{n-1}{3} Cx + \frac{n-3}{4} Dx + \frac{n-4}{5} Ex + \frac{n-5}{6} Fx$, &c which is the celebrated Binomial Series invented by the great Sir *Isaac Newton* for the raising of Powers, extracting of Roots, and the Solution of all Sort of Problems, wherein the Doctrine of Series is concerned

SUPPOSE, for Example, $\frac{1}{d+e}$ or $\overline{d+e}^{-1}$ were proposed, put $p = d$ $px = e$; then will $x = \frac{e}{p} = \frac{e}{d}$, and $n = -1$, whence $p^n = d^{-1} = A$ $nAx = -1 \times d^{-1} \times -\frac{e}{d} = -d^{-2}e = B$. $\frac{n-1}{2} Bx = -\frac{-1-1}{2} \times -d^{-2} e \times \frac{e}{d} = +d^{-3}e^2 = C$ $\frac{n-2}{3} \times Cx = \frac{-1-2}{3} \times d^{-3} e^2 \times \frac{e}{d} = -d^{-4}e^3 = D$, &c

Whence $\overline{d+e}^{-1} = d^{-1} - d^{-2}e + d^{-3}e^2 - d^{-4}e^3 + d^{-5}e^4$, &c.

Or $\frac{1}{d+e} = \frac{1}{d} - \frac{e}{dd} + \frac{ee}{d^3} - \frac{e^3}{d^4} + \frac{e^4}{d^5}$, &c

II LET us suppose the Quantity $\frac{1}{\overline{d+e}^3}$ or $\overline{d+e}^{-3}$ were given.

Put, as before, $p = d$. $e = px$, whence $x = \frac{e}{p} = \frac{e}{d}$, and $n =$

$n = -3$; consequently $p^n = d^{-3} = A$. $nAx = -3 \times d^{-1} \times \frac{e}{d} = -3d^{-4}e = B$. $\frac{n-1}{2}Bx = \frac{-3-2}{2} \times -3d^{-4}e \times \frac{e}{d} = 6d^{-5}e^2 = C$. $\frac{n-2}{3}Cx = \frac{-3-2}{3} \times 6d^{-5}e^2 \times \frac{e}{d} = -\frac{30}{3}d^{-6}e^3 = -10d^{-6}e^3 = D$, &c.

Whence $\overline{d+e}^{-3} = d^{-3} - 3d^{-4}e + 6d^{-5}e^2 - 10d^{-6}e^3$, &c.

Or $\frac{1}{\overline{d+e}^3} = \frac{1}{d^3} - \frac{e}{3d^4} + \frac{e^2}{6d^5} - \frac{e^3}{10d^6}$, &c.

III. SUPPOSE the Quantity $\frac{1}{\sqrt[3]{d+e}}$ or $\overline{d+e}^{-\frac{1}{3}}$ were given, putting $p = d$ $px = e$, whence $x = \frac{e}{d}$ and $n = -\frac{1}{3}$ we shall have $p^n = d^{-\frac{1}{3}} = A$ $nAx = -\frac{1}{3} \times d^{-\frac{1}{3}}\frac{e}{d} = -\frac{1}{3}d^{-\frac{1}{3}-1}e = -\frac{1}{3}d^{\frac{4}{3}}e = B$ $\frac{n-1}{2}Bx = \frac{-\frac{1}{3}-1}{2} \times -\frac{1}{3}d^{-\frac{4}{3}}e\frac{e}{d} = -\frac{2}{3} \times -\frac{1}{3}d^{-\frac{4}{3}-1}e^2 = +\frac{2}{9}d^{-\frac{7}{3}}e^2 = C$. $\frac{n-2}{3}Cx = \frac{-\frac{1}{3}-2}{3} \times \frac{2}{9}d^{-\frac{7}{3}}e^2 \times \frac{e}{d} = -\frac{7}{9} \times \frac{2}{9}d^{-\frac{10}{3}}e^3 = -\frac{14}{81}d^{-\frac{10}{3}}e^3 = D$, &c.

Whence $\overline{d+e}^{-\frac{1}{3}} = d^{-\frac{1}{3}} - \frac{1}{3}d^{-\frac{4}{3}}e + \frac{2}{9}d^{-\frac{7}{3}}e^2 - \frac{14}{81}d^{-\frac{10}{3}}e^3$, &c.

Or $\frac{1}{\overline{d+e}^{\frac{1}{3}}} = \frac{1}{d^{\frac{1}{3}}} - \frac{e}{3d^{\frac{4}{3}}} + \frac{2e^2}{9d^{\frac{7}{3}}} - \frac{14e^3}{81d^{\frac{10}{3}}}$, &c.

 IV. SUP-

IV. Suppose $\overline{aa+xx}|^{\frac{1}{2}}=y$. Here $p=aa$. $px=xx$, whence $x=\frac{xx}{aa}$ and $n=\frac{1}{2}$ consequently $p^n=a=A$. nAx $=\frac{1}{2}a\times\frac{xx}{aa}=\frac{1}{2}\frac{xx}{a}=B$ $\frac{n-1}{2}Bx=\frac{\frac{1}{2}-1}{2}\times\frac{1}{2}\frac{xx}{a}$ $\times\frac{xx}{aa}=-\frac{1}{4}\times\frac{1}{2}\times\frac{x^4}{a^3}=-\frac{1}{8}\frac{x^4}{a^3}=C$. $\frac{n-2}{3}Cx=$ $=\frac{\frac{1}{2}-2}{3}\times-\frac{1}{8}\frac{x^4}{a^3}\times\frac{x^2}{a^2}=-\frac{1}{2}\times-\frac{1}{8}\times\frac{x^6}{a^5}=\frac{1}{16}\frac{x^6}{a^5}=D$ $\frac{n-3}{4}Dx=\frac{\frac{1}{2}-3}{4}\times\frac{1}{16}\frac{x^6}{a^5}\times\frac{x^2}{a^2}=-\frac{5}{8}\times\frac{1}{16}\times\frac{x^8}{a^7}=-\frac{5}{128}$ $\frac{x^8}{a^7}=E$.

Whence $y=a+\frac{x^2}{2a}-\frac{x^4}{8a^3}+\frac{x^6}{16a^5}-\frac{5x^8}{128a^7}$, &c.

V. If y be supposed equal to $\overline{x-xx}|^{\frac{1}{2}}$, then $p=x$. px $=-xx$; whence $x=\frac{-xx}{p}=-\frac{xx}{x}=-x$, and $n=\frac{1}{2}$ consequently $p^n=x^{\frac{1}{2}}=A$ $nAx=\frac{1}{2}x^{\frac{1}{2}}\times-x=-\frac{1}{2}x^{\frac{3}{2}}=B$ $\frac{n-1}{2}Bx=\frac{\frac{1}{2}-1}{2}\times-\frac{1}{2}x^{\frac{3}{2}}\times-x=-\frac{1}{4}\times-\frac{1}{2}x^{\frac{3}{2}}$ $\times-x=-\frac{1}{8}x^{\frac{5}{2}}=C$.
$\frac{n-2}{3}Cx=\frac{\frac{1}{2}-\frac{4}{2}}{3}\times-\frac{1}{8}x^{\frac{5}{2}}\times-x=-\frac{1}{2}\times-\frac{1}{8}x^{\frac{5}{2}}\times-x$ $=-\frac{1}{16}x^{\frac{7}{2}}=D$, &c.

And $y=x^{\frac{1}{2}}-\frac{1}{2}x^{\frac{3}{2}}-\frac{1}{8}x^{\frac{5}{2}}-\frac{1}{16}x^{\frac{7}{2}}-\frac{5}{128}x^{\frac{9}{2}}$, &c.

VI Let

VI. Let $\frac{1}{2\sqrt{x-xx}}$, or $\frac{1}{2}\overline{x-xx}^{-\frac{1}{2}}$, be the Quantity proposed; then putting, as before, $p = x$. $px = -xx$, whence $x = -x$ and $n = -\frac{1}{2}$, we shall have $p^n = x^{-\frac{1}{2}} = A$. $nAx = -\frac{1}{2}\times x^{-\frac{1}{2}}\times -x = +\frac{1}{2}x^{-\frac{1}{2}+1} = \frac{1}{2}x^{\frac{1}{2}} = B$. $\frac{n-1}{2}Bx = \frac{-\frac{1}{2}-1}{2}\times\frac{1}{2}x^{\frac{1}{2}}\times -x = -\frac{3}{4}\times\frac{1}{2}x^{\frac{1}{2}} + x = \frac{3}{8}x^{\frac{3}{2}} = C$. $\frac{n-2}{3}Cx = \frac{-\frac{1}{2}-2}{3}\times\frac{3}{8}x^{\frac{3}{2}}\times -x = -\frac{5}{6}\times\frac{3}{8}x^{\frac{3}{2}} - x = \frac{5}{16}x^{\frac{5}{2}} = D$. $\frac{n-3}{4}Dx = \frac{-\frac{1}{2}-3}{4}\times\frac{5}{16}x^{\frac{5}{2}}\times -x = -\frac{7}{8}\times\frac{5}{16}x^{\frac{5}{2}} - x = \frac{35}{128}x^{\frac{7}{2}} = E$, &c.

Whence $\overline{x-xx}^{-\frac{1}{2}} = x^{-\frac{1}{2}} + \frac{1}{2}x^{\frac{1}{2}} + \frac{3}{8}x^{\frac{3}{2}} + \frac{5}{16}x^{\frac{5}{2}} + \frac{5}{128}x^{\frac{7}{2}}$, &c. and $\frac{1}{2\sqrt{x-xx}} = \frac{1}{2}\,\frac{1}{\sqrt{x-xx}} = \frac{1}{2}\overline{x-xx}^{-\frac{1}{2}} = \frac{1}{2}x^{-\frac{1}{2}} + \frac{1}{4}x^{\frac{1}{2}} + \frac{3}{16}x^{\frac{3}{2}} + \frac{5}{32}x^{\frac{5}{2}} + \frac{35}{256}x^{\frac{7}{2}}$, &c. $= \frac{1}{2x^{\frac{1}{2}}} + \frac{1}{4}x^{\frac{1}{2}} + \frac{3}{16}x^{\frac{3}{2}} + \frac{5}{32}x^{\frac{5}{2}} + \frac{35}{256}x^{\frac{7}{2}}$, &c. $= \frac{1}{2x^{\frac{1}{2}}} + \frac{x^{\frac{1}{2}}}{4} + \frac{3x^{\frac{3}{2}}}{16} + \frac{5x^{\frac{5}{2}}}{32} + \frac{35x^{\frac{7}{2}}}{256}$, &c.

The Excellency and Usefulness of this Series will more evidently appear, by shewing that after three or four Terms at the most are obtained, the Law of Continuation *ad Infinitum* is discovered. Thus in the fifth Example, where $\overline{x+xx}^{\frac{1}{2}}$ was the Quantity proposed, because $\overline{x-xx}^{\frac{1}{2}} = x^{\frac{1}{2}}\overline{1-x}^{\frac{1}{2}}$, and that $\overline{1+x}^{n} = 1 + nx + \frac{n}{1}\times\frac{n-1}{2}x^2 + \frac{n}{1}\times\frac{n-1}{2}\times\frac{n-2}{3}x^3 + \frac{n}{1}\times\frac{n-1}{2}\times\frac{n-2}{3}\times\frac{n-3}{4}x^4$, &c.

Therefore

Therefore $\overline{1-x}^{\frac{1}{2}} = 1 + \frac{\frac12}{1}\times\frac{-x}{1}\times\frac{\frac12}{1}+\frac{\frac12-1}{2}\times\frac{xx}{1}+\frac{\frac12}{1}\times\frac{\frac12-1}{2}\times\frac{\frac12-2}{3}\times\frac{-x^3}{1}+\frac{\frac12}{1}\times\frac{\frac12-1}{2}\times\frac{\frac12-2}{3}\times\frac{\frac12-3}{4}\times\frac{+x^4}{1}$, &c

And $\overline{1-x}^{\frac12} = 1+\frac{\frac12}{1}\times\frac{-x}{1}+\frac{\frac12}{1}\times\frac{xx}{1}+\frac{1}{2}\times\frac{-\frac12}{2}\times\frac{-\frac12}{3}\times\frac{-x^3}{1}+\frac{\frac12}{1}\times\frac{-\frac12}{2}\times\frac{-\frac12}{3}\times\frac{-\frac12}{4}\times\frac{x^4}{1}$, &c.

And $\overline{1-x}^{\frac12} = 1-\frac{1}{2}x-\frac{1\times1}{2\times4}x^2-\frac{1\times1\times3}{2\times4\times6}x^3-\frac{1\times1\times3\times5}{2\times4\times6\times8}x^4$, whence the next Step will be $\frac{1\times1\times3\times5\times7}{2\times4\times6\times8\times10}x^{10}$, &c.

And $x\overline{-xx}^{\frac12} = x^{\frac12}\,\overline{1-x}^{\frac12} = x^{\frac12}-\frac{1}{2}x^{\frac32}-\frac{1}{8}x^{\frac52}-\frac{1}{16}x^{\frac72}-\frac{5}{128}x^{\frac92}-\frac{7}{256}x^{\frac{11}{2}}$, &c

AGAIN, Suppose, as in the sixth Example, where $\frac{1}{2\sqrt{x-xx}}$ or $\frac{1}{2}\overline{x-xx}^{-\frac12}$ was the Quantity proposed, because $\frac{1}{2}\overline{x-xx}^{-\frac12} = \frac{1}{2}x^{-\frac12}\,\overline{1-x}^{-\frac12}$, and that by the former Theorem

$$\overline{1-x}^{-\frac12} = 1+\frac{-\frac12}{1}\times\frac{-x}{1}+\frac{-\frac12}{1}\times\frac{-\frac12-1}{2}\times\frac{xx}{1}+\frac{-\frac12}{1}\times\frac{-\frac12-1}{2}\times\frac{-\frac12-2}{3}\times\frac{-x^3}{1}\times\frac{-\frac12}{1}\times\frac{-\frac12-1}{2}\times\frac{-\frac12-2}{3}\times-\frac{-\frac12-3}{4}\times\frac{x^4}{1}, \text{ \&c}$$

And

And $\overline{1-x}^{-\frac{1}{2}} = 1 + \frac{-\frac{1}{2}}{1} \times \frac{-x}{1} + \frac{-\frac{1}{2}}{1} \times \frac{-\frac{1}{2}}{2} \times \frac{xx}{1} + \frac{-\frac{1}{2}}{1} \times \frac{-\frac{1}{2}}{2} \times \frac{-x^3}{3} \times \frac{-x^3}{1} + \frac{-\frac{1}{2}}{1} \times \frac{-\frac{1}{2}}{2} \times \frac{-\frac{1}{2}}{3} \times \frac{-\frac{1}{2}}{4} \times \frac{x^4}{1}$, &c

Therefore $\overline{1-x}^{-\frac{1}{2}} = 1 + \frac{1}{2}x + \frac{1 \times 3}{2 \times 4}x^2 + \frac{1 \times 3 \times 5}{2 \times 4 \times 6}x^3 + \frac{1 \times 3 \times 5 \times 7}{2 \times 4 \times 6 \times 8}x^4$, whence the next Step will be $\frac{1 \times 3 \times 5 \times 7 \times 9}{2 \times 4 \times 6 \times 8 \times 10}x^5$

and consequently $\frac{1}{2}\overline{x - xx}^{-\frac{1}{2}} = \frac{1}{2}x^{-\frac{1}{2}} \times \overline{1-x}^{-\frac{1}{2}} = x^{-\frac{1}{2}} + \frac{1}{4}x^{\frac{1}{2}} + \frac{3}{16}x^{\frac{3}{2}} + \frac{5}{32}x^{\frac{5}{2}} + \frac{35}{256}x^{\frac{7}{2}} + \frac{63}{512}x^{\frac{9}{2}}$, &c

By the same Theorem the Unciæ of the $\frac{1}{3}$ Power positive will be found to be made up of

$\frac{\frac{1}{3}}{1} \times \frac{\frac{1}{3}-1}{2} \times \frac{\frac{1}{3}-2}{3} \times \frac{\frac{1}{3}-3}{4} \times \frac{\frac{1}{3}-4}{5} \times \frac{\frac{1}{3}-5}{6} \times \frac{\frac{1}{3}-6}{7} \times \frac{\frac{1}{3}-7}{8}$, &c.

or $\frac{\frac{1}{3}}{1} \times \frac{-\frac{2}{3}}{2} \times \frac{-\frac{5}{3}}{3} \times \frac{-\frac{8}{3}}{4} \times \frac{-\frac{11}{3}}{5} \times \frac{-\frac{14}{3}}{6} \times \frac{-\frac{17}{3}}{7} \times \frac{\frac{20}{3}}{8}$, &c

Or $\frac{1}{3} \times -\frac{2}{6} \times -\frac{5}{9} \times -\frac{8}{12} \times -\frac{11}{15} \times -\frac{14}{18} \times -\frac{17}{21} \times -\frac{20}{24}$,

whence the several Unciæ will be $\frac{1}{3} - \frac{1 \times 2}{3 \times 6} + \frac{1 \times 2 \times 5}{3 \times 6 \times 9} - \frac{1 \times 2 \times 5 \times 8}{3 \times 6 \times 9 \times 12} + \frac{1 \times 2 \times 5 \times 8 \times 11}{3 \times 6 \times 9 \times 12 \times 15} - \frac{1 \times 2 \times 5 \times 8 \times 11 \times 14}{3 \times 6 \times 9 \times 12 \times 15 \times 18}$, &c and the Unciæ of the $\frac{1}{3}$ Power Negative, will be made up of $\frac{-\frac{1}{3}}{1} \times \frac{-\frac{1}{3}-1}{2} \times \frac{-\frac{1}{3}-2}{3} \times \frac{-\frac{1}{3}-3}{4} \times \frac{-\frac{1}{3}-4}{5} \times \frac{-\frac{1}{3}-5}{6}$, &c. or $\frac{-\frac{1}{3}}{1} \times \frac{-\frac{4}{3}}{2} \times \frac{-\frac{7}{3}}{3} \times \frac{-\frac{10}{3}}{4} \times \frac{-\frac{13}{3}}{5} \times \frac{\frac{16}{3}}{6}$, &c. Whence the several Coefficients will be $-\frac{1}{3} + \frac{1 \times 4}{3 \times 6} - \frac{1 \times 4 \times 7}{3 \times 6 \times 9} + \frac{1 \times 4 \times 7 \times 10}{3 \times 6 \times 9 \times 12} - \frac{1 \times 4 \times 7 \times 10 \times 13}{3 \times 6 \times 9 \times 12 \times 15}$, &c.

AFTER

After the same way the Unciæ of the $\frac{1}{4}$ Power positive will be found to be made up of $\frac{\frac{1}{4}}{1}\times\frac{\frac{1}{4}-1}{2}\times\frac{\frac{1}{4}-2}{3}\times\frac{\frac{1}{4}-3}{4}\times\frac{\frac{1}{4}-4}{5}\times\frac{\frac{1}{4}-5}{6}\times\frac{\frac{1}{4}-6}{7}$, &c. or $\frac{\frac{1}{4}}{1}\times\frac{-\frac{1}{4}}{2}\times\frac{-\frac{1}{4}}{3}\times\frac{-\frac{11}{4}}{4}\times\frac{-\frac{11}{4}}{5}\times\frac{-\frac{19}{4}}{6}\times\frac{-\frac{21}{4}}{7}$, &c or $\frac{1}{4}\times-\frac{3}{8}\times-\frac{7}{12}\times-\frac{11}{16}\times-\frac{15}{20}\times-\frac{19}{24}\times-\frac{23}{28}$, &c. whence the several Coefficients will be $\frac{1}{4}-\frac{1\times3}{4\times8}+\frac{1\times3\times7}{4\times8\times12}+\frac{1\times3\times7\times11}{4\times8\times12\times16}+\frac{1\times3\times7\times11\times15}{4\times8\times12\times16\times20}$, &c. and the Unciæ, or Coefficients of the $\frac{1}{4}$ Power Negative, will be made up of $\frac{-\frac{1}{4}}{1}\times\frac{-\frac{1}{4}-1}{2}\times\frac{-\frac{1}{4}-2}{3}\times\frac{-\frac{1}{4}-3}{4}\times\frac{-\frac{1}{4}-4}{5}\times\frac{-\frac{1}{4}-5}{6}$, &c or $\frac{-\frac{1}{4}}{1}\times\frac{-\frac{1}{4}}{2}\times\frac{-\frac{9}{4}}{3}\times\frac{-\frac{13}{4}}{4}\times\frac{-\frac{17}{4}}{5}\times\frac{-\frac{21}{4}}{6}$, &c. or $-\frac{1}{4}\times-\frac{5}{8}\times-\frac{9}{12}\times-\frac{13}{16}\times-\frac{17}{20}\times-\frac{21}{24}$; whence the several Unciæ will be $-\frac{1}{4}+\frac{1\times5}{4\times8}-\frac{1\times5\times9}{4\times8\times12}+\frac{1\times5\times9\times13}{4\times8\times12\times16}$ $-\frac{1\times5\times9\times13\times17}{4\times8\times12\times16\times20}+\frac{1\times5\times9\times13\times17\times20}{4\times8\times12\times16\times20\times24}$, &c And by comparing the Unciæ of these several Powers together, may the Rule for finding the Unciæ of higher Powers be found, without having Regard to the general Theorem, the Law being very obvious

Let us now suppose the Trinomial Root $a+b+c$ to be raised to n Power, putting $b+c$ in the room of x in the former Series, we shall have $\overline{a+b+x}^{n}=a^{n}+na^{n-1}\overline{b+c}^{1}$ $+\frac{n}{1}\times\frac{n-1}{2}a^{n-2}\overline{b+c}^{2}+\frac{n}{1}\times\frac{n-1}{2}\times\frac{n-2}{3}a^{n-3}\overline{b+c}^{3}$ &c

&c. and by substituting the several Powers of $b+x$ in their respective Places, instead of the Roots themselves, we shall have

$$\overline{a+b+c}^n = a^n + na^{n-1}b + \frac{n}{1}\times\frac{n-1}{2}a^{n-2}b^2 + \frac{n}{1}\times\frac{n-1}{2}\times\frac{n-2}{3}a^{n-3}b^3 +$$

$$na^{n-1}c \qquad \frac{n}{1}\times\frac{n-1}{1}a^{n-2}bc \qquad \frac{n}{1}\times\frac{n-1}{2}\times\frac{n-2}{1}a^{n-3}b^2c$$

$$\frac{n}{1}\times\frac{n-1}{2}a^{n-2}c^2 \qquad \frac{n}{1}\times\frac{n-1}{1}\times\frac{n-2}{2}a^{n-3}bcc$$

$$\frac{n}{1}\times\frac{n-1}{2}\times\frac{n-1}{3}a^{n-3}c^3$$

$$\frac{n}{1}\times\frac{n-1}{2}\times\frac{n-2}{3}\times\frac{n-3}{4}a^{n-4}b^4 +, \&c$$

$$\frac{n}{1}\times\frac{n-1}{2}\times\frac{n-2}{3}\times\frac{n-3}{1}a^{n-4}b^3c$$

$$\frac{n}{1}\times\frac{n-1}{2}\times\frac{n-2}{1}\times\frac{n-3}{2}a^{n-4}b^2c^2$$

$$\frac{n}{1}\times\frac{n-1}{1}\times\frac{n-2}{2}\times\frac{n-3}{3}a^{n-4}bc^3$$

$$\frac{n}{1}\times\frac{n-1}{2}\times\frac{n-2}{3}\times\frac{n-3}{4}a^{n-4}c^4$$

Whence the Law of Continuation is obvious.

But if in the room of $\overline{a+b+c}^n$ we assume $\overline{a+bz+czz}^n$, and rank the several Members of the Powers of $bz+czz$ under the respective Powers of z, in the first or uppermost Line, in a regular and successive Order, we shall have

$$\overline{a+bz+czz}^n = a^n + na^{n-1}bz + \frac{n}{1}\times\frac{n-1}{2}a^{n-2}b^2z^2 + \frac{n}{1}\times\frac{n-1}{2}\times\frac{n-2}{3}a^{n-3}b^3z^3 +$$

$$\frac{n}{1}a^{n-1}c \qquad \frac{n}{1}\times\frac{n-1}{1}a^{n-2}bc$$

$$\frac{n}{1}\times\frac{n-1}{2}\times\frac{n-2}{3}\times\frac{n-3}{4}a^{n-4}b^4z^4 + \frac{n}{1}\times\frac{n-1}{2}\times\frac{n-2}{3}\times\frac{n-3}{4}\times\frac{n-4}{5}a^{n-5}b^5z^5$$

$$\frac{n}{1}\times\frac{n-1}{2}\times\frac{n-2}{1}a^{n-3}bbc \qquad \frac{n}{1}\times\frac{n-1}{2}\times\frac{n-2}{3}\times\frac{n-3}{1}a^{n-4}b^3c$$

$$\frac{n}{1}\times\frac{n-1}{2}a^{n-3}cc \qquad \frac{n}{1}\times\frac{n-1}{1}\times\frac{n-2}{2}a^{n-3}bcc$$

$$\frac{n}{1}\times\frac{n-1}{2}\times\frac{n-2}{3}\times\frac{n-3}{4}\times\frac{n-4}{5}\times\frac{n-5}{6}a^{n-5}b^6z^6 + \frac{n}{1}\times\frac{n-1}{2}\times\frac{n-2}{3}\times\frac{n-3}{4}\times\frac{n-4}{5}\times\frac{n-5}{6}\times\frac{n-6}{7}a^{n-7}b^7z^7$$

$$\frac{n}{1}\times\frac{n-1}{2}\times\frac{n-2}{3}\times\frac{n-3}{4}\times\frac{n-4}{1}a^{n-5}b^4c \qquad \frac{n}{1}\times\frac{n-1}{2}\times\frac{n-2}{3}\times\frac{n-3}{4}\times\frac{n-4}{5}\times\frac{n-5}{1}a^{n-6}b^5c$$

$$\frac{n}{1}\times\frac{n-1}{2}\times\frac{n-2}{1}\times\frac{n-3}{2}a^{n-4}b^2c^2 \qquad \frac{n}{1}\times\frac{n-1}{2}\times\frac{n-2}{3}\times\frac{n-3}{1}\times\frac{n-4}{2}a^{n-5}b^3c^2$$

$$\frac{n}{1}\times\frac{n-1}{2}\times\frac{n-2}{3}a^{n-3}c^3 \qquad \frac{n}{1}\times\frac{n-1}{1}\times\frac{n-2}{2}\times\frac{n-3}{3}a^{n-4}bc^3$$

AGAIN, if the Quadrinomial $\overline{a+bz+cz^2+dz^3}^n$ were propofed, by putting cz^2+dz^3 in the room of cz^2, in the former Cafe, and the feveral Powers of that in the room of the feveral Powers of this, ranging each under its refpective Power of z, we fhall have

$$\overline{a+bz+cz^2+dz^3}^n = a^n + na^{n-1}bz + \frac{n}{1}\times\frac{n-1}{2}a^{n-2}b^2z^2 + \frac{n}{1}\times\frac{n-1}{2}\times\frac{n-2}{3}a^{n-3}b^3z^3 +$$

$$\frac{n}{1}a^{n-1}c \qquad \frac{n}{1}\times\frac{n-1}{1}a^{n-2}bc$$

$$\frac{n}{1}a^{n-1}d$$

$+ \frac{n}{1}$

$$\frac{n}{1}\times\frac{n-1}{2}\times\frac{n-2}{3}\times\frac{n-3}{4}\,a^{n-4}\,b^4\,z^4$$
$$\frac{n}{1}\times\frac{n-1}{2}\times\frac{n-2}{1}\,a^{n-3}\,b^2\,c$$
$$\frac{n}{1}\times\frac{n-1}{1}\,a^{n-2}\,b\,d$$
$$\frac{n}{1}\times\frac{n-1}{2}\,a^{n-2}\,c\,c$$

$$+\frac{n}{1}\times\frac{n-1}{2}\times\frac{n-2}{3}\times\frac{n-3}{4}\times\frac{n-4}{5}\,a^{n-5}\,b^5\,z^5$$
$$\frac{n}{1}\times\frac{n-1}{2}\times\frac{n-2}{3}\times\frac{n-3}{1}\,a^{n-4}\,b^3\,c$$
$$\frac{n}{1}\times\frac{n-1}{2}\times\frac{n-2}{1}\,a^{n-3}\,b^2\,d$$
$$\frac{n}{1}\times\frac{n-1}{1}\times\frac{n-2}{2}\,a^{n-3}\,b\,c\,c$$
$$\frac{n}{1}\times\frac{n-1}{1}\,a^{n-2}\,c\,d$$

$$\frac{n}{1}\times\frac{n-1}{2}\times\frac{n-2}{3}\times\frac{n-3}{4}\times\frac{n-4}{5}\times\frac{n-5}{6}\,a^{n-6}b^6z^6$$
$$\frac{n}{1}\times\frac{n-1}{2}\times\frac{n-2}{3}\times\frac{n-3}{4}\times\frac{n-5}{1}\,a^{n-5}b^4\,c$$
$$\frac{n}{1}\times\frac{n-1}{2}\times\frac{n-2}{3}\times\frac{n-3}{1}\,a^{n-4}b^3\,d$$
$$\frac{n}{1}\times\frac{n-1}{2}\times\frac{n-2}{1}\times\frac{n-3}{2}\,a^{n-4}\,b^2\,d^2$$
$$\frac{n}{1}\times\frac{n-1}{1}\times\frac{n-2}{1}\,a^{n-3}\,b\,c\,d$$
$$\frac{n}{1}\times\frac{n-1}{2}\times\frac{n-2}{3}\,a^{n-3}\,c$$
$$\frac{n}{1}\times\frac{n-1}{2}\,a^{n-2}\,d\,d$$

$$+\frac{n}{1}\times\frac{n-1}{2}\times\frac{n-2}{3}\times\frac{n-3}{4}\times\frac{n-4}{5}\times\frac{n-5}{6}\times\frac{n-6}{7}\,a^{n-7}b^7\,z^7$$
$$\frac{n}{1}\times\frac{n-1}{2}\times\frac{n-2}{3}\times\frac{n-3}{4}\times\frac{n-4}{5}\times\frac{n-5}{1}\,a^{n-6}\,b^5\,c$$
$$\frac{n}{1}\times\frac{n-1}{2}\times\frac{n-2}{3}\times\frac{n-3}{4}\times\frac{n-4}{1}\,a^{n-5}\,b^4\,d$$
$$\frac{n}{1}\times\frac{n-1}{2}\times\frac{n-2}{3}\times\frac{n-3}{1}\times\frac{n-4}{2}\,a^{n-5}b^3\,c^2$$
$$\frac{n}{1}\times\frac{n-1}{2}\times\frac{n-2}{1}\times\frac{n-3}{1}\,a^{n-4}\,b^2\,c\,d$$
$$\frac{n}{1}\times\frac{n-1}{1}\times\frac{n-2}{2}\times\frac{n-3}{3}\,a^{n-4}\,b\,d^3$$
$$\frac{n}{1}\times\frac{n-1}{1}\times\frac{n-2}{2}\,a^{n-3}\,b\,d^2$$
$$\frac{n}{1}\times\frac{n-1}{2}\times\frac{n-2}{1}\,a^{n-3}\,c^2\,d\;.$$

AND after the ſame manner, by a continual Subſtitution of the Binomial itſelf, and its ſeveral Powers, or the Trinomial itſelf, and its ſeveral Powers, &c. in the room of the laſt Term, we ſhall have ſo many Theorems for the raiſing of any Number of Terms to any given Power.

THUS, if the Quantity $a + bz + cz^2 + dz^3 + ez^4 + fz^5 + gz^6 + hz^7$, &c. were propoſed, then $\overline{a + bz + cz^2 + dz^3 + ez^4 + fz^5 + gz^6 + hz^7}$, &c. $= a^n + na^{n-1}bz + n \times \frac{n-1}{2}a^{n-2}b^2z^2 +$

$$\phantom{n \times \frac{n-1}{2}} na^{n-1}c$$

$$\frac{n}{1} \times \frac{n-1}{2} \times \frac{n-2}{3}a^{n-3}b^3z^3 + \frac{n}{1} \times \frac{n-1}{2} \times \frac{n-2}{3} \times \frac{n-3}{4}a^{n-4}b^4z^4 + \frac{n}{1} \times \frac{n-1}{2} \times \frac{n-2}{3} \times \frac{n-3}{4} \times \frac{n-4}{5}a^{n-5}b^5z^5$$

$$\frac{n}{1} \times \frac{n-1}{1}a^{n-2}bc \qquad \frac{n}{1} \times \frac{n-1}{2} \times \frac{n-2}{1}a^{n-3}b^2c \qquad \frac{n}{1} \times \frac{n-1}{2} \times \frac{n-2}{3} \times \frac{n-3}{1}a^{n-4}b^3c$$

$$\frac{n}{1}a^{n-1}d \qquad \frac{n}{1} \times \frac{n-1}{1}a^{n-2}bd \qquad \frac{n}{1} \times \frac{n-1}{2} \times \frac{n-2}{1}a^{n-3}b^2d$$

$$\frac{n}{1}a^{n-1}e \qquad \frac{n}{1} \times \frac{n-1}{1} \times \frac{n-2}{2}a^{n-3}bc^2$$

$$\frac{n}{1} \times \frac{n-1}{1}a^{n-2}be$$

$$\frac{n}{1} \times \frac{n-1}{1}a^{n-2}cd$$

$$\frac{n}{1}a^{n-1}f$$

$$\frac{n}{1} \times$$

$$\frac{n}{1}\times\frac{n-1}{2}\times\frac{n-2}{3}\times\frac{n-3}{4}\times\frac{n-4}{5}\times\frac{n-5}{6}a^{n-6}b^{6}z^{6}$$
$$\frac{n}{1}\times\frac{n-1}{2}\times\frac{n-2}{3}\times\frac{n-3}{4}\times\frac{n-4}{1}a^{n-5}b^{4}c$$
$$\frac{n}{1}\times\frac{n-1}{2}\times\frac{n-2}{3}\times\frac{n-3}{1}a^{n-4}b^{3}d$$
$$\frac{n}{1}\times\frac{n-1}{2}\times\frac{n-2}{1}\times\frac{n-3}{2}a^{n-4}b^{2}c^{2}$$
$$\frac{n}{1}\times\frac{n-1}{2}\times\frac{n-2}{1}a^{n-3}b^{2}e$$
$$\frac{n}{1}\times\frac{n-1}{1}\times\frac{n-2}{1}a^{n-3}bcd$$
$$\frac{n}{1}\times\frac{n-1}{1}a^{n-2}bf$$
$$\frac{n}{1}\times\frac{n-1}{2}\times\frac{n-2}{3}a^{n-3}c^{3}$$
$$\frac{n}{1}\times\frac{n-1}{1}a^{n-2}ce$$
$$\frac{n}{1}\times\frac{n-1}{2}a^{n-2}dd$$
$$\frac{n}{1}a^{n-1}g$$

$$+\frac{n}{1}\times\frac{n-1}{2}\times\frac{n-2}{3}\times\frac{n-3}{4}\times\frac{n-4}{5}\times\frac{n-5}{6}\times\frac{n-6}{7}a^{n-7}b^{7}z^{7}$$
$$\frac{n}{1}\times\frac{n-1}{2}\times\frac{n-2}{3}\times\frac{n-3}{4}\times\frac{n-4}{5}\times\frac{n-5}{1}a^{n-6}b^{5}c$$
$$\frac{n}{1}\times\frac{n-1}{2}\times\frac{n-2}{3}\times\frac{n-3}{4}\times\frac{n-4}{1}a^{n-5}b^{4}d$$
$$\frac{n}{1}\times\frac{n-1}{2}\times\frac{n-2}{3}\times\frac{n-3}{1}\times\frac{n-4}{2}a^{n-5}b^{3}c^{2}$$
$$\frac{n}{1}\times\frac{n-1}{2}\times\frac{n-2}{3}\times\frac{n-3}{1}a^{n-4}b^{3}e$$
$$\frac{n}{1}\times\frac{n-1}{2}\times\frac{n-2}{1}\times\frac{n-3}{1}a^{n-4}b^{2}cd$$
$$\frac{n}{1}\times\frac{n-1}{2}\times\frac{n-2}{1}a^{n-3}b^{2}f$$
$$\frac{n}{1}\times\frac{n-1}{1}\times\frac{n-2}{2}\times\frac{n-3}{3}a^{n-4}bc^{3}$$
$$\frac{n}{1}\times\frac{n-1}{1}\times\frac{n-2}{1}a^{n-3}bce$$
$$\frac{n}{1}\times\frac{n-1}{1}\times\frac{n-2}{2}a^{n-3}bdd$$
$$\frac{n}{1}\times\frac{n-1}{1}a^{n-2}bg$$
$$\frac{n}{1}\times\frac{n-1}{2}\times\frac{n-2}{1}a^{n-3}c^{2}d$$
$$\frac{n}{1}\times\frac{n-1}{1}a^{n-2}cf$$
$$\frac{n}{1}\times\frac{n-1}{1}a^{n-2}de$$
$$\frac{n}{1}a^{n-1}h$$

FROM this Disposition of the several Products belonging to the same Power of z, in a successive Order, the one under the other, it is observable, that the several Products belonging to any Power of z are formed by multiplying those which belong to the next lower Degree of the Power of z, or those which immediately precede, by b, and dividing by a. Those which immediately precede the last, or which belong to the Power of z, less by 2, by multiplying by c, and dividing by a. Those which immediately precede the last, or which belong to the Power of z, less by 3, by multiplying by d, and dividing by a, *&c.* and rejecting the same Products when they arise again. And hence arises not only the Law of Continuation of any Number of Terms *ad Infinitum*, but of raising an infinite Multinomial to any given Power, for by multiplying each Side of the former Equation by z^n, we shall have

$$az^1 + bz^2 + cz^3 + dz^4 + ez^5 + fz^6 + gz^7 + hz^8, \&c = a^n z^n + n a^{n-1} b z^{n+1} +$$

$$\begin{array}{llll}
\frac{n}{1} \times \frac{n-1}{2} a^{n-2} b^2 z^{n+2} & + \frac{n}{1} \times \frac{n-1}{2} \times \frac{n-2}{3} a^{n-3} b^3 z^{n+3} & + \frac{n}{1} \times \frac{n-1}{2} \times \frac{n-2}{3} \times \frac{n-3}{4} a^{n-4} b^4 z^{n+4} & \\
\quad \frac{n}{1} a^{n-1} c & \quad \frac{n}{1} \times \frac{n-1}{1} a^{n-2} bc & \quad \frac{n}{1} \times \frac{n-1}{2} \times \frac{n-2}{1} a^{n-3} b^2 c & \\
\quad \&c. & \quad \frac{n}{1} a^{n-1} d & \quad \frac{n}{1} \times \frac{n-1}{1} a^{n-2} bd & \\
 & & \quad \frac{n}{1} \times \frac{n-1}{2} a^{n-2} c & \\
 & & \quad \frac{n}{1} a^{n-1} e &
\end{array}$$

Which is the infinite Multinomial Theorem first published by that excellent *Analyst* Mr *Abraham De Moivre*, in *Philos Transact* Numb. 230, the Application of which Theorem to Practice is very easy.

FOR let us suppose it were required to find the Cube Root of the Infinite Multinomial $1 - \frac{1}{2}x^2 - \frac{1}{8}x^4 - \frac{1}{16}x^6$, *&c* or $\overline{1 - \frac{1}{2}x^2 - \frac{1}{8}x^4 - \frac{1}{16}x^6, \&c}^{\frac{1}{3}}$ here $a = 1 . b = -\frac{1}{2}x^2 . c = -\frac{1}{8}x^4 . d = \frac{1}{16}x^6$, *&c.* and $n = \frac{1}{3}$; whence $a = 1 . n a^{n-1} b = \frac{1}{3} \times -\frac{1}{2}x^2 = -\frac{1}{6}x^2$.

$\frac{n}{1} \times$

$$\left.\begin{array}{l} \times\frac{n-1}{2}a^{n-2}b^2 = \frac{1}{3}\times-\frac{1}{3}\times\frac{1}{4}x^4 = -\frac{1}{36}x^4 \\ \frac{n}{1}\quad a^{n-1}e = \frac{1}{3}\times-\frac{1}{8}\times\quad x^4 = -\frac{1}{24}x^4 \end{array}\right\} = -\frac{5}{72}x^4$$

$$\left.\begin{array}{l} \times\frac{n-1}{2}\times\frac{n-2}{3}a^{n-3}b^3 = \frac{1}{3}\times-\frac{1}{3}\times-\frac{5}{9}\times-\frac{1}{8}x^6 = -\frac{5}{648}x^6 \\ \frac{n}{1}\times\frac{n-1}{1}a^{n-2}bc = \frac{1}{3}\times-\frac{2}{3}\times-\frac{1}{2}\times-\frac{1}{8}x^6 = -\frac{2}{144}x^6 \\ \frac{n}{1}\quad a^{n-1}d = \frac{1}{3}\times-\frac{1}{16}x^6 = -\frac{1}{48}x^6 \end{array}\right\} = -\frac{55}{1296}x^6$$

Whence $1-\frac{1}{2}x^2-\frac{1}{8}x^4-\frac{1}{16}x^6$, &c. $=1-\frac{1}{6}x^2-\frac{5}{72}x^4-\frac{55}{1296}x^6$, &c. the same as was investigated in Page 21 And proceeding after the same way, the Root of any infinite Multinomial may be found

WHOSOEVER considers the Nature of Powers, and the Manner of their Generation, will readily perceive that the Sum of the Letters that make up each Product of any Power, is the same, and equal to the Index of the same Power, or n, that the Sum of the several Products is equal to the Sum of the Combinations that can be made of the Quantity n thus taken, and that the Uncia, Coefficient, or Number prefixed to each Product, shews the Alternations, Variations or Permutations of the same Product Thus the Sum of the Letters that make up each Member, or Product, in the fourth Power is 4, the Sum of the several Products in the Quadrinomial is equal to $\frac{n}{1}\times\frac{n+1}{2}\times\frac{n+2}{3}\times\frac{n+3}{4}=35$, where n in this Case represents the Number of Terms in the Root as 2 in the Binomial, 3 in the Trinomial, 4 in the Quadrinomial, &c and the Uncia, Coefficient, or Number prefixed to any one of the Factors suppose $abcd$ is $\frac{n}{1}\times\frac{n-1}{1}\times\frac{n-2}{1}\times\frac{n-3}{1}$, or $\frac{n}{1}\times\frac{n-1}{1}\times\frac{n-2}{1}=24$ To $abdd$, another Member, is $\frac{n}{1}\times\frac{n-1}{1}\times\frac{n-2}{1}\times\frac{n-3}{2}$, or $\frac{n}{1}\times\frac{n-1}{1}\times\frac{n-2}{2}=12$,

&c

&c. and in like manner the Sum of the Letters that make up each Product in the sixth Power is 6, the Sum of the several Products of the Quadrinomial, raised to the sixth Power, is $\frac{n}{1} \times \frac{n+1}{2} \times \frac{n+2}{3} \times \frac{n+3}{4} \times \frac{n+4}{5} \times \frac{n+5}{6} = 84$, and the Uncia, or Number prefixed to any Product, suppose $a\,a\,b\,c$, is $\frac{n}{1} \times \frac{n-1}{2} \times \frac{n-2}{1} \times \frac{n-3}{1}$, or $\frac{n}{1} \times \frac{n-1}{1} = 12$, and after the same way may the Uncia to any Term, and the Number of Terms, as well as the Terms themselves, in any Power of any Multinomial be found. And from these Considerations alone may the Theorem for the Binomial, Trinomial, &c. Series be readily investigated, whence the Reason of all the former Processes will more evidently appear.

By the Help of the general Theorem for raising of an Infinite Multinomial to any given Power, or for extracting any Root out of the same, may the Root of an Infinite Equation be extracted, which is called the Reversion of Series.

For Example, Suppose $t = a + \frac{1}{3}a^3 + \frac{2}{15}a^5 + \frac{17}{315}a^7$, &c.

$$\text{Then } t^3 = a^3 + a^5 + \frac{11}{15}a^7, \&c.$$

$$\text{and } t^5 = a^5 + \frac{5}{3}a^7, \&c.$$

$$\text{and } t^7 = a^7, \&c.$$

$$\text{Whence } t - \frac{1}{3}t^3 = a - \frac{1}{5}a^5 - \frac{4}{21}a^7, \&c.$$

$$\text{and } t - \frac{1}{3}t^3 + \frac{1}{5}t^5 = a + \frac{1}{7}a^7, \&c.$$

$$\text{and } t - \frac{1}{3}t^3 + \frac{1}{5}t^5 - \frac{1}{7}t^7, \&c. = a$$

$$\text{Whence } a = t - \frac{1}{3}t^3 + \frac{1}{5}t^5 - \frac{1}{7}t^7, \&c.$$

Or,

Put $a = At + Bt^3 + Ct^5 + Dt^7$, &c.

$$\left.\begin{array}{ll} \text{then } \frac{1}{3}a^3 = & \frac{1}{3}A^3t^3 + A^2Bt^5 + A^2Ct^7, \text{ \&c.} \\ & \qquad\qquad\qquad AB^2t^7, \text{ \&c} \\ \text{and } \frac{2}{15}a^5 = & \frac{2}{15}A^5t^5 + \frac{2}{3}A^4Bt^7, \text{ \&c} \\ \text{and } \frac{17}{315}a^7 = & \frac{17}{315}A^7t^7, \text{ \&c} \end{array}\right\} = t + 0t^3 + 0t^5, \text{ \&c.}$$

Whence $At = t$. $B + \frac{1}{3}A = 0$, also $C + A^2B + \frac{2}{15}A^5 = 0$,

and $A = 1$ $B = -\frac{1}{3}A = -\frac{1}{3}$ $C = -A^2B - \frac{2}{15}A^5$

$C = +\frac{1}{3} - \frac{2}{15} = \frac{1}{5}$

and $D + A^2C + AB^2 + \frac{2}{3}A^4B + \frac{17}{315}A^7 = 0$,

and $D = -A^2C - AB^2 - \frac{2}{3}A^4B - \frac{17}{315}A^7$

and $D = -\frac{1}{5} - \frac{1}{9} + \frac{2}{9} - \frac{17}{315} = \frac{1}{7}$

Wherefore $a = t - \frac{1}{3}t^3 + \frac{1}{5}t^5 - \frac{1}{7}t^7$, &c the same as was before found.

AGAIN, Suppose $z = x + \frac{1}{2}x^2 + \frac{1}{3}x^3 + \frac{1}{4}x^4 + \frac{1}{5}x^5$, &c

Then $z^2 = x^2 + x^3 + \frac{11}{12}x^4 + \frac{5}{6}x^5$, &c

And $z^3 = x^3 + \frac{3}{2}x^4 + \frac{7}{4}x^5$, &c.

And $z^4 = x^4 + 2x^5$, &c

And $z^5 = x^5$, &c

Whence $z - \frac{1}{2}z^2 = x - \frac{1}{6}x^3 - \frac{5}{24}x^4 - \frac{13}{60}x^5$, &c

and $z - \frac{1}{2}z^2 + \frac{1}{6}z^3 = x + \frac{1}{24}x^4 + \frac{3}{40}x^5$, &c.

and $z - \frac{1}{2}z^2 + \frac{1}{6}z^3 - \frac{1}{24}z^4 = x - \frac{1}{120}z^5$, &c.

and $z - \frac{1}{2}z^2 + \frac{1}{6}z^3 - \frac{1}{24}z^4 + \frac{1}{120}z^5$, &c $= x$.

Wherefore $x = z - \frac{1}{2}z^2 + \frac{1}{6}z^3 - \frac{1}{24}z^4 + \frac{1}{120}z^5$, &c.

Or, Put $x = Az + Bz^2 + Cz^3 + Dz^4 + Ez^5$, &c

Then $\frac{1}{2}x^2 = \frac{1}{2}A^2z^2 + ABz^3 + ACz^4 + ADz^5$, &c $+ \frac{1}{2}B^2z^4 + BCz^5$, &c.

and $\frac{1}{3}x^3 = + \frac{1}{3}A^3z^3 + A^2Bz^4 + A^2Cz^5$, &c $+ AB^2z^5$, &c.

and $\frac{1}{4}x^4 = + \frac{1}{4}A^4z^4 + A^3Bz^5$, &c

and $\frac{1}{5}x^5 = + \frac{1}{5}A^5z^5$

$= z + 0z^2 + 0z^3$, &c.

Whence $Az = z$ $A = 1$

$B + \frac{1}{2}A = 0$. $B = -\frac{1}{2}A = -\frac{1}{2}$,

$C + AB + \frac{1}{3}A^3 = 0$ · $C = -AB - \frac{1}{3}A^3 = \frac{1}{2} - \frac{1}{3} = +\frac{1}{6}$

$D + AC + \frac{1}{2}B^2 + A^2B + \frac{1}{4}A^4 = 0$.

$D = -AC - \frac{1}{2}B^2 - A^2B - \frac{1}{4}A^4 = -\frac{1}{6} - \frac{1}{8} + \frac{1}{2} - \frac{1}{4} = -\frac{1}{24}$

$E + AD + BC + A^2C + AB^2 + A^3B + \frac{1}{5}A = 0$ ·

$E = -AD - BC - A^2C - AB^2 - A^3B - \frac{1}{5}A^5$ . .

$$E = \frac{1}{24} + \frac{1}{12} - \frac{1}{6} - \frac{1}{4} + \frac{1}{2} - \frac{1}{5} = + \frac{1}{120}.$$

Whence $x = z - \frac{1}{2}z^2 + \frac{1}{6}z^3 - \frac{1}{24}z^4 + \frac{1}{120}x^5$, &c as before.

And universally, If $az + bz^2 + cz^3 + dz^4 + ez^5 + fz^6$, &c $= gy + hy^2 + iy^3 + ky^4 + ly^5 + my^6$, &c. Then

$$z = \frac{g}{a}y + \frac{h - bAA}{a}y^2 + \frac{i - 2bAB - cA^3}{a}y^3 + \frac{k - bB^2 - 2bAC - 3cA^2B - dA^4}{a}y^4 + \frac{l - 2bBC - 2bAD - 3cAB^2 - 3cA^2C - 4dA^3B - eA^5}{a}y^5$$

Whence A is $= \frac{g}{a}$. $B = \frac{h - bAA}{a}$. $C = \frac{i - 2bAB - cA^3}{a}$, &c.

Li

LET us now suppose the former Equation $z = x + \frac{1}{2}x^2 + \frac{1}{3}x^3 + \frac{1}{4}x^4 + \frac{1}{5}x^5$, &c. and put $x + \frac{1}{2}x^2 + \frac{1}{3}x^3 + \frac{1}{4}x^4 + \frac{1}{5}x^5$, &c. $= z + o z^2 + o z^3 + o z^4 + o z^5$, &c.

Then $a = 1 . b = \frac{1}{2}$ $c = \frac{1}{3} . d = \frac{1}{4}$, &c $g = 1 . h = o$ $i = o . k = o$, &c.

and $\frac{g}{a} = 1 = A$ $\frac{h - bAA}{a} = -\frac{1}{2} = B$ $\frac{i - 2baB - cA^3}{a} = \frac{1}{6} = C$,

and $\frac{k - bB^2 - 2bAC - 3A^2B - dA^4}{a} = -\frac{1}{24} = D$, &c.

Whence $x = z - \frac{1}{2}z^2 + \frac{1}{6}z^3 - \frac{1}{24}z^4$, &c. the same as was before investigated.

SECT. III.

Of the Nature of FLUXIONS, *and the Generation of* Mathematical Quantities.

BY *Fluxions* are to be underſtood the Velocities of the Increments of Variable or Indeterminate Quantities, conſider'd not as actually generated, but *Quatenus naſcentia*, as ariſing, or beginning to be generated And to form a juſt and adequate Notion of them in the Mind, we are to conſider Mathematical Quantities not as made up of an infinite Number of very ſmall conſtituent Parts, but as generated or deſcribed by a continued uninterrupted Motion or regular Flux.

A LINE is deſcribed, and in that Deſcription is generated, not by the Appoſition of Parts, but by the continual Motion of a Point A Surface is generated by the uninterrupted Motion of a Line, and a Solid by the conſtant Motion of a Superficies An Angle by the Rotation of one of its Legs And the Quantities thus generated in equal Spaces of Time, become equal, greater or leſſer, according as the Celerities of the Motions by which they were generated, are equal, greater or leſſer

A————C

B————D

FOR Example, If the Point A move or be carried forward with an equal and uniform Motion from A towards C, according to the Direction of the Line A C, and the Point B, move or be carried forward with an equal and uniform Motion from B towards D, according to the Direction of the Line B D, and the Velocity of the Point A be equal to the Velocity of the Point B, the Line A C, generated by the Point A, will be equal to the Line B D, generated by the Point B in the ſame Time If the Velocity of the Point A be double to the Velocity of the Point

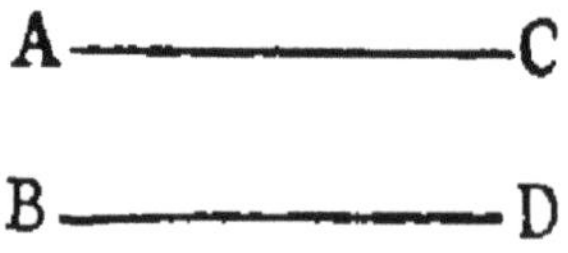

B,

B, the Line A C, generated by the Point A, will be double to the Line B D, generated by the Point B in the same Time, and if the Velocity of the Point A be triple of the Velocity of the Point B, the Line A C, described by the Point A, in any Space of Time will be triple of the Line B D, described by the Point B in the same Part of Time, and universally if U represent the Velocity of the Point A, and *u* the Velocity of the Point B, the Line described by the Point A will be to the Line described by the Point B, in any Time *t*, as U to *u*, and these Velocities U and *u*, with which the generating, or describing Points are carried, are called the *Fluxions* of the Lines A C and B D, as the Lines A C and B D, thus described, are called the *Fluents*

AGAIN, if, as in the following Figure, the whole Line A B be supposed to be carried along the Line B D from B towards D, constantly perpendicular to B D, and parallel to itself, and at the same time the Point A be imagined to move according to the Direction of the Line A B, it will by this compound Motion, one according to the Direction A C, and the other according to the Direction A B, describe either a Right Line, or a Curve Line, according as the Velocities of it in each Direction are adjusted or proportioned to each other, as will the Line A B, for the same Reason, describe a Rectilineal or a Curvilineal Superficies

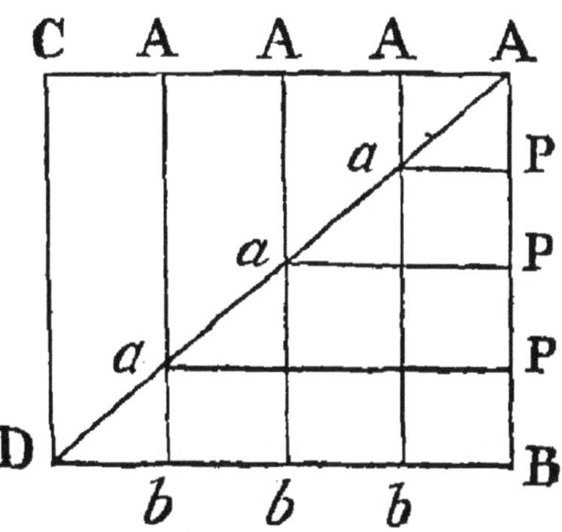

IF the Points A and B move with an equable and uniform Velocity, that is, if in the Time the Point A with an equable Velocity move to P, the Point B is carried with an uniform Velocity to *b*, so that the Space A P, described in any given Time by the Point A, is to the Space described by the Point B in the same Time, as the whole Space A B

A B deſcribed by the Point A in a certain Time, to the whole Space B D, deſcribed by the Point B, in the ſame Time, the Point A, by this Compound Motion, will deſcribe the Right Line A *a* D, as will the whole Line A B generate the Parallelogramick Space A B D C, while the ſame Line A B, diminiſhing according to the Velocity of the Point A, deſcribes the Triangular Space A B D

For inaſmuch as in the ſame Time that the Line A B is ſuppoſed, with an uniform Velocity, to have moved into the Place A *b*, the Point A is ſuppoſed to have travelled with an equable Velocity through the Space A *a* equal to A P, it is manifeſt that the Point A will be found in *a*, and becauſe A P is in every Point P to the whole Line A B, as *a* P or A A is to the whole Line B D or A C, the Points *a a a* will be in a ſtreight Line, and conſequently the Point A, by the Compound Motion, will deſcribe the Right Line A *a a* D in the ſame Time as the whole Line A B ſhall have generated the Parallelogram A B D C, and the ſame Line A B diminiſhing in the Ratio of the Velocity of the Point A, ſhall have deſcribed the Triangle A B D But if in the Time that the Point B, by the uniform Motion of the Line A B, moves over equal Spaces B *b*, *b b*, *&c.* in equal Times, the Point A moves through Spaces A *a*, A *a*, *&c.* equal to A P, A P, *&c*, which ſhall be to each other in a duplicate Ratio of the Spaces B *b*, B *b*, *&c* run through by the Point B in the ſame Time, the Point A will, by this Compound Motion, deſcribe the Parabolick Curve A *a a a* D, as will the whole Line A B, the Parallelogramick

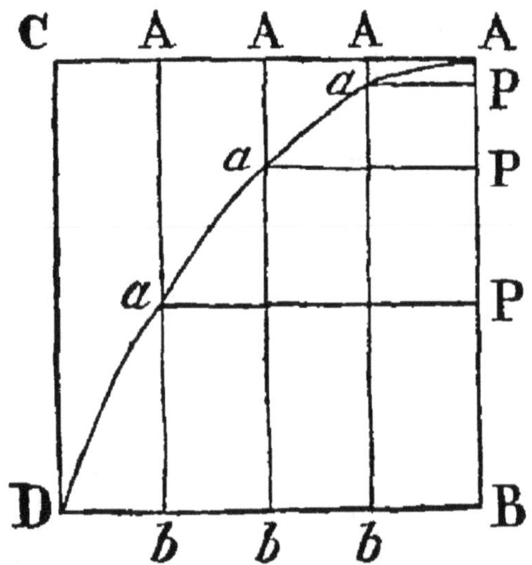

Space

Space A B D C, and the Line *a b*, *a b*, the Parabolick Space A B D *a* A

For because it is as A B : A P :: B D² : P *a*², wheresoever the Point P be taken, the Curve A *a a a* D will be a Parabola

Or, If while the Point B, by the uniform Motion of the Line B A along the Line D B describes equal Spaces B *b*, *b b*, *b b*, &c in equal Times, the Point A descends through Spaces A P, A P, A P, &c. which shall be to each other in a Subduplicate Ratio of the Spaces B *b*, B *b*, B *b*, &c the Curve described by this Compound Motion of the Point A, will be a Parabola Convex towards A B, and the Space A B D is the Supplemental Part wherein the Lines P *a*, P *a*, P *a*, which, in the former Case, were the Abscissa, now become the Ordinates, and the Lines A P, A P, A P, which before were equal to the Ordinates, become now the Abscissa But if instead of imagining the Line A B to be carried along the Line B D parallel to itself, we conceive the same Line A B to revolve about the Point B, fixed as a Centre, whilst the Point A moves in the Direction A B, from A towards B, as before, then the Point A, by these two Motions, will describe some one of the Radial or Spiral Curves, and as all Curves whatsoever arise from the different Velocities of one or both of the Points A and B, it will be easy for the Reader, from hence, to carry his Imagination so far as to conceive readily how any one, or all, of the infinite Variety of Curves may be generated

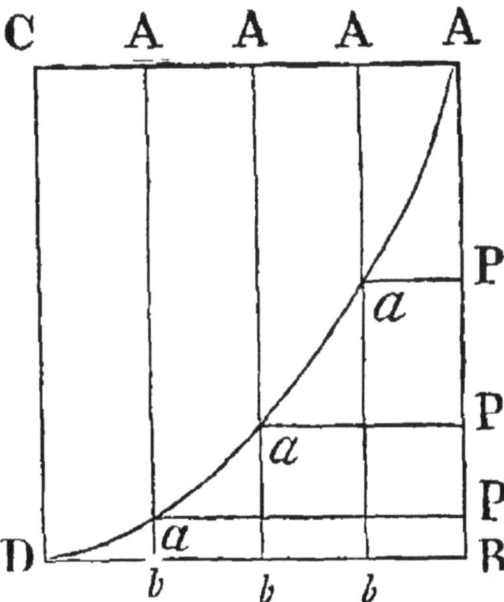

FROM the Generation of Curves, thus explain'd, the Nature of *Fluxions* will more evidently appear.

FOR let A P *p* D represent any given Curve, A B its Axis, P M, *p m* Ordinates applied, and draw the Lines P *b*, *p b* parallel to the Axis A B. Now inasmuch as the Points P and *b*, *p* and *b* represent the several Positions of the Points A and B in the regular and orderly Formation of the Curve, so the Lines P *b*, *p b*, which represent the several Distances of these Points asunder at those several Moments of

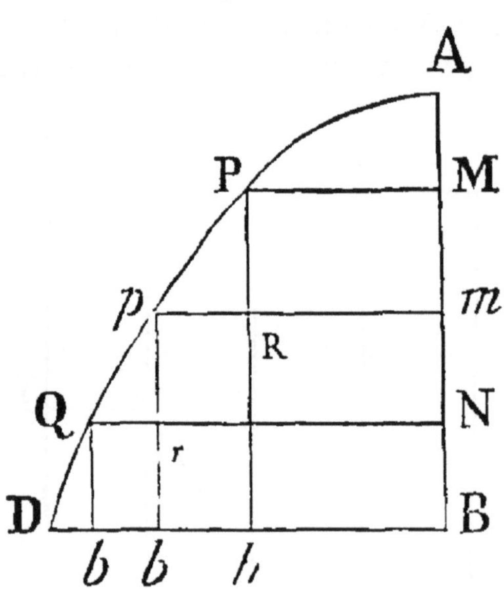

Time, are very properly and significantly called the several flowing Values of the Line A B; and as there is no imaginable Moment of Time wherein the Points A and B are supposed to be at Rest, so there is no imaginable Point of Time wherein the Line A B continues of the same Length, but is constantly in a State of Change, and flowing into a new Value; and, for the same Reason, the Ordinates P M, *p m*, *&c.* equal in Length to the Distances B *b*, B *b*, the Spaces run through by the Point B, being in a continual Flux and Change, are called the several flowing Values of the Base B D.

IN the Generation or Formation of any Curve, if one of the Points B, for Example, move with an equable and uniform Motion, the other Point A must necessarily move with an accelerated Motion (according to such Degrees of Acceleration as the Nature of the Curve required; for if the Velocities of the generating Points were equable, the Path described would be a streight Line) and consequently the Velocity of the generating Point A must be variable in every Point of the Curve. For as as the Motion of the Point A towards B is a continued uninterrupted Motion, so being at the same time an accelerated one, the Acceleration itself must be without the least Intermission and for the Acceleration to be without Intermission, is to undergo infinite and indeterminate Variations Again, if the unequal Particles of the Curve P*p* and *p* Q are generated in equal Particles of Time, there must be infinite Variations of Velocity of the generating Point A, between the Points P and *p*, as also between the Points *p* and Q and as the Point B may be conceived to move with an accelerated Motion towards D, the Velocity of the Point B, in every conceivable Part of the Line B D, must be accelerated, and consequently there must be infinite Variations of Velocity between the Points *p* and R, and Q and *r*, while those Increments *p* R, Q *r*, of the Ordinates *p m*, Q N are generated

INASMUCH therefore as an infinite Variety of Velocities are requisite to the Production or Formation of any Increment or generated Quantity, such as P *p* or *p* R, *&c* how small soever, so, in order to compare these Increments together, it is absolutely necessary to consider them in their arising State, or before they begin to be, and those Velocities with which they thus arise, or begin to be, are what are meant by their *Fluxions* So that *Fluxions* are not therefore the Velocities of the Increments considered as actually generated, but as arising or beginning to be generated, and are accurately and exactly, in the first Ratio of the Increments, consider'd as arising, or in the first Moment of their Generation

SO that the genuine Sense and Meaning of finding the *Fluxions* of flowing or determinate Quantities, is to find the Velocities with which they arise or begin to be generated in the first Moments of Formation And the same way of Reasoning obtains, whether we consider the first or last Ratios of the Velocities of the Incremental Parts that is, whether we consider them in their first Ratios, as arising or beginning to be, or whether we consider them in their last Ratios, as vanishing and ceasing to be.

FROM what has been said it is manifest, that the Progression of *Fluxions* is without End, that is, that there are *Fluxions* of *Fluxions*, and *Fluxions* of *Fluxions*, &c. *ad Infinitum*

FOR as there is a continual Acceleration or perpetual Mutation of Velocity in every Part of the Figure, so the small Increments do every where arise, or begin to be generated with variable and different Degrees of Velocity and as these Mutations are without Bounds or Limits, it is very evident that the Series of Mutation itself must be infinite

THESE Considerations of the Velocities of the Incremental Parts, as arising, &c or of the Decremental Parts, as vanishing, &c are not confin'd to Geometrical Quantities only, but may be extended in Arithmetick to Facts, Quotients, Roots, &c and to all Quantities in general, which may be consider'd as Indeterminate and Variable, and in a perpetual Flux or Change

AND although *Fluxions* are, accurately speaking, in the first Ratio of their *nascent Augments*, or in the last Ratio of their *evanescent Decrements*, yet there are certain Right Lines of a finite Length, to which they may be shewn to be Proportional, and by which they may be expounded

THUS the *Fluxions* of the Areas A B C, A B D G, described by the uniform Motion of the Ordinate B C, B D, along the Base A B, are to each other as the generating or describing Ordinates B C, B D, and may be expounded by them, inasmuch as these Ordinates are as their nascent Augments

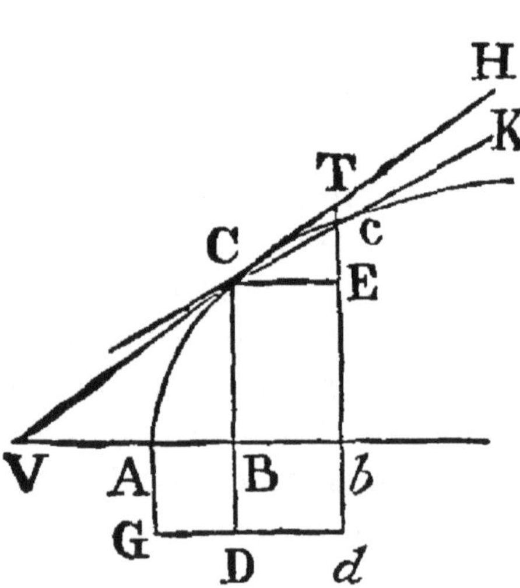

LET us suppose the Ordinate BC to move out of its first Place BC, and to

to come into a new Place *b c*, and compleat the Parallelogram BCE*b*, and let the Right Line VTH be drawn to touch the Curve in the Point C, and to cut the Right Lines BA and *b c*, produced in V and T.

INASMUCH therefore as the little Lines B*b*, or CE, *c*E and C*c*, are the nascent Augments of the Abscis AB, the Ordinate BC, and the Curve Line AC, and that the Sides of the Triangle CET are, in the first Ratio of these nascent Augments, the *Fluxions* of AB, BC, and AC are as the Sides CE, ET and CT of the Triangle CET, and may therefore be expounded by them, or, which is the same thing, by the Sides of the Triangle VBC, which is similar to it.

AND the same Consequence will follow, if the *Fluxions* are taken in the last Ratio of their evanescent Parts. For having drawn the Line C*c*, and produced it to K, let the Right Line *b c* return back again into its former Place CB, then will the Points C and *c* coincide, and the Right Line CK coincide with the Tangent CH, and the Triangle CE*c*, in its evanescent Form, will become similar to the Triangle CET: wherefore the Sides CE, E*c* and C*c*, in their evanescent State, will be to each other as the Sides CE, ET and CT of the Triangle CET, that is, as the *Fluxions* of the Lines AB, BC, and AC.

AN exact Coincidence of the Points C and *c*, in order to obtain the ultimate Ratios of the Lines CE, E*c*, and C*c*, is of the greatest Consequence; for if the Distance between them be never so small, the Right Line CK will be distant from the Tangent CH by a small Interval, and consequently the Triangles formed thereby will cease to be similar.

BY the same Method of Reasoning, if the Circle described about the Centre B, with the Radius BC, be carried with an uniform Motion along the Abscis AB, and at Right Angles to it, the *Fluxion* of the generated Solid ABC will be as the generating Circle, and the *Fluxion* of its Superficies, as the Circumference of the generating Circle, and the *Fluxion* of the Curve conjunctly: for in the same Time that the Solid

ABC is generated by the Motion of the generating Circle along the Abſciſs AB, in the ſame Time the Superficies is generated by the Motion of the Perimeter of the ſame Circle along the Arch AC, as ſhall be explain'd more at large hereafter.

SECT. IV.

Of the Notation of FLUXIONS.

CONSTANT or determinate Quantities, that is, ſuch as never increaſe or decreaſe, but perpetually remain the ſame, are uſually, for the ſake of Diſtinction, and to avoid Confuſion, denoted by the former Letters of the Alphabet, ſuch as a, b, c, d, &c.

INDETERMINATE or flowing Quantities, that is, ſuch Quantities as are conſtantly increaſing or decreaſing by a perpetual and regular Flux or Motion, are commonly expreſſed by the latter Letters of the Alphabet, ſuch as u, x, y, z, and their *Fluxions*, or Celerities of Increaſe or Decreaſe, by the ſame Letters, with a Tittle over the Heads, thus $\dot{v}$, $\dot{x}$, $\dot{y}$, $\dot{z}$ repreſent the *Fluxions* of the Quantities v, x, y, z: And inaſmuch as theſe *Fluxions* may be conſider'd as Fluents, and conſequently have their *Fluxions* of Celerity, and Increaſe or Decreaſe, theſe are uſually denoted by the ſame Letters with two Points, or Tittles, over the Head, thus $\ddot{v}$, $\ddot{x}$, $\ddot{y}$, $\ddot{z}$ are the *Fluxions* of $\dot{v}$, $\dot{x}$, $\dot{y}$, $\dot{z}$, and after the ſame manner the *Fluxions* of theſe, conſidered as Fluents, are denoted by the ſame Letters with three Tittles, or Points, over their Heads, thus $\dddot{v}$, $\dddot{x}$, $\dddot{y}$, $\dddot{z}$, and the *Fluxions* of theſe with four Points, or Tittles, thus, $\ddddot{v}$, $\ddddot{x}$, $\ddddot{y}$, $\ddddot{z}$, &c. and theſe are called firſt, ſecond, third and fourth *Fluxions*.

THUS

THUS $v, \dot{x}, y, z,$ which are the first *Fluxions* of $v, x, y, \dot{z},$ are the second *Fluxions* of $v, x, y, z,$ and $v, x, y, z,$ which are the third *Fluxions* of $v, x, y, z,$ are the second *Fluxions* of $v, x, y, z,$ and the third *Fluxions* of $v, x, y, z.$ In like manner v, x, y, z are the first *Fluxions* of $v, \dot{x}, y, z,$ the second *Fluxions* of $v, x, y, z,$ the third *Fluxions* of $v, x, y, \dot{z},$ and fourth *Fluxions* of $v, x, y, z,$ &c.

AND the *Fluxions* of Fractions, as well as their second, third, fourth, &c. *Fluxions*, are denoted by 1, 2, 3 or 4, &c. Points placed horizontally in the Break of the Line that separates the Numerator from the Denominator.

THUS, $\frac{az+zz}{a-z}, \frac{az+zz}{a-z}, \frac{az+zz}{a-z},$ and $\frac{az+zz}{a-z}$ are first, second, third and fourth *Fluxions* of the Quantity $\frac{az+zz}{a-z}.$

IN like manner if the Quantity $az+zz$ be a Root, or Surd Quantity, then its first, second, third and fourth, &c. *Fluxion* is expressed by one, two, three, four, &c. Points in the Break of the Vinculum.

THUS, $\sqrt[n]{az+zz}, \sqrt[n]{az+zz}, \sqrt[n]{az+zz}, \sqrt[n]{az+zz},$ denote the first, second, third and fourth *Fluxions* of the Quantity $\sqrt[n]{az+zz},$ or $\overline{az+zz}^{\frac{1}{n}}$ and after the same manner may the first, second, third, fourth, &c. *Fluxions* of any other Quantity of the same Kind be expressed.

AS v, x, y, z are the *Fluxions* of $\dot{v}, \dot{x}, \dot{y}, z,$ and these again the *Fluxions* of $v, x, y, z,$ so these Quantities v, x, y, z may be considered as the *Fluxions* of a superior Order of Quantities, which (as the first *Fluxions* are denoted by a Point, or Tittle, so these) are expressed by a Dash over the Head, after this

this manner, $\overset{\prime}{v}$, $\overset{\prime}{x}$, $\overset{\prime}{y}$, $\overset{\prime}{z}$; and these again may be considered as the Fluxions of other Quantities, which are expressed by two little Dashes over the Head, as $\overset{\prime\prime}{v}$, $\overset{\prime\prime}{x}$, $\overset{\prime\prime}{y}$, $\overset{\prime\prime}{z}$, and these again as the Fluxions of $\overset{\prime\prime\prime}{v}$, $\overset{\prime\prime\prime}{x}$, $\overset{\prime\prime\prime}{y}$, $\overset{\prime\prime\prime}{z}$, denoted by three Strokes, &c. and these again as the Fluxions of $\overset{\prime\prime\prime\prime}{v}$, $\overset{\prime\prime\prime\prime}{x}$, $\overset{\prime\prime\prime\prime}{y}$, $\overset{\prime\prime\prime\prime}{z}$, *ad Infinitum, Neque enim novit Natura limitem*

AND as the Fluxions of Fractions, or Surd Quantities, are expressed by one, two, three, four, or more Points in the Break of the Line, or Vinculum, so these Fluents are denoted by one, two, three, four, or more little Strokes or Lines in the same Break, or Vinculum

THUS, $\sqrt{az\overset{\prime}{+}zz}$ is the Fluent of $\sqrt{az+zz}$, $\sqrt{az\overset{\prime\prime}{+}zz}$ is the Fluent of $\sqrt{az\overset{\prime}{+}zz}$, and $\sqrt{az\overset{\prime\prime}{+}zz}$ is the Fluent of $\sqrt{az\overset{\prime}{+}zz}$, as $\sqrt{az\overset{\prime\prime\prime\prime}{+}zz}$ is the Fluent of $\sqrt{az\overset{\prime\prime\prime}{+}zz}$, &c or, which is the same thing, $\sqrt{az+zz}$ is the Fluxion of $\sqrt{az\overset{\prime}{+}zz}$, as $\sqrt{az\overset{\prime}{+}zz}$ is the Fluxion of $\sqrt{az\overset{\prime}{+}zz}$, and $\sqrt{az\overset{\prime\prime}{+}zz}$ is the Fluxion of $\sqrt{az\overset{\prime\prime\prime}{+}zz}$, as $\sqrt{az\overset{\prime\prime\prime}{+}zz}$ is the Fluxion of $\sqrt{az\overset{\prime\prime\prime\prime}{+}zz}$, &c

WHENCE it comes to pass that, &c. $\overset{\prime\prime\prime\prime}{z}$, $\overset{\prime\prime\prime}{z}$, $\overset{\prime\prime}{z}$, $\overset{\prime}{z}$, z, $\dot{z}$, z, $\dot{z}$, z, &c or, &c. $\sqrt{az\overset{\prime\prime\prime\prime}{+}zz}$, $\sqrt{az\overset{\prime\prime\prime}{+}zz}$, $\sqrt{az\overset{\prime\prime}{+}zz}$, $\sqrt{az\overset{\prime}{+}zz}$, $\sqrt{az+zz}$, $\sqrt{az+zz}$, $\sqrt{az+zz}$, $\sqrt{az+zz}$, $\sqrt{az+zz}$, &c or, &c $\frac{az+zz}{a-z}\overset{\prime\prime\prime\prime}{}$, $\frac{az+zz}{a-z}\overset{\prime\prime\prime}{}$, $\frac{az+zz}{a-z}\overset{\prime\prime}{}$, $\frac{az+zz}{a-z}\overset{\prime}{}$, $\frac{az+zz}{a-z}$, $\frac{az+zz}{a-z}$, $\frac{az+zz}{a-z}$, $\frac{az+zz}{a-z}$, $\frac{az+zz}{a-z}$, &c are each of them Series of Flu-

ents,

ents, or Fluxional Quantities, every Term being the Fluent of the subsequent Quantity or Term immediately following, as it is the Fluxion of the Quantity that immediately precedes, or is next removed above it in the Order of the Series, as is abundantly manifest from what has been said

AND it is to be farther noted, that every prior Term in this Series is the Area of a Curvilinear Figure, whose Ordinate is the Quantity immediately following, and the Abscis z. Thus $\sqrt{az + zz}$ is the Area of a Curve, whose Ordinate is $\sqrt{ax + zz}$, and Abscis z.

SECT. V.

Of the Algorithm *of* FLUXIONS.

PROPOSITION I

To find the Fluxions of Quantities added, or subtracted

SOLUTION

IN the room of every Quantity substitute its Fluxion, and connect them with the Signs of their respective Quantities, and the Sum will be the Fluxion required

DEMONSTRATION

BECAUSE, by the former Section, $\dot{x}$ is the Fluxion of x, and $\dot{y}$ the Fluxion of y, therefore $\dot{x} + \dot{y}$ is the Fluxion of $x + y$, as is $\dot{x} - \dot{y}$ the Fluxion of $x - y$, for if while x increases, y diminishes, and as the Fluxion of x is Positive, the Fluxion of y must

must be Negative, and for the same reason the Fluxion of $x - y + z$ will be $\dot{x} - \dot{y} + \dot{x}$, and the Fluxion of $a + x + y + v$ will be $\dot{x} + \dot{y} + \dot{v}$, for a being supposed, by the former way of Notation, to be a constant Quantity never encreasing nor diminishing, cannot undergo any Alteration or Change, and has therefore no Fluxion, and consequently vanishes in the Operation In like manner the Fluxion of $x + a + y + b - v$ is $\dot{x} + \dot{y} - \dot{v}$, and after the same manner may the Fluxion of any Aggregate, whether Sum or Difference, be found. *Q. E. D*

PROPOSITION II

To find the Fluxions of the Product of any Number of Flowing Quantities, multiplied into one another

SOLUTION

MULTIPLY the Fluxion of every particular Flowing Quantity by the Product of all the other Quantities, and add the several Products together, and the Sum will be the Fluxion required

DEMONSTRATION

LET $xy = v$ be a Quantity proposed, and let o represent a Quantity infinitely small; then if $\dot{x}$ $\dot{y}$ represent the Velocities of the Increments of the Flowing Quantity x and y, $\dot{x}$o and $\dot{y}$o will represent the Increments themselves, generated in the first Moment of Time, and consequently the Quantities themselves x and y, are become, after they began to flow, $x + \dot{x}o$, and $y + \dot{y}o$. These therefore being multiplied into each other, will produce $xy + y\dot{x}o + x\dot{y}o + \dot{y}\dot{x}oo = v + \dot{v}o$, from which taking away the Original Equation $xy = v$, and dividing each of the remaining Terms by o, there will remain $y\dot{x} + x\dot{y} + \dot{y}\dot{x}o = \dot{v}$ Imagine the Quantity o to be infinitely

finitely diminished, or, which is the same thing, the Quantity xy is drawn back again into its arising State; then the Quantity $\dot{x}\dot{y}o$, in this Case, into which o is multiplied, will vanish, whence we shall have $\dot{x}y + \dot{y}x = \dot{v}$ for the Fluxion of the Quantity proposed.

Again, Suppose it were required to find the Fluxion of the Quantity zxy, put this equal to v, and let o, as in the former Case, represent an infinite small Quantity, then will $\dot{z}o$, $\dot{x}o$ and $\dot{y}o$ represent the nascent Augments of the Quantities z, x and y, and consequently in the same Time that z flows into or becomes $z + \dot{z}o$, x flows into or becomes $x + \dot{x}o$, and y becomes $y + \dot{y}o$, these therefore multiplied successively into each other, will produce $zxy + zyo\dot{x} + zxo\dot{y} + yxo\dot{z} + \dot{z}oo\dot{x}y + \dot{x}oo\dot{y}z + \dot{y}oo\dot{z}x + ooo\dot{z}\dot{x}\dot{y} = v + \dot{v}o$, from which, as before, taking away the original Equation $zxy = v$, and dividing the remaining Terms by o, we shall have $zy\dot{x} + zx\dot{y} + yx\dot{z} + \dot{z}o\dot{x}y + \dot{y}o\dot{z}x + \dot{x}o\dot{z}y + oo\dot{z}\dot{x}\dot{y} = \dot{v}$, but when the Quantity zxy was arising, or beginning to be, the Quantity o had no Place. And as the Fluxions themselves are the Velocities with which the Quantities arise, or begin to be, so all the Terms into which the Quantity o is multiplied will vanish, whence we shall have $zy\dot{x} + zx\dot{y} + xy\dot{z} = \dot{v}$ for the Fluxion of the Quantity zxy.

After the same way of Reasoning the Fluxion of $vxyz$ will be found to be $\dot{v}xyz + v\dot{x}zy$, $vyz\dot{x} + xyz\dot{v}$, of axy, will be $a\dot{x}y + ay\dot{x}$, for the Quantity a being a constant or fix'd Quantity, the Products that would arise from the Multiplication, by the momentaneous Augment of a, if it were a Fluent, will vanish. *Q. E. D.*

PROPOSITION III.

To find the Fluxions of Quantities divided one by the other, or of Fractions.

SOLUTION.

Multiply the Fluxion of the Numerator by the Denominator, and from the Product subtract the Fluxion of the Denominator, multiplied into the Numerator, then divide the Remainder by the Square of the Denominator, and the last Quote, or Fraction, thence resulting, will be the Fluxion of the Quantity proposed.

DEMONSTRATION.

FOR let $\frac{z}{x}$ be the Fraction proposed, and suppose $\frac{z}{x} = v$, then will $z = xv$, and $z + o\dot{z} = xv + vo\dot{x} + xo\dot{v} + oo\dot{x}\dot{v}$, and because $z = xv$, taking away this Equation from the former, we shall have $o\dot{z} = vo\dot{x} + xo\dot{v} + oo\dot{x}\dot{v}$, and dividing each Term by o, there will arise $\dot{z} = v\dot{x} + x\dot{v} + o\dot{x}\dot{v}$, but because the infinite small Quantity o, when $\frac{z}{x}$ was in its arising State, had no Place, therefore the Term $o\dot{x}\dot{v}$ vanishes, and consequently $\dot{z} = v\dot{x} + x\dot{v}$, whence, by Reduction, $\dot{v} = \frac{\dot{z} - v\dot{x}}{x}$, and substituting $\frac{z}{x}$ in the room of v, we shall have $\dot{v} = \frac{\dot{z}}{x} - \frac{z}{x} \times \frac{\dot{x}}{x} = \frac{\dot{z}}{x} - \frac{z\dot{x}}{xx} = \frac{x\dot{z} - z\dot{x}}{xx}$ for the Fluxion required, or because the Fluxion $z = xv$, by the former Rule is $\dot{z} = x\dot{v} + v\dot{x}$, whence $x\dot{v} = \dot{z} - v\dot{x}$, and consequently

quently $\dot{v} = \frac{\dot{z} - v\dot{x}}{x}$. Putting therefore $\frac{z}{x}$ in the room of v, we shall have $\dot{v} = \frac{\dot{z}}{x} - \frac{z}{x} \times \frac{\dot{x}}{x} = \frac{\dot{z}}{x} - \frac{z\dot{x}}{xx} = \frac{x\dot{z} - z\dot{x}}{xx}$ therefore for the Fluxion of $\frac{z}{x}$.

Again, Suppose it be required to find the Fluxion of $\frac{x}{a+x}$, put $\frac{x}{a+x} = v$, then is $x = va + vx$, and consequently $\dot{x} = a\dot{v} + \dot{v}x + \dot{x}v$, and by Transposition $\dot{x} - v\dot{x} = a\dot{v} + x\dot{v}$, and by Division $\dot{v} = \frac{\dot{x} - v\dot{x}}{a+x}$, and putting $\frac{x}{a+x}$ in the room of v, we shall have $\dot{v} = \frac{\dot{x}}{a+x} - \frac{x}{a+x} \times \frac{\dot{x}}{a+x} = \frac{a\dot{x} + x\dot{x} - x\dot{x}}{aa + 2ax + xx} = \frac{a\dot{x}}{aa + 2ax + xx} = \frac{a\dot{x}}{\overline{a+x} \times \overline{a+x}}$ for the Fluxion of the Quantity $\frac{x}{a+x}$ proposed.

Again, Suppose the Quantity $\frac{1}{x}$ be proposed, put as before $\frac{1}{x} = v$, then will $1 = vx$, and consequently $0 = \dot{v}x + \dot{x}v$, whence $x\dot{v} = -v\dot{x}$, and $\dot{v} = \frac{-v\dot{x}}{x}$, putting therefore $\frac{1}{x}$ in the room of v, we shall have $\dot{v} = \frac{-\dot{x}}{x} \times \frac{1}{x} = \frac{-\dot{x}}{xx}$ for the Fluxion of $\frac{1}{x}$, after the same manner the Fluxion of $\frac{a}{x}$ will be found to be $\frac{-a\dot{x}}{xx}$. *Q. E. D.*

PROPOSITION IV.

To find the Fluxions of Powers.

SOLUTION.

MULTIPLY the given Power by its Exponent, then lessen the Index of the Power by Unity, and lastly, multiply the Quantity thus produced by the Fluxion of the Root, and the last Product will be the Fluxion of the given Power.

DEMONSTRATION.

LET xx be the Power proposed, and suppose it equal to z, then by the second Proposition $\dot{x}x + x\dot{x} = \dot{z}$, that is $2x\dot{x} = \dot{z}$. In like manner the Fluxion of x^3 will be $\dot{x}xx + x\dot{x}x + xx\dot{x}$, equal to $3xx\dot{x}$, or $3x^2\dot{x}$, and for the same Reason the Fluxion of x^4 will be $\dot{x}xxx + x\dot{x}xx + xx\dot{x}x + xxx\dot{x}$, equal to $4xxx\dot{x}$, or $4x^3\dot{x}$, where if m be put for the Index of the Power, we shall have $mx^{m-1}\dot{x}$ for the Fluxion required.

AGAIN, Suppose $x^{\frac{1}{2}}$ be the Power proposed, put it equal to v, then will $x^{\frac{1}{2}} = v$, and $x = vv$, whence $\dot{x} = 2v\dot{v}$, and $\dot{v} = \frac{\dot{x}}{2v}$, substituting therefore $x^{\frac{1}{2}}$ in the room of v, we shall have $\frac{\dot{x}}{2x^{\frac{1}{2}}} = \frac{1}{2}x^{-\frac{1}{2}}\dot{x}$ by Section the first. In like manner if $x^{\frac{1}{3}}$ be the Power proposed, putting this equal to v, we shall have $vvv = x$, whence $3vv\dot{v} = \dot{x}$, and $\dot{v} = \frac{\dot{x}}{3vv}$, substituting therefore $x^{\frac{2}{3}}$ in the room of vv, to which it is equal by by Section the first, we shall have $\dot{v} = \frac{\dot{x}}{3x^{\frac{2}{3}}} = \frac{1}{3} x^{-\frac{2}{3}} \dot{x}$, by the same Section, and for the same Reason, if $x^{\frac{1}{n}} = v$ be the Power proposed, we shall have $x = v^{n}$, whence $\dot{x} = n v^{n-1} \dot{v}$, and $\dot{v} = \frac{\dot{x}}{n v^{n-1}} = \frac{\dot{x}}{n x^{1-\frac{1}{n}}}$, (putting $x^{\frac{1}{n}}$ in the room of v) equal to $\frac{1}{n} x^{\frac{1}{n}-1} \dot{x}$, the Fluxion required.

Again, Suppose it be required to find the Fluxion of $x^{\frac{2}{3}}$, putting this equal to v, there will arise $x^{2} = v^{3}$, and $2 x \dot{x} = 3 v^{2} \dot{v}$, whence $\dot{v} = \frac{2 x \dot{x}}{3 v^{2}} = \frac{2 x \dot{x}}{3 x^{\frac{4}{3}}}$ by substituting $x^{\frac{4}{3}}$ in the room of v^{2}, to which it is equal by Section the first, whence $\dot{v} = \frac{2}{3} x \dot{x}^{-\frac{4}{3}} = \frac{2}{3} x^{-\frac{1}{3}} \dot{x}$, for the Fluxion of $x^{\frac{2}{3}}$; by the same way of Reasoning the Fluxion of $x^{\frac{1}{4}}$, will be $\frac{1}{4} x^{\frac{1}{4}-1} \dot{x} = \frac{1}{4} x^{-\frac{3}{4}} \dot{x}$, and the Fluxion of $x^{\frac{3}{4}}$ will be $\frac{3}{4} x^{-\frac{1}{4}} \dot{x}$, and if we put $\frac{m}{n}$ for the Index of the Power of x, we shall have $x^{\frac{m}{n}} = v$, and $x^{m} = v^{n}$, whence $m x^{m-1} \dot{x} = n v^{n-1} \dot{v}$, and $\dot{v} = \frac{m x^{m-1} \dot{x}}{n v^{n-1}}$, and putting x^{m}, and $x^{\frac{m}{n}}$ in the room of v^{n}, we shall have $\dot{v} = \frac{m x^{m-1} \dot{x}}{n x^{m-\frac{m}{n}}} = \frac{m}{n} x^{m-1-m+\frac{m}{n}} \dot{x} = \frac{m}{n} x^{\frac{m}{n}-1} \dot{x}$ by the first Section for the Fluxion of $x^{\frac{m}{n}}$.

Again, Suppose it be required to find the Fluxion of x^{-3}, or $\frac{1}{x^{3}}$, assume it equal to v, then will $1 = v x^{3}$, and $0 = \dot{v} x^{3} + 3 x^{2} \dot{x} v$, whence $\dot{v} x^{3} = -3 x^{2} \dot{x} v$, and $\dot{v} = \frac{-3 x^{2} \dot{x} v}{x^{3}} = \frac{-3 \dot{x} v}{x} = \frac{-3 \dot{x}}{x} v = \frac{-3 \dot{x}}{x} \frac{1}{x^{3}} = \frac{-3 \dot{x}}{x^{4}}$

by,

by substituting $\frac{1}{x}$ in the room of v, whence $\dot{v} = -1x^{-1-1}\dot{x}$ will be the Fluxion of $\frac{1}{x}$, or x^{-1}.

Again, Let $x^{-\frac{1}{3}}$, or $\frac{1}{x^{\frac{1}{3}}}$, be the Quantity proposed, suppose it, as before, equal to v, then is $1 = vx^{\frac{1}{3}}$, and $0 = \dot{v}x^{\frac{1}{3}} + \frac{1}{3}x^{\frac{1}{3}-1}\dot{x}v$, and $\dot{v}x^{\frac{1}{3}} = -\frac{1}{3}x^{\frac{1}{3}-1}\dot{x}v$, whence $\dot{v} = \frac{-\frac{1}{3}x^{\frac{1}{3}-1}\dot{x}v}{x^{\frac{1}{3}}} = -\frac{1}{3}x^{-1}\dot{x}v = -\frac{1}{3}x^{-\frac{1}{3}-1}\dot{x}$ (by putting $x^{-\frac{1}{3}}$ in the room of v) will be the Fluxion required, and if instead of $\frac{1}{3}$ we put $\frac{m}{n}$, we shall have $x^{-\frac{m}{n}}$, or $\frac{1}{x^{\frac{m}{n}}} = v$, whence $1 = vx^{\frac{m}{n}}$ and $0 = \dot{v}x^{\frac{m}{n}} + \frac{m}{n}x^{\frac{m}{n}-1}\dot{x}v$, and by Transposition $\dot{v}x^{\frac{m}{n}} = -\frac{m}{n}x^{\frac{m}{n}-1}\dot{x}v$, whence $\dot{v} = -\frac{m}{n}\frac{x^{\frac{m}{n}-1}}{x^{\frac{m}{n}}}\dot{x}v = -\frac{m}{n}x^{-1}\dot{x}v = -\frac{m}{n}x^{-\frac{m}{n}-1}\dot{x}$, by substituting $x^{-\frac{m}{n}}$ in the Room of v for the Fluxion of the Quantity $x^{-\frac{m}{n}}$, and universally let m represent any Number, whether Positive or Negative, whole Number or Fraction, and put $x^m = v$. Let o represent a Quantity infinitely small: then will $o\dot{x}$ and $o\dot{v}$ be the Increments of the Quantities x and v generated in the same Moment of Time, and consequently while x flows into, or becomes $x + o\dot{x}$, the Quantity x^m flows into, or becomes $\overline{x+o\dot{x}}^m$, and in the same Time that x^m becomes $\overline{x+o\dot{x}}^m$, the Quantity v becomes

$v+o\dot{v}$

$v + o\dot v$. But by Section II. $\overline{x+o\dot x}^{m} = x^m + m x^{m-1} o \dot x + \frac{mm-m}{2} x^{m-2} oo\dot x\dot x + \frac{m^3-3m^2+2m}{6} x^{m-3} o^3 \dot x^3$, &c $= v + o\dot v$. Taking away therefore the original Equation $x^m = v$, and dividing each of the remaining Terms by o, we shall have $m x^{m-1}\dot x + \frac{mm-m}{2} x^{m-2} o\dot x\dot x + \frac{m^3-3m^2+2m}{6} x^{m-3} oo\dot x^3$, &c $= \dot v$. But because when the Quantities x^m and v were in their arising, or evanescent State, the Quantity o was nothing, therefore the Terms $\frac{mm-m}{2} x^{m-2} o\dot x\dot x$, &c into which it is multiplied will vanish, whence we shall have $m x^{m-1}\dot x = \dot v$ for the Fluxion of the Quantity x^m. *Q. E. D.*

As there is scarce any Example can be proposed, but what will fall under some one or other of the preceding Propositions, so, from what has been said, it will be easy to find the Fluxion of any Quantity proposed, howsoever complicated.

Thus the Fluxion $x^m z^n$ will be $z^n m x^{m-1}\dot x + x^m n z^{n-1}\dot z$, of $x^m z^n y^p$, will be $x^m z^n p y^{p-1}\dot y + x^m y^p n z^{n-1}\dot z + z^n y^p m x^{m-1}\dot x$, of $\overline{x^m z^n}^{q}$ will be $q\,\overline{x^m z^n}^{q-1} \times z^n m x^{m-1}\dot x + x^m n z^{n-1}\dot z$, and of $\frac{x^m}{z^n}$, will be $\frac{z^n m x^{m-1}\dot x - x^m n z^{n-1}\dot z}{z^{n+n} \text{ or } z^{2n}}$.

In like manner the Fluxion of $\sqrt{2rx-xx}$, or $\overline{2rx-xx}^{\frac12}$ will be $\frac12\overline{2rx-xx}^{\frac12-1} \times 2r\dot x - 2x\dot x = \frac12\overline{2rx-xx}^{-\frac12} \times 2r\dot x - 2x\dot x = \frac{r\dot x - x\dot x}{\sqrt{2rx-xx}}$, also the Fluxion of $\overline{ay-xx}^{3} = 3\overline{ay-xx}^{2} \times a\dot y - 2x\dot x = 3a^3y^2\dot y - 6a^2x^2y\dot y$

+ 3a

$+ 3ax^{4}\dot{y} - 6a^{2}y^{2}x\dot{x} + 12ayx^{3}\dot{x} - 6x^{5}\dot{x}$, and the Fluxion of $\overline{xy+yy}^{\frac{1}{2}}$ is $\frac{1}{2}\overline{xy+yy}^{-\frac{1}{2}} \times x\dot{y} + y\dot{x} + 2y\dot{y}$ $= \frac{x\dot{y}+y\dot{x}+2y\dot{y}}{2\sqrt{xy+yy}}$.

AND that $\frac{x\dot{y}+y\dot{x}+2y\dot{y}}{2\sqrt{xy+yy}}$, in the former Example, is the Fluxion of $\sqrt{xy+yy}$, is evident from *Proposition* II and IV, for by *Proposition* II. the Fluxion of $xy+yy$, the Root is $x\dot{y}+y\dot{x}+2y\dot{y}$, and by the fourth *Proposition* the Fluxion of the $\frac{1}{2}$ Power of $xy+yy$ is found first by multiplying the Power $\overline{xy+yy}^{\frac{1}{2}}$ by the Index, whence arises $\frac{1}{2}\overline{xy+yy}^{\frac{1}{2}}$ Secondly, by lessening the Index by Unity, whence arises $\frac{1}{2}\overline{xy+yy}^{\frac{1}{2}-1}$ or $\frac{1}{2}\overline{xy+yy}^{-\frac{1}{2}}$ and Thirdly, by multiplying of this Quantity by $x\dot{y}+y\dot{x}+2y\dot{y}$, the Fluxion of the Root before found, whence we shall have $\frac{1}{2}\overline{xy+yy}^{-\frac{1}{2}} \times x\dot{y} + y\dot{x} + 2y\dot{y}$, or by *Section* I. $\frac{x\dot{y}+y\dot{x}+2y\dot{y}}{2\sqrt{xy+yy}}$ for the Fluxion of $\sqrt{xy+yy}$, and by the same way of Reasoning we shall have $r\dot{x} - x\dot{x} \times \overline{2rx-xx}^{-\frac{1}{2}}$ or $\frac{r\dot{x}-x\dot{x}}{\sqrt{2rx-xx}}$ for the Fluxion of $\sqrt{2rx-xx}$. But the Fluxions of any of the former Examples may be easily Investigated, without having Recourse to the general Rule for Powers

FOR put $\sqrt{xy+yy} = v$, then will $xy+yy = vv$, and $x\dot{y}+y\dot{x}+2y\dot{y} = 2v\dot{v}$, by *Proposition* II. whence by by Division $\dot{v} = \frac{x\dot{y} + \dot{y}x + 2y\dot{y}}{2v}$, and substituting $\sqrt{xy+yy}$, in the room of v, we shall have $\frac{x\dot{y}+\dot{y}x+2y\dot{y}}{2\sqrt{xy+yy}}$ for the Fluxion of $\sqrt{xy+yy}$.

AGAIN, put $\sqrt{2rx - xx} = v$, then will $2rx - xx = vv$, and $2r\dot{x} - 2x\dot{x} = 2v\dot{v}$, whence $r\dot{x} - x\dot{x} = v\dot{v}$, and $\dot{v} = \frac{r\dot{x} - x\dot{x}}{v}$, and by Substitution, $\dot{v} = \frac{r\dot{x} - x\dot{x}}{\sqrt{2rx-xx}}$ the Fluxion of $\sqrt{2rx-xx}$

AGAIN, put $x^m z^n = v$, then will $\overline{x+o\dot{x}}^m \times \overline{z+o\dot{z}}^n = v + o\dot{v}$, but by *Section* II, $\overline{x+o\dot{x}}^m = x^m + mx^{m-1}o\dot{x} + \frac{mm-m}{2}x^{m-2}oo\dot{x}\dot{x}$, &c. and $\overline{z+o\dot{z}}^n = z^n + nz^{n-1}o\dot{z} + \frac{nn-n}{2}z^{n-2}oo\dot{z}\dot{z}$, &c. these being therefore multiplied into each other, will produce $x^m z^n + z^n m x^{m-1} o\dot{x} + x^m n z^{n-1} o\dot{z} + nz^{n-1}o\dot{z} \times mx^{m-1}o\dot{x} + nz^{n-1}o\dot{z} \times \frac{mm-m}{2} x^{m-2}oo\dot{x}\dot{x} + mx^{m-1}o\dot{x} \times \frac{nn-n}{2}z^{n-2}oo\dot{z}\dot{z} + \frac{nn-n}{2} z^{n-2}oo\dot{z}\dot{z} \times \frac{mm-m}{2}x^{m-2}oo\dot{x}\dot{x}$, &c $= v + o\dot{v}$, from which taking away the original Equation $x^m z^n = v$, and dividing the Remainder by o, and making the Terms after this Division, in which o is found to vanish, we shall have $z^n m x^{m-1}\dot{x} + x^m z^{n-1}\dot{z} = \dot{v}$, for the Fluxion of the Quantity $x^m z^n$ proposed.

AND by the same Method of Investigation may the Fluxion of any other Quantity of the same Kind be found

THIS Independent Method of finding the Fluxions of Quantities, howſoever complicated, is no leſs Inſtructive and Entertaining to the Mind, than it is general and uſeful, and ought to be well underſtood by the Learner, ſince it will not only make him very ready in all future Operations, but aſſiſt him in many Caſes where the narrow Compaſs of the Rule may ſeem to render it not quite ſo applicable.

THE Fluxions of Surd, or irrational Quantities, may yet be more ſimply expreſſed, and render'd more fit for uſe, by ſubſtituting the actual Roots or Powers of the Surd Quantities themſelves, in the room of the Surd Quantities with the Radical Sign Thus the Fluxion of $\overline{r-x}^{2}$, which, by the former Expreſſion, is $2\times\overline{r-x}^{1}\times\dot{x}$, will be $2r\dot{x}-2x\dot{x}$, of $\overline{r-x}^{3}$, which is $3\times\overline{r-x}^{2}\times\dot{x}$, by ſquaring the Quantity $r-x$, will be found to be $3rr\dot{x}-6rx\dot{x}+3x^{2}\dot{x}$, and the Fluxion of $\overline{r-x}^{\frac{3}{2}}$ or $\sqrt{\overline{r-x}^{3}}$, which, by the former Expreſſion, is $\frac{3}{2}\overline{r-x}^{\frac{1}{2}}\dot{x}$ by extracting the Square Root of $\overline{r-x}$, which is $r^{\frac{1}{2}}-\frac{1}{2}\frac{x}{r^{\frac{1}{2}}}-\frac{1}{8}\frac{x^{2}}{r^{\frac{3}{2}}}-\frac{1}{16}\frac{x^{3}}{r^{\frac{5}{2}}}-\frac{5}{128}\frac{x^{7}}{r^{\frac{7}{2}}}$, &c. will be $\frac{3}{2}\times r^{\frac{1}{2}}\dot{x}-\frac{1}{2}\frac{x\dot{x}}{r^{\frac{1}{2}}}-\frac{1}{8}\frac{x^{2}\dot{x}}{r^{\frac{3}{2}}}-\frac{1}{16}\frac{x^{3}\dot{x}}{r^{\frac{5}{2}}}-\frac{5}{128}\frac{x^{4}\dot{x}}{r^{\frac{7}{2}}}$, &c or $\frac{3r^{\frac{1}{2}}\dot{x}}{2}-\frac{3x\dot{x}}{4r^{\frac{1}{2}}}-\frac{3x^{2}\dot{x}}{16r^{\frac{3}{2}}}-\frac{3x^{3}\dot{x}}{32r^{\frac{5}{2}}}-\frac{15x^{4}\dot{x}}{256r^{\frac{7}{2}}}$, &c

AND after the ſame manner may the Fluxion of any other Irrational Quantity be expreſſed, as will appear more fully in the Sequel of this Work.

SECT.

SECT. VI.

Of the Operations in Second, Third, Fourth, &c. FLUXIONS.

ALTHOUGH the Nature of Fluxions in general has been sufficiently explained in the third Section, yet, as we are now going to treat of the Operations in second, third, *&c* Fluxions, it may not be amiss, in this Place, to speak of them in a more particular manner, that so the Reader may have a clear and distinct Conception of them, and thereby be better enabled to see the Reason of every Step that is taken

NOW in the Generation of the Flowing Line A B, if the generating Point A moves with an uniform Velocity, that is, if it describe equal Portions of the flowing

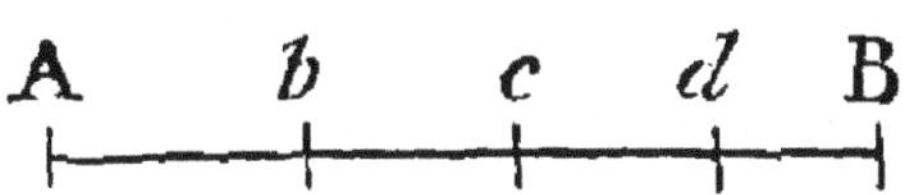

Line A B, in equal Times, then this Velocity or Fluxion of the flowing Line A B, will be a constant Quantity, and the Line A B will have only a first Fluxion, and no second Fluxion, and let this first Fluxion be represented by A *b* But if, when the generating Point in flowing and arriving at some Place, suppose at *b*, it increases or decreases its Velocity, then that Increase or Decrease of Velocity is called a Fluxion of a Fluxion, or a second Fluxion, and the Part A *b* of the Line A B, which represents the first Fluxion, will now become a flowing Quantity, and have a first Fluxion, which we will represent by *b c*, whence the flowing Line A B will have a first and second Fluxion, but no third Fluxion, and *b c* will represent this second Fluxion of the Line A B, and if when the generating Point A, in flowing, arrives at some other Place, suppose at *c*, it again alters or changes its Velocity, the Alteration or

Change, in this Case, is called a third Fluxion; and *b c*, which before was a constant Quantity, and represented the second Fluxion of A B, becomes now a flowing Quantity, and will have a first Fluxion, which we will represent by *c d*, and consequently in this Case *c d*, which is a first Fluxion of *b c*, is a second Fluxion of A *b*, and a third Fluxion of A B, whence the flowing Line A B will have a first, a second, and a third Fluxion, but no fourth Fluxion And again, if when the generating Point A shall arrive at a third Place, suppose at *d*, it shall again alter or change its Velocity, then this new Alteration or Change of its Velocity, is called a fourth Fluxion, that is, a first Fluxion of *c d*, which now becomes a flowing Quantity, a second Fluxion of *b c*, a third Fluxion of A *b*, and a fourth Fluxion of the flowing Line A B, so that the flowing Line A B in its present State, will have a first, a second, a third, and a fourth Fluxion, but no fifth Fluxion, and as the Velocity of the generating Point A may alter or change in every conceivable Point of the flowing Line A B, it is abundantly manifest, that the Progression of Fluxions, is without End, that is, there are fifth, sixth, seventh, eighth, &c Fluxions, *ad Infinitum.* Wherefore

As second, third, fourth, &c Fluxions arise from the same Cause, and are generated after the same manner as first Fluxions are, so the Rules deliver'd in the former Section for finding the first Fluxions, will serve to find the second, third and fourth, &c Fluxions, or, as the Inventor himself tells us, to find the second, third, fourth, &c Fluxions, we have nothing more to do than to repeat the Operations over again

FOR as $\dot{x}$ is the Fluxion of x, and $\dot{y}$ the Fluxion of y, so the Fluxion of $\dot{x}$ is $\ddot{x}$, and the Fluxion of $\dot{y}$ is $\ddot{y}$; whence $\ddot{x} + \ddot{y}$ will be the Fluxion of $\dot{x} + \dot{y}$, or the second Fluxion of $x + y$ In like manner, because $\dot{x}$ is the Fluxion of x, as $\dot{y}$ is the Fluxion of y, therefore $\dot{x} + \dot{y}$, which is the Fluxion of $x + y$

$\dot{x} + y$ will be the second Fluxion of $\dot{x} + \dot{y}$, and the third Fluxion of $x + y$, as will $x + y$, the Fluxion of $x + y$, be the fourth Fluxion of $x + y$, and for the same Reason $\dot{x} - y + z$, which is the Fluxion of $x - \dot{y} + \dot{z}$, will be the second Fluxion of $x - y + z$, as will $x - y + z$, which is the second Fluxion of $x - y + z$, or first Fluxion of $\dot{x} - y + z$, be the third Fluxion of $x - y + z$, also $x - y + z$, which is the first Fluxion of $x - y + z$, and the second Fluxion of $x - y + z$, and the third Fluxion of $\dot{x} - \dot{y} + \dot{z}$, be the fourth Fluxion of $x - y + z$ And the same will hold good in finding the first, second, third, *&c.* Fluxions of any Aggregate whatsoever

AGAIN, as $x y + y x$ is the Fluxion of $x y$, so $\dot{x} y + \dot{y} \ddot{x}$ is the Fluxion of $\dot{x} y$, for assume $x y = v$, then will x, by flowing, become $\dot{x} + o x$, as will y become $\dot{y} + y o$, and v, $\dot{v} + v o$, multiplying therefore the two former Quantities together, we shall have $y \dot{x} + \dot{y} o x + \dot{x} y o + o o y x = \dot{v} + o \dot{v}$, taking away therefore the original Equation $x \dot{y} = v$, and dividing the remaining Terms by o, and making those afterward to vanish, in which the Quantity o is found, we shall have $\dot{y} x + z x$ for the Fluxion of the Fluxionary Quantity $x \dot{y}$, or second Fluxion, and by the same way of Reasoning $\dot{x} y z + \dot{x} \dot{z} y + \dot{y} \dot{z} x$ will be the Fluxion of $\dot{x} \dot{y} \dot{z}$, or second Fluxion of that Quantity, of which $\dot{x} \dot{y} \dot{z}$ is the first Fluxion, as will $x y z + x z y + y z x$ be the Fluxion of $x y z$, or third Fluxion of that Quantity, of which $x y z$ is the second Fluxion.

AGAIN, as $2 x \dot{x}$ is the Fluxion of $x x$, so by substituting $2 x + 2 o \dot{x}$ in the room of $2 x$, and $\dot{x} + o x$ in the room of of $\dot{x}$, we ſhall have $2\dot{x}\dot{x}+2x\ddot{x}$ for the Fluxion of $2x\dot{x}$, or ſecond Fluxion of xx, and by putting $\dot{x}+o\ddot{x}$ in the room of $\dot{x}$, and $\ddot{x}+o\dddot{x}$ in the Place of $\ddot{x}$, and $x+o\dot{x}$ in the room of x, we ſhall have $6\dot{x}\ddot{x}+2x\dddot{x}$ for the third Fluxion of x^2, and by the ſame Method of Inveſtigation we ſhall find that as $3x^2\dot{x}$ is the firſt Fluxion of x^3, ſo $6x\dot{x}\dot{x}+3xx\ddot{x}$ will be the ſecond Fluxion, $18x\dot{x}\ddot{x}+6\dot{x}^3+3x^2\dddot{x}$ the third Fluxion, *&c.* Alſo as $4x^3\dot{x}$ is the firſt Fluxion of x^4, ſo $12xx\dot{x}\dot{x}+4xxx\ddot{x}$ will be the ſecond, $24x\dot{x}\dot{x}\dot{x}+36xx\dot{x}\ddot{x}+4xxx\dddot{x}$ will be the third, *&c* and univerſally if n repreſent the Power of x, and $\dot{v}$, $\ddot{v}$, $\dddot{v}$, its firſt, ſecond, third, *&c* Fluxion, then will $nx^{n-1}\dot{x}=\dot{v}$ be its firſt Fluxion $\overline{nn-n}\,x^{n-2}\dot{x}^2+nx^{n-1}\ddot{x}=\ddot{v}$, its ſecond Fluxion $\overline{n^3-3n^2+2n}\,x^{n-3}\dot{x}^3+\overline{3nn-3n}\,x^{n-2}\dot{x}\ddot{x}+nx^{n-1}\dddot{x}=\dddot{v}$, its third, and $\overline{n^4-6n^3+11n^2-6n}\,x^{n-4}\dot{x}^4+\overline{6n^3-18n^2+12n}\,x^{n-3}\dot{x}^2\ddot{x}+\overline{3nn-3n}\,x^{n-2}\ddot{x}^2+\overline{4nn-4n}\,x^{n-2}\dot{x}\dddot{x}+nx^{n-1}\ddddot{x}=\ddddot{v}$, its fourth Fluxion, *&c.*

AGAIN, as $\dfrac{\dot{y}x-x\dot{y}}{xx}$ is the Fluxion of $\dfrac{y}{x}$, ſo $\dfrac{\ddot{y}x-x\ddot{y}}{xx}$ will be the Fluxion of $\dfrac{\dot{y}}{x}$; for aſſuming $\dfrac{\dot{y}}{x}=v$, we ſhall have $\dot{y}=xv$ and $\ddot{y}=\dot{x}v+x\dot{v}$, whence $\ddot{y}-\dot{x}v=x\dot{v}$, and $\dot{v}=\dfrac{\ddot{y}-\dot{x}v}{x}$, and putting $\dfrac{\dot{y}}{x}$ in the room of v, we ſhall have $\dfrac{\ddot{y}x-\dot{x}\dot{y}}{xx}=\dot{v}$, for the ſecond Fluxion of $\dfrac{y}{x}$.

IN like manner as $\dfrac{\dot{x}yz+y\dot{x}z-xy\dot{z}}{zz}$ is the Fluxion of $\dfrac{xy}{z}$, ſo $\dfrac{z\dot{x}y+\dot{z}yx-\dot{x}yz}{zz}$ will be the Fluxion of $\dfrac{xy}{\dot{z}}$; for

for putting this equal to v, we shall have $\frac{x\dot{y}}{z} = \dot{v}$, whence $\dot{x}y = \dot{z}\dot{v}$, and $\dot{x}y + \dot{y}x = \dot{z}\dot{v} + z\dot{v}$, whence $z\dot{v} = \dot{x}y + \dot{y}x - \dot{z}v$, and $\dot{v} = \frac{\dot{x}y + \dot{y}x - \dot{z}v}{z}$, and substituting $\frac{x\dot{y}}{z}$ in the room of $\dot{v}$, there will arise $\frac{\dot{x}y + \dot{y}x}{z} - \frac{\dot{z}}{z} \times \frac{x\dot{y}}{z} = \frac{z\dot{x}y + z\dot{y}x - x\dot{y}\dot{z}}{zz} = \dot{v}$, the 2d Fluxion of that Quantity, of which $\frac{x\dot{y}}{z}$ is the first Fluxion, as was asserted. After the same manner of Investigation, we shall have $\frac{z\dot{x}x + z\dot{z}x - zz\dot{x}}{xx}$ for the Fluxion of $\frac{zz}{x}$, and $\frac{2z\dot{z}x - zz\dot{x}}{xx}$ for the Fluxion of $\frac{z^2}{x}$, and $-\frac{\dot{x}}{xx}$ for the Fluxion of $\frac{1}{x}$ and $\frac{-\dot{z}}{z^2}$ for the Fluxion of $\frac{1}{z}$.

AGAIN, as $3x^2\dot{x}$ is the Fluxion of x^3, so $3\dot{x}^2\ddot{x}$ will be the Fluxion of $\dot{x}^3$, for put $\dot{x} + o\ddot{x}$ in the room of $\dot{x}$, then will $\dot{x}^3 = \dot{x}^3 + 3\dot{x}\dot{x}o\ddot{x} + 3\dot{x}oo\ddot{x}\ddot{x} + ooo\ddot{x}\ddot{x}\ddot{x}$; taking away $\dot{x}^3$ from each Side of the Equation, dividing the Remainder by o, and making the Terms $3\dot{x}o\ddot{x}\ddot{x}$ and $oo\ddot{x}\ddot{x}\ddot{x}$ to vanish, we shall have $3\dot{x}\dot{x}\ddot{x}$ for the Fluxion of $\dot{x}^3$, and for the same Reason $4\dot{x}^3\ddot{x}$ will be the Fluxion of $\dot{x}^4$, as will $5\dot{x}^4\ddot{x}$ be the Fluxion of $\dot{x}^5$; in like manner $\frac{1}{2}\dot{x}^{-\frac{1}{2}}\ddot{x}$ will be the Fluxion of $\dot{x}^{\frac{1}{2}}$, and $\frac{2}{3}\dot{x}^{-\frac{1}{3}}\ddot{x}$, the Fluxion of $\dot{x}^{\frac{2}{3}}$, and universally if n be put for the Index, or Exponent, of any Quantity $\dot{x}$, its Fluxion will be $n\dot{x}^{n-1}\ddot{x}$.

AND

AND the Law obtains in the superior Orders of Quantities: Thus the Fluxion of $\overset{\prime\prime\prime\prime}{z}{}^m$ is $m\overset{\prime\prime\prime}{z}{}^{m-1}\overset{\prime\prime\prime}{z}$, of $\overset{\prime\prime\prime}{z}{}^m$ is $m\overset{\prime\prime\prime}{z}{}^{m-1}\overset{\prime\prime}{z}$, of $\overset{\prime\prime}{z}{}^m$ is $m\overset{\prime\prime}{z}{}^{m-1}\overset{\prime}{z}$, of $\overset{\prime}{z}{}^m$ is $m\overset{\prime}{z}{}^{m-1}z$, of $\overset{\prime}{z}\overset{\prime}{x}\overset{\prime}{y}$ is $\overset{\prime}{z}\overset{\prime}{x}y+\overset{\prime}{z}\overset{\prime}{y}x+\overset{\prime}{x}\overset{\prime}{y}z$ of $\frac{\overset{\prime\prime}{z}}{\overset{\prime}{x}}$ is $\frac{\overset{\prime}{z}\overset{\prime}{x}-x\overset{\prime\prime}{z}}{\overset{\prime}{x}\overset{\prime}{x}}$,

and of $\frac{\overset{\prime}{z}\overset{\prime}{x}}{\overset{\prime}{y}}$ is $\frac{\overset{\prime}{z}x\overset{\prime}{y}+\overset{\prime}{x}z\overset{\prime}{y}-\overset{\prime}{z}\overset{\prime}{x}y}{\overset{\prime}{y}\overset{\prime}{y}}$, &c

WHEN we proceed to find second, third and fourth Fluxions, &c if any Quantity in an Equation, suppose z, flow uniformly for its first Fluxion, which is a constant Quantity, put 1, for its second, &c Fluxion put 0, then will the Fluxionary Equation be more concisely expressed, some of its Terms being shortned, and others quite vanishing. Thus the Equation $z\ y^3 - z^4 + a^4 = 0$, whose first Fluxion is $z\ y^3 + 3\ z\ y\ y^2 - 4\ \dot{z}\ z^3 = 0$, second Fluxion $zy^3 + 6\ zyy^2 + 3\ zy\ y^2 + 6\ z\ y^2 y - 4\ zz^3 - 12\ z^2 z^2 = 0$, and its third Fluxion $z\ y^3 + 9\ z\ y\ y^2 + 9\ z\ yy^2 + 18\ z\ y^2\ y + 3\ z\ y\ y^2 + 18\ z\ y\ y\ y + 6\ zy^3 - 4\ z\ z^3 - 36\ z\ z\ z - 24\ z^3\ z = 0$, by supposing z to flow uniformly, will have its first Fluxion $y^3 + 3\ z\dot{y}\ y^2 - 4\ z^3 = 0$, its second Fluxion $6\ y\ y^2 + 3\ z\ y\ y^2 + 6\ z\ y^2\ y - 12\ z^2 = 0$, and its third Fluxion $9\ \dot{y}\ y^2 + 18\ y^2\ y + 3\ z\ y\ y^2 + 18\ z\ y\ y\ y + 6\ zy^3 - 24\ z = 0$, by which means the first Fluxion is more simply expressed, two Terms vanish in the second Fluxion, and four in the third

BY a Quantity flowing uniformly, as has been already explained, we are to understand a Quantity whose Increments, generated in equal Particles of Time, are equal, or that the flowing Quantity, in equal Particles of Time, be equally augmented.

IN

In Equations of the same kind with the former, we are to conceive that the Fluxions in each of the Terms are all of the same Order, that is, all of the first Order, or first Fluxions, as $\dot{x}, y, \dot{z}$, or all of the second Order, that is, second Fluxions, or Rectangles, or Squares of first Fluxions, as y, $\dot{y}^2$, $\dot{y}\dot{z}$, $\dot{z}^2$, or all of the third Order, that is, third Fluxions, or third Powers of first Fluxions, Rectangles of second Fluxions multiplied into first Fluxions, or Squares of second Fluxions into first Fluxions, as $y, y\,y, y\,z, y^3, y^2\,z, y\,z^2, z^3$, &c. and when any one or more Terms are wanting, they must be supplied by the Fluxions, or Powers of some Fluxion of a Quantity flowing uniformly. Thus in the last Equation $9\,y\,y^2 + 18\,y^2\,y + 3\,z\,y\,y^2 + 18\,z\,y\,y\,y + 6\,z\,y^3 - 24\,z^3 = 0$, because the two first Terms are of the second Order, and the three middle ones of the third. To make them all of the same kind, let us suppose z to flow uniformly, then multiplying the first and second Terms by $\dot{z}$, and the last by $\dot{z}^3$, we shall have a new Equation $9\,z\,y\,y^2 + 18\,z\,y^2\,y + 3\,z\,y\,y^2 + 18\,y\,y\,y + 6\,z\,y^3 - 24\,z^3\,\dot{z} = 0$, compleat of the third Order In like manner by multiplying the fiιst Term of the second Equation by z, and the last by z^2, we shall have $6\,z\,y\,y^2 + 3\,z\,y\,y^2 + 6\,z\,y^2\,y - 12\,z^2\,z^2 = 0$, an Equation of the second Order compleat, and by multiplying the first and last Terms of the first Equation by $\dot{z}$, we shall have $\dot{z}\,y^3 + 3\,z\,\dot{y}\,y^2\,4\,z\,z^3 = 0$, an Equation compleat of the first Order

As it is left at Discretion to suppose which of the flowing Quantities we will to flow uniformly, so it is necessary, in order to reduce the Equation as low as possible, to choose that Quantity that will strike out most Terms, and that must be that Quantity whose second or third Fluxions, &c occur oftenest Thus in the Equation of the third Order, because the second and third Fluxion of z are found in four of the Terms.

IF we suppose *z* to flow uniformly, we shall lose four Terms, whereas if we should pitch upon *y*, we should lose but three, because the inferior Fluxions of *y* are found in but three of the Terms

IF a Quantity flow uniformly, its first Power will have a first Fluxion, and no second Fluxion, its second Power will have a first and second Fluxion, and no third Fluxion; its third Power will have a first, second and third Fluxion, and no fourth Fluxion, its fourth Power will have a first, second, third and fourth Fluxion, and no fifth Fluxion, and so on infinitely And the Order of the standing, or fix'd Fluxion, will be of the same Denomination with the Order of the Power of the uniformly flowing Quantity. Thus, if *x* be supposed to flow uniformly, then will $x = 1$, $x = 0$, and $x = 0$, &c.

IF $x^n = v$, and $n = 1$, then $\dot{v} = n x^{n-1} x = 1 \dot{x}$, and $\dot{v} = n n - n x^{n-2} \dot{x}^2$, &c. $= 1 \times 1 - 1 = 0$. If $n = 2$, then $v = n x^{n-1} x = 2 x \dot{x}$, and $v = n n - n x^{n-2} x^2 + n x^{n-1} x = 2 x^2 + 2 x \dot{x}$, and $\ddot{v} = n^3 - 3 n^2 + 2 n x^{n-3} \dot{x}^3 = 2^3 - 3 \times 2^2 + 2 \times 2 = 0$. If $n = 3$, then $v = n x^{n-1} x = 3 x^2 \dot{x}$ $v = n n - n x^{n-2} x^2 + n x^{n-1} \ddot{x} = 6 x x^2 + 3 x^2 x$ $v = n^3 - 3 n^2 + 2 n x^{n-3} x^3 + 3 n^2 - 3 n x^{n-2} x x + n x^{n-1} x = 6 x^3 + 18 x x x + 3 x^2 x$, and $v = n^4 - 6 n^3 + 11 n^2 - 6^n$, &c $= 3^4 - 6 \times 3^3 + 11 \times 3^2 - 6 \times 3$, &c $= 0$; and the same Consequence will arise in carrying the Operation as high as you please

AND hence it will follow, that if the Quantity *x* be supposed to flow uniformly, that is, while *x* in flowing becomes $x + o$, x^n becomes $\overline{x + o}^n$, that the first, second, third, fourth Fluxions, &c. of the Quantity x^n will be as the respective Terms of an infinite Series formed by raising of the Quantity $\overline{x + o}^n$ to the same Power *n*.

FOR

I

For it has already been ſhewn, that the firſt, ſecond, third, *&c.* Fluxions of the Quantity x^n are expreſſed by the Terms $n x^{n-1} \dot{x}$, $\overline{nn-n}\, x^{n-2} \dot{x}^2$, $\overline{n^3-3n^2+2n}\, x^{n-3} \dot{x}^3$, that is, becauſe $\dot{x}$, $\dot{x}^2$, $\dot{x}^3$, *&c* $= 1$, by the Terms $n x^{n-1}$. $\overline{nn-n}\, x^{n-2}$. $\overline{n^3-3n^2+2n}\, x^{n-3}$, *&c* and becauſe by the Law of infinite Series $\overline{x+o}^n = x^n + n x^{n-1} o + \frac{nn-n}{2} x^{n-2} o^2 + \frac{nnn-3nn+2n}{6} x^{n-3} o^3$, *&c.* and o being a ſtanding Quantity, and the Powers of x the ſame in the reſpective Terms on each Side, therefore by comparing the correſpondent Terms together we ſhall find $n x^{n-1} o . n x^{n-1}$ $o . 1$, and $\frac{nn-n}{2} x^{n-2} oo$ $\overline{nn-n}\, x^{n-2}$ $\because \frac{1}{2} oo$ 1, and $\frac{n^3-3n^2+2n}{6} x^{n-3} o^3$ $\overline{n^3-3nn+2n}\, x^{n-3}$. $\frac{1}{6} o^3$ 1, and the ſame will follow of the reſt of the Terms *ad infinitum.*

In all the preceding Operations about finding the Fluxions of flowing Quantities, we have ſuppoſed that while one of the flowing Quantities, ſuppoſe x, increaſes, that the Quantities z, y, *&c* increaſe alſo, that is, that while x, for Example, in flowing becomes $x + o\dot{x}$, that z and y, *&c.* by flowing become $z + o\dot{z}$, and $y + o\dot{y}$, *&c.* but if it ſo happen that while one of them, as ſuppoſe x, increaſes, the others z and y, *&c* decreaſe, that is, by flowing become $z - o\dot{z}$, and $y - o\dot{y}$, we muſt conſider the Fluxions of theſe as negative Quantities, in Compariſon of the Fluxions of thoſe which increaſe at the ſame time, and conſequently we muſt change the Signs of thoſe Terms wherein the negative Fluxions are found. Thus in taking the Fluxions of this Product x, y, z, if we ſuppoſe x to increaſe, that is, becomes $x + o\dot{x}$, while y and z decreaſe, or become $y - o\dot{y}$, and $z - o\dot{z}$, the Fluxion of

xyz, which, in the Case of supposing them all increasing, would be $yzx + z\dot{y} + yzx$, will, in this Case, become $yzx - xzy - xyz$ And the same must be observed in all other Cases, the Reason of all which is very evident.

SECT. VII.

Of the FLUXIONS *of Exponential Quantities, that is, of such Quantities, or Powers, whose Exponents themselves are variable or flowing Quantities.*

THE Fluxions of Exponential Quantities may readily and easily be found by the Help of the Logarithmick Series, and to this End it is necessary to premise, that the Fluxion of any Logarithm is equal to the Fluxion of the absolute Number or Quantity whose Logarithm it is, divided by the same Number. Thus, if $x + 1$ represent any given Quantity, I say the Fluxion of the Logarithm of this Quantity will be $\frac{x}{x+1}$

DEMONSTRATION.

FOR inasmuch as the Logarithm of $1 + x$ is $x - \frac{1}{2}x^2 + \frac{1}{3}x^3 - \frac{1}{4}x^4 + \frac{1}{5}x^5 - \frac{1}{6}x^6$, *&c.* its Fluxion will be $\dot{x} - x\dot{x} + x^2\dot{x} - x^3\dot{x} + x^4\dot{x} - x^5\dot{x}$, *&c.* that is, $\dot{x} \times 1 - x + x^2 - x^3 + x^4 - x^5$, *&c.* equal to $x \times \frac{1}{x+1} = \frac{x}{x+1}$.

And

And that $\frac{1}{x+1}$ is equal to $1 - x + x^2 - x^3 + x^4 - x^5$, &c. will evidently appear by multiplying $1 - x + x^2 - x^3 + x^4 - x^5$, &c. by $x + 1$, or dividing 1 by $x + 1$, as has been sufficiently shewn in the second Section *Q. E. D.*

HENCE the Fluxion of the Logarithm of $xx + yy$, which is express'd after this manner, $L\ \overline{xx+yy}$ is $\frac{2x\dot{x} + 2y\dot{y}}{xx+yy}$, and the Fluxion of the Logarithm of $ax^2 + x^3$, or $L.\overline{ax^2+x^3}$ is $\frac{2ax\dot{x} + 3\dot{x}x^2}{ax^2 + x^3} = \frac{2a\dot{x} + 3x\dot{x}}{ax + xx}$, and the Fluxion of the Logarithm of $ax^n + x^m$, or of $L\ \overline{ax^n + x^m}$ is $\frac{nax^{n-1}\dot{x} + mx^{m-1}\dot{x}}{ax^m + x^m}$; also the Fluxion of the Logarithm of $\overline{z^m+z^n}^p$, or $L\ \overline{z^m+z^n}^p$ is equal to

$$\frac{\overline{z^m + x^n}^{p-1} \times pmz^{m-1}\dot{z} + pnx^{n-1}\dot{x}}{\overline{z^m + x^n}^p}$$

$$= \frac{pmz^{m-1}\dot{z} + pnx^{n-1}\dot{x}}{\overline{z^m + x^n}^1}.$$

AND after the same way may the Fluxion of the Logarithm of any Power of a given Quantity be determined

AGAIN, the Fluxions of the Powers of Logarithms are found after the manner taught in *Section* V, for finding the Fluxions of other Powers. Thus, if the Quantity $\overline{a+x}$ were given, and it were required to find the Fluxion of the m Power of its Logarithm, I say, that $\dot{L}:^{m}\overline{a+x}$ is $mL^{m-1}\overline{a+x} \times \frac{\dot{x}}{a+x}$ for $L.^{m-1}\overline{a+x}$ is the Power of the flowing Quantity less by Unity, and $mL^{m-1}\overline{a+x}$ is the same Quantity multiplied by its Exponent, and because the Fluxion of $L\ \overline{a+x}$ the

the Root is $\frac{\dot{x}}{a+x}$, this therefore multiplied by the former Quantity $m\,L^{m-1}\,\overline{a+x}$, will give $m\,L^{m-1}\,\overline{a+x}\times\frac{\dot{x}}{a+x}$ for the Fluxion of the m Power of the Logarithm of $\overline{a+x}$, alſo the Fluxion of $L^{m}\,\overline{a+x}^{n}$ will be $m\,L^{m-1}\,\overline{a+x}^{n}\times\frac{n\dot{x}}{a+x}$; for the Fluxion of $L\,\overline{a+x}^{n}$ is $\frac{n\times\overline{a+x}^{n-1}\,\dot{x}}{\overline{a+x}^{n}} = \frac{n\dot{x}}{a+x}$, and the Fluxion of $L^{m}\,\overline{a+x}^{n}$ is $m\,L^{m-1}\,\overline{a+x}^{n}\times\frac{n\dot{x}}{a+x}$.

In like manner the Fluxion of the $-m$ Power of the Logarithm of $\overline{a+x}^{n}$ will be $-m\,L^{-m-1}\,\overline{a+x}^{n}\times\frac{n\dot{x}}{a+x} = \frac{-m}{L^{m+1}\,\overline{a+x}^{n}}\times\frac{n\dot{x}}{a+x}$.

Hence the Fluxions of the Logarithms of any Powers of the ſame Quantity are one to another, as the Exponents of thoſe Powers, that is, $L.\dot{\overline{1+x}} : L\,\dot{\overline{1+x}}^{n} :: 1 : n$.

For $L\,\dot{\overline{1+x}} = \frac{\dot{x}}{1+x}$, and $L\,\dot{\overline{1+x}}^{n} = \frac{n\dot{x}}{1+x}$.

And $\frac{\dot{x}}{1+x} : \frac{n\dot{x}}{1+x} :: 1 . n$.

Whence it follows, that the Fluxions of the Logarithms of any Powers of the ſame Quantity are in Proportion one to another as thoſe Logarithms themſelves.

Hence

HENCE the Fluxion of the Logarithm of the Root is $\frac{1}{2}$ the Fluxion of the Logarithm of the Square, and $\frac{1}{3}$ of the Fluxion of the Logarithm of the Cube, *&c.*

HENCE we are taught how to find the Fluxions of Exponential Quantities, that is, such Quantities whose Exponents are indeterminate or flowing Quantities, and these are of several Orders or Degrees, according as the Exponents themselves are more or less involved If the Exponent be a simple Quantity, as z^{y}, it is called an Exponential of the first or lowest Degree, but when the Exponent itself is an Exponential of the first Degree, as $z^{y^{x}}$, it is called an Exponential of the second Degree In like manner if the Exponent itself be an Exponential of the second Degree as $z^{y^{x^{0}}}$, it is called an Exponential of the third Degree, *&c*

THESE things being premised, let it be required to find the Fluxion of a^{x}, where a is supposed to be a constant and determinate Quantity

PUT $a^{x}=y$, then $\dot{y}$ will be equal to the Fluxion of a^{x}, and because $a^{x}=y$, therefore L $a^{x}=$ L y, but from the Nature of the Logarithms L $a^{x}=x$ L a, wherefore x L $a=$ L y, and consequently $\dot{x}$ L $a+x$ L $\overline{a}=$ L $\overline{y}$, but L $\dot{\overline{a}}=\frac{\dot{a}}{a}=0$, because the Quantity a is a constant Quantity, and therefore its Fluxion nothing; and L $\overline{y}=\frac{\dot{y}}{y}$, therefore $\dot{x}$ L $a=\frac{\dot{y}}{y}$, and yL $a\dot{x}=\dot{y}=a^{x}$ L $a\dot{x}$, because $y=a^{x}$, and consequently a^{x} L $a\dot{x}$ is the Fluxion of a^{x}.

AGAIN, if it be required to find the Fluxion of z^{y}, where y is supposed to be a flowing Quantity

PUT $z^{y}=v$, then will L $\cdot z^{y}=$ L v, and yL $z=$ L v, whence L. $z\dot{y}+y$L. $\overline{z}=$L $\dot{\overline{v}}$, that is, L $z\dot{y}+y\frac{\dot{z}}{z}=\frac{\dot{v}}{v}=\frac{\dot{v}}{z^{y}}$

because

because $v = z^y$, and consequently $z^y\,L:z\dot{y} + y z^{y-1}\dot{z} = \dot{v} =$ the Fluxion of z^y.

AGAIN, Let it be required to find the Fluxion of z^{y^x}.

PUT $z^{y^x} = v$, then $L\ z^{y^x} = L.v$, and $y^x L\cdot z = L\ v$, and taking the Fluxion of each, we shall have $\overline{y^x}\ L:z + y^x\ L:\bar{z} = L\ \bar{v}$, but $\overline{y^x}$ the Fluxion of y^x, is equal to $y^x L\ y\dot{x} + x y^{x-1}\dot{y}$, also $L\ \bar{z} = \frac{\dot{z}}{z}$, and $L:\bar{v} = \frac{\dot{v}}{v}$; wherefore substituting these Values in the former Equation, we shall have $L.z y^x L\ y\dot{x} + L z x y^{x-1}\dot{y} + y^x\frac{\dot{z}}{z} = \frac{\dot{v}}{v} = \frac{\dot{v}}{z^{y^x}}$; and multiplying each Term by z^{y^x}, we shall have $z^{y^x} L:z\,y^x L:y\,\dot{x} + z^{y^x} L.z x y^{x-1}\dot{y} + y^x z^{y^x-1}\dot{z} = \dot{v}$, for the Fluxion of z^{y^x}. And by the same way of proceeding may the Fluxion of any other Quantity of the same Kind be found.

SECT. VIII.

Of the Inverse Method of FLUXIONS.

HOW from given Fluxions to find the Fluents, or flowing Quantities themselves, is a Problem no less difficult than it is useful, and in some Cases almost impossible; and could it be compleatly and universally solved, it would, in a manner, render the Science of Geometry compleat, and set Bounds to farther Improvement.

THE great Author, in his Treatiſe of the Quadrature of Curves, tells us, that in order to find the Fluents of given Fluxions, we may aſſume a Fluent at Pleaſure, and that this Aſſumption, which muſt be gather'd from the Conſideration of the Nature of the Fluxion itſelf, muſt be corrected by putting the Fluxion of the aſſumed Fluent equal to the Fluxion propoſed, and comparing the homologous Terms together. And after you have found the Fluents of the given Fluxions (if you doubt the Truth of it) collect the Fluxions of the Fluents found, and compare them with the Fluxions at firſt given If they come out equal, the Concluſion is right, if not, you muſt correct your Fluents, ſo as to make their Fluxions come out equal to the Fluxions originally propoſed

NOW as the Fluxions of flowing Quantities are expreſſed by the ſame Letters by which the Fluents themſelves are, with a Tittle or Point over them, ſo the Fluents of theſe are again reſtored, by ſetting them down without it.

AGAIN, the Fluent of the Fluxion $b\dot{x} \pm c\dot{y} \pm d\dot{z}$, will be $bx \pm cy \pm dz \pm a$, where a denotes a conſtant Quantity of no determinate Value, but taken at Pleaſure.

FOR as a Fluent may be either an Expreſſion compoſed of flowing Quantities only, or may have beſides ſome conſtant Quantities connected to it by the Signs of $+$ and $-$, and as theſe conſtant Quantities, in bringing out the Fluxion by the direct Method, vaniſh and are loſt, their Fluxions being equal to nothing, ſo 'tis neceſſary that the Fluent ſhould be expreſſed after ſuch a general manner, that it may repreſent indifferently any of all thoſe various conſtant Quantities with which the flowing Quantities themſelves might have been compounded, unleſs it be known for certain that there are no ſuch Quantities to be connected, and then the Fluent of the former Fluxion will be ſimply $bx \pm cy \pm dz$; and in either Caſe, if the Fluxions of theſe Fluents be taken by the direct Method, we ſhall have the Fluxionary Expreſſion firſt given, which ſhews that the Aſſumptions are true.

AGAIN, Suppose it were required to find the Fluent of this Expression $x\dot{y} + y\dot{x}$, assume it equal to $Axy \pm a$; where A represents any indeterminate Quantity, then by the direct Method the Fluxion of $Axy \pm a$ will be $Ax\dot{y} + Ay\dot{x}$, and comparing this with the Fluxion first given $x\dot{y} + y\dot{x}$, we shall find $A = 1$, whence xy is the Fluent required

AGAIN, Suppose the Fluxionary Expression $xy\dot{z} + yz\dot{x} + zx\dot{y}$ were given by assuming $Axyz \pm a$ for its Fluent, and proceeding after the former manner, we shall find $A = 1$, whence xyz will be the Fluent required, and hence arises this Rule for finding the Fluents of such Fluxionary Products, where the Fluxion of each particular flowing Quantity is multiplied into the Product of the rest of the Fluent Quantities.

RULE.

SUBSTITUTE instead of each Fluxion its respective flowing Quantity, and adding all the Terms together, divide that Sum by the Number of Terms, and the Quote will give the Fluent.

HENCE the Fluent of $vxy\dot{z} + vxz\dot{y} + vyz\dot{x} + vzx\dot{y}$ will be found to be $vxyz$, by substituting $vxyz$ in the room of $\dot{v}\dot{x}\dot{y}\dot{z}$ in the respective Terms, and dividing the Sum of the Terms $vxyz + vxzy + vyzx + yzxv$, or $4vxyz$ by 4, the Number of Terms, and after the same way may the Fluent of any such Fluxionary Expression be found.

AGAIN, Suppose the Fluxionary Quantity, whose Fluent is required, were $\pm n x^{\pm n-1} \dot{x}$, assume $Ax^{\pm n} \pm a^{\pm n}$ for the Fluent itself, then will its Fluxion, by the direct Method, be $\pm nAx^{\pm n-1}\dot{x}$ Put this equal to the given Fluxion, and we shall have $\pm nAx^{\pm n-1}\dot{x} = \pm n x^{\pm n-1}\dot{x}$, whence, by comparing the homologous Terms together, we shall find $\pm n A = \pm n$, and $A = \frac{\pm n}{\pm n} = 1$, whence the Fluent will be $x^{\pm n} \pm a^{\pm n}$, and after the same manner the Fluent of $\pm mbz^{\pm m-1}\dot{z}$ will be found to be $bz^{\pm m} \pm a^{\pm m}$, and by comparing these Fluents with their respective Fluxions, we may infer this general Rule for finding the Fluents of all Fluxionary Expressions that involve some Power of the flowing Quantity.

I. Divide the given Fluxion by the Fluxion of the Root.

II Multiply the Quotient by the Root itself.

III Divide the Quantity thus produced by the Index thus increased

Or, which is the same thing, reject the Fluxion of the Root, and increase the Index of the Power by Unity, and divide the Quantity thus elevated by the Index thus increased, and the Quantity thus produced in either way will be the Fluent required.

Thus if the Fluxion $\pm nx^{\pm n-1}\dot{x}$ were proposed, by dividing first by the Fluxion of the Root, or, which is the same thing, by rejecting the Fluxion of the Root, we shall have $\pm nx^{\pm n-1}$, and by multiplying this Quantity by x, the Root itself, or, which is the same thing, by increasing the Index of the Power by Unity, there will arise $\pm nx^{\pm n-1}x$, or $\pm nx^{\pm n}$, and by dividing this Product, or Quantity, thus elevated by the new, or increased Index, we shall have $x^{\pm n}$ for the Fluent of the given Fluxion.

And by comparing this, as well as the former Methods, with the Methods for finding the Fluxions from given Fluents, it will appear, that the Fluents of simple Fluxions, or such as are not involved under a Vinculum, are obtained by Operations just retrograde, or contrary to those whereby the Fluxions are brought out from their Fluents, so that Multiplication

depressing of Powers of flowing Quantities, and putting in Fluxionary Letters in the direct Operation, are, in the Inverse Operation, to be answer'd by Division, by the same Quantities as the Multiplication was made, by the Elevation of the flowing Quantities, just as much as they were depressed, and by leaving out the same Fluxionary Letters as were in the former Operations put in; and hence the Fluent of $2x\dot{x}$ will be found to be x^2, of $4x^3\dot{x}$ to be x^4, of $x\dot{x}$ to be $\frac{1}{2}x^2$, of $x^3\dot{x}$ to be $\frac{1}{4}x^4$, of $\frac{1}{2}x^{-\frac{1}{2}}\dot{x}$ to be $x^{\frac{1}{2}}$, of $\frac{3}{2}x^{\frac{1}{2}}\dot{x}$ to be $x^{\frac{3}{2}}$, of $\frac{5}{2}x^{\frac{3}{2}}\dot{x}$ to be $x^{\frac{5}{2}}$, of $\frac{x^2\dot{x}}{\sqrt{rx}}$ or $r^{-\frac{1}{2}}x^{-\frac{1}{2}}\times x^2\dot{x}$, or $r^{-\frac{1}{2}}x^{\frac{3}{2}}\dot{x}$ to be $\frac{2}{5}r^{-\frac{1}{2}}x^{\frac{5}{2}}$, or $\frac{2\sqrt{x^5}}{5\sqrt{r}}$ of $\overline{n+1}\,x^n\dot{x}$ to be x^{n+1}, of $\frac{1}{n}x^{\frac{1-n}{n}}\dot{x}$ to be $x^{\frac{1}{n}}$ of $\frac{n}{m}x^{\frac{n-m}{m}}\dot{x}$ to be $x^{\frac{n}{m}}$ of $-nx^{-n-1}\dot{x}$ to be x^{-n} or $\frac{1}{x^n}$ of $\frac{x^n\dot{x}}{px^{\frac{1}{m}}}$ or $\frac{x^{\frac{nm-1}{m}}\dot{x}}{p}$ to be $\frac{mx^{\frac{nm-1+m}{m}}}{\overline{nm+m-1}\times p}$ or $\frac{mx^{\frac{nm+m-1}{m}}}{nmp+mp-p}$, of $x^n\dot{x}\sqrt{rx}$, or $x^n\dot{x}\,\overline{rx}^{\frac{1}{2}}$ or $x^n\dot{x}\times r^{\frac{1}{2}}\times x^{\frac{1}{2}}$, or $x^{\frac{2n+1}{2}}\dot{x}\times r^{\frac{1}{2}}$ to be $\frac{2x^{\frac{2n+1+2}{2}}r^{\frac{1}{2}}}{2n+1+2}$ or $\frac{2x^{\frac{2n+3}{2}}r^{\frac{1}{2}}}{2n+3}$ or $\frac{2x^{\frac{2n+3}{2}}\sqrt{r}}{2n+3}$, of $\frac{x^n\dot{x}}{\sqrt{px}}$ or $x^n\dot{x}\,\overline{px}^{-\frac{1}{2}}$, or $x^n\dot{x}\times p^{-\frac{1}{2}}\times x^{-\frac{1}{2}}$, or $x^{\frac{2n-1}{2}}\dot{x}p^{-\frac{1}{2}}$ to be $\frac{2x^{\frac{2n-1+2}{2}}p^{-\frac{1}{2}}}{2n-1+2}$, or $\frac{2x^{\frac{2n+1}{2}}p^{-\frac{1}{2}}}{2n+1}$, or $\frac{2x^{\frac{2n+1}{2}}}{\overline{2n+1}\sqrt{p}}$, &c.

AND the same Rules will hold good in finding the Fluents of Expressions however compounded, where the Terms consist of certain Powers of the flowing Quantities multiplied into their respective Fluxions.

THUS

THUS the Fluent of the Expression $b\dot{v}v \pm cx^2\dot{x} \pm dy^3\dot{y} + rz^4\dot{z}$, will be $\frac{1}{2}bv^2 \pm \frac{1}{3}cx^3 \pm \frac{1}{4}dy^4 \pm \frac{1}{5}rz^5 \pm a^n$; of the Expression $my^{\pm n}x^{m-1}\dot{x} \pm nx^m y^{\pm n-1}\dot{y}$, will be $x^m y^{\pm n} \pm a^{m\pm n}$; of the Expression $\frac{ny^m x^{n-1}\dot{x} - mx^n y^{m-1}\dot{y}}{y^{2m}}$, or $\overline{ny^m x^{n-1}\dot{x} - mx^n y^{m-1}\dot{y}} \times y^{-2m}$, or $ny^{-m}x^{n-1}\dot{x} - mx^n y^{-m-1}\dot{y}$, will be $x^n y^{-m}$, or $\frac{x^n}{y^m} \pm a^m$, &c.

AGAIN, if the Fluxional Expression be affected with a Vinculum, that is, if there be some Compound Surd Quantity multiplied into a Fluxion, yet if the Fluxion standing before the Radical Sign be the Fluxion of the Quantity contain'd under the Radical Sign, the Fluent, in this Case, may be found by the general Rules for Powers already given.

THUS, for Example, if the Fluxion propofed be $a\dot{x}\sqrt{ax-aa}$ or $a\dot{x}\times\overline{ax-aa}^{\frac{1}{2}}$, because the Fluxion $a\dot{x}$ standing before the Radical Sign, is the Fluxion of $ax-aa$, the Quantity standing under it, we must raise the Quantity $\overline{ax-aa}^{\frac{1}{2}}$ to $\overline{ax-aa}^{\frac{3}{2}}$, a Power whose Exponent is greater by Unity, and divide the Quantity $\overline{ax-aa}^{\frac{3}{2}}$, thus elevated, by $\frac{3}{2}$, the Index thus increas'd, and the Quotient $\frac{2}{3}\overline{ax-aa}^{\frac{3}{2}}$, or $\frac{2ax-2aa}{3}\times\overline{ax-aa}^{\frac{1}{2}}$, or $\frac{2}{3}\overline{ax-aa}\sqrt{ax-aa}$ will be its Fluxion, or by putting z in the room of $\overline{ax-aa}^{\frac{1}{2}}$, the Surd Part of the fluxionary Quantity given, we shall have $ax-aa=zz$, and $a\dot{x}=2z\dot{z}$, whence $a\dot{x}\times\overline{ax-aa}^{\frac{1}{2}}=2z^2\dot{z}$, and consequently $=\frac{2}{3}\overline{ax-aa}^{\frac{3}{2}}$, or $\frac{2}{3}\overline{ax-aa}\times\overline{ax-aa}^{\frac{1}{2}}=\frac{2}{3}z^3$ for the Fluent of the given Fluxion, the same as was before determined.

AFTER

After the ſame manner of proceeding we ſhall find the Fluent of $\frac{r\dot{x} - x\dot{x}}{\sqrt{2rx - xx}}$, or $r\dot{x} - x\dot{x} \times \overline{2rx - xx}^{-\frac{1}{2}}$ to be $\overline{2rx - xx}^{\frac{1}{2}}$, or $\sqrt{2rx - xx}$, of $x\dot{x} + a\dot{x}\sqrt{x + a}$, or $x\dot{x} + a\dot{x} \times \overline{x + a}^{\frac{1}{2}}$, or $\dot{x} \times \overline{a + x}^{\frac{3}{2}}$ to be $\frac{2}{5}\overline{a + x}^{\frac{5}{2}}$ or $\frac{2xx + 4ax + 2aa}{5}\overline{a + x}^{\frac{1}{2}}$ of $2x\dot{x} \times \overline{xx + aa}^{\frac{1}{2}}$ to be $\frac{2}{3}\overline{xx + aa}^{\frac{3}{2}}$, or $\frac{2xx + 2aa}{3} \times \overline{xx + aa}^{\frac{1}{2}}$, of $\dot{x}\,\overline{a + x}^{\frac{n}{m}}$ to be $\frac{m}{n + m}\overline{a + x}^{\frac{n + m}{m}}$, and the Fluent of $mx^{m-1}\dot{x} \times \overline{x^m + a^p}^{n}$ to be $\frac{1}{n + 1}\overline{x^m + a^p}^{n+1}$, &c.

And although the fluxionary Expreſſions without the Vinculum be not the Fluxions of the Quantity contained under the Vinculum, yet if it has a given Ratio to it, the Fluent may, notwithſtanding, be had in finite Terms.

Thus, if the fluxionary Quantity $x\dot{x} \times \overline{xx + aa}^{\frac{1}{2}}$ were given, where $x\dot{x}$, the Fluxion without the Vinculum, is to the Quantity contained under the Vinculum as 1 to 2. If we put $\overline{xx + aa}^{\frac{1}{2}} = z$, we ſhall have $zz = xx + aa$, and by the direct Method $2z\dot{z} = 2x\dot{x}$; whence $z\dot{z} = x\dot{x}$, and $z^2\dot{z} = x\dot{x} \times \overline{xx + aa}^{\frac{1}{2}}$, and conſequently $\frac{1}{3}z^3$, the flowing Value of $z^2\dot{z}$, will be equal (by ſubſtituting $xx + aa$ in the room of zz, and $\overline{xx + aa}^{\frac{1}{2}}$ in the room of z) to $\frac{1}{3}xx + aa \times \overline{xx + aa}^{\frac{1}{2}}$, the Fluent of the given Fluxion.

In like manner, to find the Fluent of $x^{m-1}\dot{x} \times \overline{x^m + a^q}^{n}$, where the Fluxion $x^{m-1}\dot{x}$, without the Vinculum, is to the

the Fluxion $m x^{m-1} \dot{x}$, of the Quantity under the Vinculum, as 1 to m If we put, as before, $\overline{x^m + a^q}^{n} = z^n$, we shall have $\overline{x^m + a^q} = z$, and by the direct Method $m x^{m-1} \dot{x} = \dot{z}$, whence $x^{m-1} \dot{x} = \frac{\dot{z}}{m}$, and $x^{m-1} \dot{x} \times \overline{x^m + a^q}^{n} = \frac{z^n \dot{z}}{m}$, and

$\frac{1}{nm+m} \overline{x^m + a^q}^{n+1} = \frac{1}{nm+m} z^{n+1}$ will be the Fluent required.

But if the Fluxion without the Vinculum be neither the Fluxion of the Quantity contained under it, nor bears any Proportion to it, yet, notwithstanding, in many Forms of Expressions, the Fluent may be had in finite Terms.

Thus, if the Fluxion $x^m \dot{x} \times \overline{a + x}^{\frac{1}{n}}$ were the Expression proposed, if the Exponent m be an Integer, the Fluent of the Expression may be had in finite Terms.

For put $a + x = z$, then $z - a = x$, and $\overline{z - a}^{m} = x^m$, also $\overline{x + a}^{\frac{1}{n}} = z^{\frac{1}{n}}$, and $\dot{x} = \dot{z}$, whence $x^m \dot{x}\, \overline{a + x}^{\frac{1}{n}} = \overline{z - a}^{m}$ $\dot{z} z^{\frac{1}{n}}$, but by the Law of Infinite Series $\overline{z - a}^{m} = z^m - m z^{m-1}$ $a + \frac{m^2 - m}{2} z^{m-2} a^2 - \frac{m^3 - 3m^2 + 2m}{6} z^{m-3} a^3$, &c whence

$z^{\frac{1}{n}} \dot{z}\, \overline{z - a}^{m} = z^{\frac{nm+1}{n}} \dot{z} - m z^{\frac{nm-n+1}{n}} \dot{z} a + \frac{m^2 + m}{2}$ $z^{\frac{nm-2n+1}{n}} \dot{z} a^2 - \frac{m^3 - 3m^2 + 2m}{6} z^{\frac{nm-3m+1}{n}} \dot{z} a^3$, &c and consequently the flowing Quantity of this Series, by the Rules already given, will be $\frac{n}{nm+n+1} z^{\frac{nm+n+1}{n}}$ $- \frac{n}{nm+1} z^{\frac{nm+1}{n}} a + \frac{nmm - nm}{2nm - 2n + 2} z^{nm-n+1} a^2 -$

$-\frac{nm^3-3nm^2+2nm}{6nm-12n+6}z^{\frac{nm-2n+1}{n}}a^3$, &c. whence by substituting $a+x$ in the room of z, we shall find the Fluent of the given Fluxion $x^m\dot{x}\sqrt[n]{a+x}$ to be $\frac{n}{nm+n+1}\overline{a+x}^{\frac{nm+n+1}{n}}-\frac{n}{nm+1}\overline{a+x}^{\frac{nm+1}{n}}a+\frac{nm^2-nm}{2nm-2n+1}\overline{a+x}^{\frac{nm-2n+1}{n}}a^2-\frac{nm^3-3nm^2+2nm}{6nm-12n+6}\overline{a+x}^{\frac{nm-2n+1}{n}}a^3$, &c. which Series will terminate when the Power of a becomes equal to m, the Index of x^m Power.

And although the flowing Part of the Quantity under the Vinculum be raised to some Power, yet even this, in many Cases, may have its Fluent expressed in finite Terms.

As suppose, for Example, that the Fluxion proposed were $x^m\dot{x}\,\overline{aa+xx}^{\frac{1}{n}}$. Put $\overline{aa+xx}^{\frac{1}{n}}=z^{\frac{1}{n}}$, then will $aa+xx=z$, and $xx=z-aa$, whence $x=\overline{z-aa}^{\frac{1}{2}}$, and $x^m=\overline{z-aa}^{\frac{m}{2}}$; again, $2x\dot{x}=\dot{z}$, and $\dot{x}=\frac{\dot{z}}{2x}=\frac{\dot{z}}{2\sqrt{z-aa}^{\frac{1}{2}}}$; whence $x^m\dot{x}\times\overline{aa+xx}^{\frac{1}{n}}=\overline{z-aa}^{\frac{m}{2}}\times\frac{\dot{z}}{2\sqrt{z-aa}}z^{\frac{1}{n}}=\frac{z^{\frac{1}{n}}\dot{z}\,\overline{z-aa}^{\frac{m}{2}}}{2\sqrt{z-aa}}$ equal by Division to $\frac{1}{2}z^{\frac{1}{n}}\dot{z}\,\overline{z-aa}^{\frac{m-1}{2}}$, and consequently if the Expression $\frac{m-1}{2}$ be an Integer, which will always happen when m is an odd Number, the Fluent will be had in finite Terms, according to the manner taught in the former Example, but if the Expression $\frac{m-1}{2}$ be a Fraction, as will happen when m is an even Number, then the Fluent will be expressed by an Infinite Series.

And in all other Cases, when the flowing Part of the Quantity under the Vinculum is raised to some Power, and the Fluxional Expression without the Vinculum is only the Fluxion of the Root, in such Cases the Fluent itself will run up into an Infinite Series. For Example,

If the Fluxion proposed were $\dot{x} \times \overline{aa + xx}|^{\frac{1}{n}}$, if we put, as before, $\overline{aa + xx}|^{\frac{1}{n}} = z^{\frac{1}{n}}$, then $aa + xx = z$, and $xx = z - aa$, and $x = \sqrt{z - aa}$, also $2x\dot{x} = \dot{z}$, and $\dot{x} = \frac{\dot{z}}{2x} = \frac{\dot{z}}{2\sqrt{z - aa}}$

whence $\dot{x} \times \overline{aa + xx}|^{\frac{1}{2}} = z^{\frac{1}{n}} \dot{z}\, 2 \times \overline{z - aa}|^{\frac{1}{2}}$, which because the Power of $2 \times \overline{z - aa}|^{\frac{1}{2}}$ is a Fraction, the Series arising from the Expression $2 \times \overline{z - aa}|^{\frac{1}{2}}$, will never terminate but run on infinitely, as is abundantly manifest from the Laws of Infinite Series, so that if it were required to find the Fluent of this Expression $\dot{x} \times \overline{aa + xx}|^{\frac{1}{2}}$, we must throw the Expression $\overline{aa + xx}|^{\frac{1}{2}}$ into an Infinites Series, which, according to the Method taught in *Section* II, will be $a + \frac{xx}{2a} - \frac{x^4}{8a^3} + \frac{x^6}{16a^5} - \frac{5x^8}{128a^7} + \frac{7x^{10}}{256a^9}$ &c. and multiplying this Series by $\dot{x}$, we shall have $a\dot{x} + \frac{x^2\dot{x}}{2a} + \frac{x^4\dot{x}}{8a^3} - \frac{x^6\dot{x}}{16a^5} - \frac{5x^8\dot{x}}{128a^7} + \frac{7x^{10}\dot{x}}{256a^9}$, &c whence the Fluent Quantity, according to the former Rules for Powers, will be $ax + \frac{x^3}{6a} - \frac{x^5}{40a^3} + \frac{x^7}{112a^5} - \frac{5x^9}{1152a^7} + \frac{7x^{11}}{2816a^9}$, &c.

After the same manner the Fluent of $\dot{x} \times \overline{rr - xx}|^{\frac{1}{2}}$ will

be

be found to be $rx + \frac{x^3}{6r} + \frac{x^5}{40r^3} + \frac{x^7}{112r^5} + \frac{5x^9}{1152r^7}$, &c.
and the Fluent of $\frac{rr\dot{x}}{r+x}$, or $rr\dot{x} \times \overline{r+x}|^{-1}$ will be $rx - \frac{x^2}{2} + \frac{x^3}{3r} - \frac{x^4}{4r^2}$, &c. For $\overline{r+x}|^{-1} = r^{-1} - \frac{x}{r^2} + \frac{x^2}{r^3} - \frac{x^3}{r^4}$, &c. and consequently $r^2 \times \overline{r+x}|^{-1} = r - x + \frac{x^2}{r} - \frac{x^3}{r^2}$, &c. and $rr\dot{x} = r\dot{x} - x\dot{x} + \frac{x^2\dot{x}}{r} - \frac{x^3\dot{x}}{r^2}$, &c whence the flowing Quantity will be $rx - \frac{x^2}{2} + \frac{x^3}{3r} - \frac{x^4}{4r^2}$, &c. as was to be shewn.

AGAIN, Suppose it were required to find the Fluent of this general Expression $bx^p\dot{x} \times \overline{c+dx^n}|^m$, by assuming $Abx^{p-n+1} + Bbx^{p-2n+1} + Cbx^{p-3n+1}$, &c. $\times \overline{c+dx^n}|^{m+1}$ for the Fluent of the given fluxionary Expression $bx^p\dot{x} \times \overline{c+dx^n}|^m$ we shall have $\overline{p-n+1} \times Abx^{p-n}\dot{x} + \overline{p-2n+1} \times Bbx^{p-2n}\dot{x} + \overline{p-3n+1} \times Cbx^{p-3n}\dot{x}$, &c. $\times \overline{c+dx^n}|^{m+1} + \overline{m+1} \times \overline{c+dx^n}|^{m+1} \times ndx^{n-1}\dot{x} \times Abx^{p-n+1} + Bbx^{p-2n+1} + Cbx^{p-3n+1}$, &c $= bx^p\dot{x} \times \overline{c+dx^n}|^m$, and by the Rules for Reduction of Equations, we shall find $A = \frac{b}{\overline{mn+p+1} \times d}$
$B = \frac{\overline{n-p-1} \times Acb}{\overline{mn+p-n+1} \times d}$. $C = \frac{\overline{2n-p-1} \times Bcb}{\overline{mn+p-2n+1} \times d}$, &c. consequently $\frac{1}{mn+p+1} \times \frac{b}{d}$ $(=A)$ $\times x^{p-n+1} + \frac{n-p-1}{mn+p-n+1} \times \frac{bc}{d} \times A (=B) \times x^{p-2n+1} + \frac{2n-p-1}{mn+p-2n+1}$ $\times$

$\times \frac{bc}{d} \times B (= C) \times x^{p-3n+1}$, &c. $\times \overline{c + dx^n}^{m+1}$, will be the Fluent of $bx^p \dot{x} \times \overline{c + dx^n}^m$; whence the Fluents of former Expressions may be found. Thus if the Expression $a\dot{x} \times \overline{ax - aa}^{\frac{1}{2}}$, in Page 85, were proposed by assuming $a\dot{x} \times \overline{ax - aa}^{\frac{1}{2}} = bx^p \dot{x} \times \overline{c + dx^n}^m$, and comparing the homologous Terms together, we shall find $b = a$. $p = 0$. $d = a$. $n = 1$ $m = \frac{1}{2}$. $c = -aa$; and by substituting these several Values of b, p, d, &c in the general Fluent $\frac{1}{mn + p + 1} \times \frac{b}{d} \times x^{p-n+1}$, &c. $\times \overline{c + dx^n}^{m+1}$ in the room of b, p, d, &c. we shall have $\frac{1}{1 \times \frac{1}{2} + 0 + 1} \times \frac{a}{a} \times x^{0-1+1} \times \overline{ax - aa}^{\frac{1}{2}+1} = \frac{2}{3} \overline{ax + aa}^{\frac{3}{2}}$ for the Fluent of $a\dot{x} \times \overline{ax - aa}^{\frac{1}{2}}$, the same as was before determined.

Again, if the Expression $mx^{m-1}\dot{x} \times \overline{x^m + a^p}^n$ were proposed, by putting it equal to $bx^p \dot{x} \times \overline{c + dx^n}^m$, and comparing the homologous Terms together, we shall have $b = m$. $p = m - 1$ $c = a^p$ $n = m$. $d = 1$. $m = n$, and by putting m, $m - 1$, a^p, &c. the several Values of b, p, c, &c in the general Fluent $\frac{1}{mn + p + 1} \times \frac{b}{d} \times x^{p-n+1}$, &c $\times \overline{c + dx^n}^{m+1}$ in the room of b, p, c, &c we shall have $\frac{1}{mn + m - 1 + 1}$ $\times \frac{m}{1} x^{m-1-m+1} \times \overline{x^m + a^p}^{n+1} = \frac{m}{mn + n} \times \overline{x^m + a^p}^{n+1}$ $= \frac{1}{n+1} \times \overline{x^m + a^p}^{n+1}$ for the Fluent of $mx^{m-1}\dot{x} \times \overline{x^m + a^p}^n$, the same as was found in Page 86.

After the same manner may the Fluents of other fluxionary Expressions of the same Kind be found, by the Help of the general Fluent.

The Rules hitherto deliver'd for finding the Fluents from first Fluxions, will hold good in finding the Fluents of second, third, fourth Fluxions, &c. (which likewise may be augmented or diminished, and for the same Reasons as the Fluents of the first Fluxions were, by Quantities that have no second, third, fourth, &c Fluxions), and the same Laws will obtain in all the superior Orders of Quantities.

Several other Methods might be shewn, for finding of Fluents from given Fluxions, but these that are exhibited are general, and the fittest for the Purpose.

The End of the First Part.

FLUXIONS.

PART II.

CONTAINING

The Use of the Direct METHOD of FLUXIONS.

In SIX SECTIONS.

SECT.

SECTION I.

Contains the Use of Fluxions *in drawing Tangents to Curves.*

SECT. II.

Contains the Use of Fluxions *in the Solution of Problems* de Maximis & de Minimis.

SECT. III.

Contains the Use of Fluxions *in the Invention of Points of Inflection and Retrogression.*

SECT. IV.

Contains the Use of Fluxions *in finding the Evoluta of a given Curve.*

SECT. V.

Contains the Use of Fluxions *in finding the Caustick Curves by Reflection.*

SECT. VI.

Contains the Use of Fluxions *in finding the Caustick Curves by Refraction.*

FLUXI-

FLUXIONS.

SECT. I.

Of the Use of FLUXIONS *in drawing of Tangents to Curves.*

PROPOSITION.

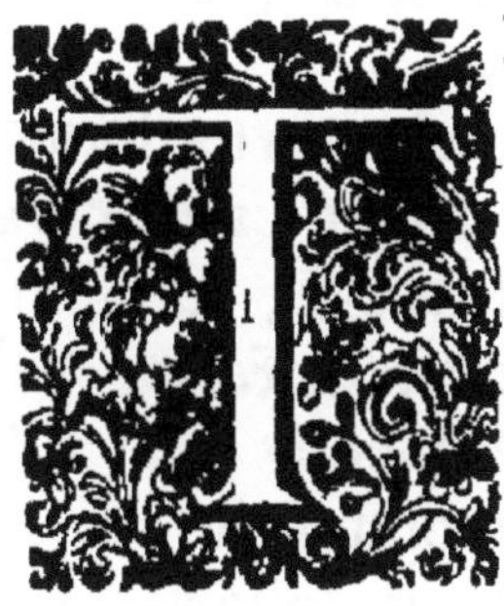

HE Fluxion of the Ordinate is to the Fluxion of the Absciſſe, as the Ordinate is to the Subtangent

IN the adjacent Figure, let A C *c* represent a Curve, A its Vertex, A B the Absciſſe, B C the Ordinate, V C a Tangent to the Curve in the Point C, and V B the Subtangent. I ſay, that the Ordinate B C is to the

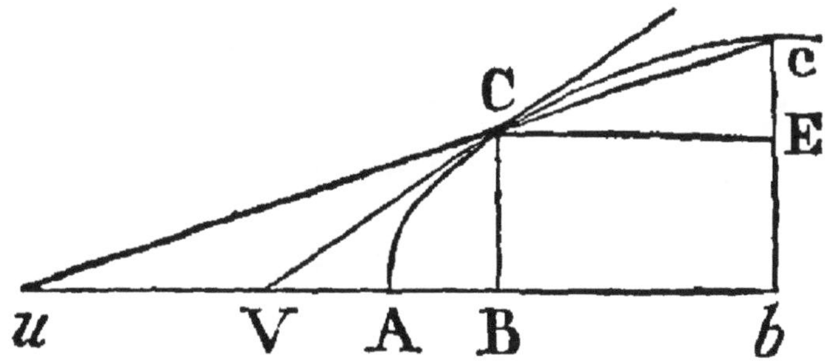

Subtangent V B, as the Fluxion of the Ordinate B C is to the Fluxion of the Absciſſe A B.

DEMON-

DEMONSTRATION.

CONCEIVE the Ordinate B C to flow uniformly, and move 'till it come into the Place *b c*, and draw C E parallel to A B.

IT is manifest, by *Section* III, that C E and *c* E are in the first Ratio of the nascent Increments of A B and B C, generated in the first Moment of Time, for while A B flowed into or became A *b*, B C flowed into or became *b c*.

DRAW C*c* subtending the Arch C *c*, and produce it 'till it cut the Abscisse produced in the Point *u*, then will the Triangles E C *c*, and *c b u* be similar.

AND it will be as $cE \quad EC \quad cb \quad bv$;
That is, as $cE \quad EC \,.\, cE + Eb \quad bB + Bu$;
For $cb = cE + Eb$, and $bu = bB + Bu$;
Also $Eb = CB$, and $Bb = CE$,
Wherefore $cE \,.\, EC : \ cE + CB \,.\, EC + Bu$.

IMAGINE the Ordinate *b c* to return back into its former Place, and become B C, at which time the Right Lines *c* C *u*, and V C, will be coincident, the Increments *c* E, E C will vanish, and the Triangle *c* E C, in its evanescent Form, will be similar to the Triangle C B V, and consequently *c* E · E C :. C B B V, which was the thing to be demonstrated.

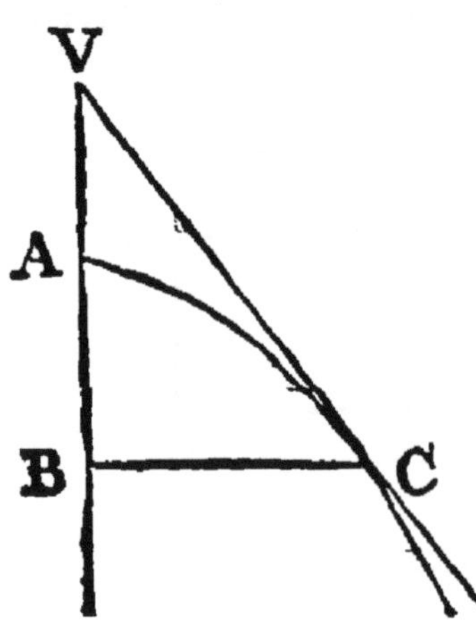

WHENCE it follows, supposing x to represent the Abscisse AB of any Curve A C, y the Ordinate B C, and t the Subtangent BV, that $\dot{y} \quad \dot{x} \,.\, y \quad t$; whence $t\dot{y} = x\dot{y}$, and $t = \frac{x\dot{y}}{\dot{y}}$; and hence arises this general Rule for drawing of Tangents to Curves.

First,

First, Find the fluxionary Value of the Absciffe, from the Equation expreffing the Nature of the Curve

Secondly, Multiply this fluxionary Value by y, the Ordinate

Thirdly, Divide this laft Product by $\dot{y}$, the Fluxion of the fame Ordinate

Or, which is the fame thing,

IN the room of $\dot{y}$, in the fluxionary Value of the Subtangent, fubftitute the Fluent itfelf, and the Refult, in either way, will be the Value of the Subtangent in the Terms of the Equation firft given

AND hence we are taught how to draw a Tangent to any Point in a Curve, the Equation, expreffing the Nature of the Curve, being firft given Thus in

EXAMPLE I

LET it be required to draw a Tangent CV to any Point C, taken in the Circumference of a Circle DCA

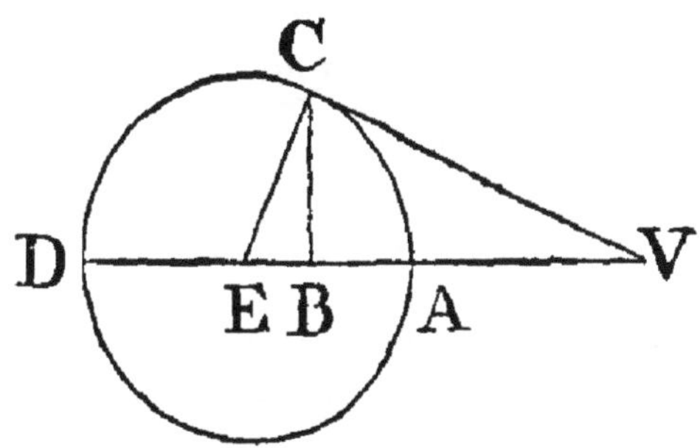

PUT $BC = y$ $AB = x$. $DA = 2r$, then will $DB = 2r - x$, and $EB = r - x$, and becaufe from the Nature of the Circle, $BD \times BA = BC^2$, therefore $\overline{2r - x} \times x = yy$; that is, $2rx - xx = yy$, and by finding the Fluxions of the Quantities on each Side of the Equation, we fhall have $2r\dot{x} - 2x\dot{x} = 2y\dot{y}$; whence (by dividing each Side by 2) we fhall have $r\dot{x} - x\dot{x} = y\dot{y}$, and $\dot{x} = \frac{y\dot{y}}{r - x}$, whence t the Subtangent, which is equal to $\dot{x} \times \frac{y}{\dot{y}}$ will be equal to $\frac{yy}{r - x}$, confequently $r - x : y :: y : t$; that is, becaufe $r - x = EB$,

and

and $BC = y$, it will be as EB BC: $BC \cdot BV$, consequently CV must be perpendicular to CE, that is EC, the Perpendicular to the Tangent, will always fall in the Centre: Whence it follows, that if from E, the Centre of the Circle, to any Point C in the Circumference, the Right Line E C be drawn, the Right Line C V, perpendicular to it, will touch the Circle in the Point C, which was the thing to be done.

EXAMPLE II.

LET it be required to draw a Tangent C V to any Point C, taken in the Periphery of an Ellipsis D C A

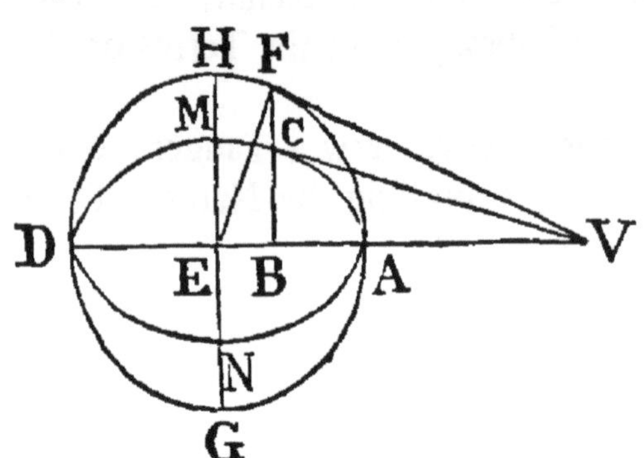

IN the adjacent Figure put $AB = x$ $BC = y$. $AD = 2a$, and the Parameter $= 1$, then will $DB = 2a - x$, and because, by the Property of the Ellipsis $DB \times BA$ BC^2 . DA to the Parameter, it will be as $\overline{2a - x} \times x$ yy $2a$ 1, whence $2ax - xx = 2ayy$, and taking the Fluxions of the Quantities on each Side of the Equation, we shall have $2a\dot{x} - 2x\dot{x} = 4ay\dot{y}$, whence $a\dot{x} - x\dot{x}$ $= 2ay\dot{y}$, and $\dot{x} = \dfrac{2ay\dot{y}}{a - x}$, consequently $t = \dfrac{2ayy}{a - x}$, and putting $2ax - xx$ in the room of $2ayy$, to which it is equal, we shall have $t = \dfrac{2ax - xx}{a - x}$, but $2ax - xx = FB$ in the circumscribing Circle, and $a - x = EB$ in the same Circle, and because in the Circle EB BF BF BV, therefore the Length of the Subtangent is the same in the Ellipsis, as in the circumscribing Circle, whence to draw a Tangent to any Point in the Ellipsis, having first circumscribed a Circle about the Ellipsis, produce the Ordinate B C in the Ellipsis, 'till it cut the Circumference

cumference of the circumscribed Circle in F, and draw F V perpendicular to E F, where this Line F V cuts the Axis of the Ellipsis produced in V, it will give the Extremity V of the Elliptical Subtangent, or the Point to which, if a Line be drawn to the given Point C, it will be a Tangent to the Ellipsis in that Point, which was the thing to be done. And universally if m represent the Exponent of the Power of AB, and n the Exponent of the Power of B D, then $\overline{2a-x}^{n} \times x^{m} = 2ay^{m+n}$, consequently $mx^{m-1}\dot{x} \times \overline{2a-x}^{n} - n \times \overline{2a-x}^{n-1}\dot{x} \times x^{m} = \overline{m+n}\, 2ay^{m+n-1}\dot{y}$, wherefore $\dot{x} = \dfrac{\overline{m+n}\, 2ay^{m+n-1}\dot{y}}{mx^{m-1} \times \overline{2a-x}^{n} - n \times \overline{2a-x}^{n-1} \times x^{m}}$

and $t = \dot{x} \times \dfrac{y}{\dot{y}} = \dfrac{\overline{m+n} \times 2ay^{m+n}}{mx^{m-1} \times \overline{2a-x}^{n} - n \times \overline{2a-x}^{n-1}\, x^{m}}$

and by substituting $\overline{2a-x}^{n} \times x^{m}$ in the room of $2ay^{m+n}$, we shall have $t = \dfrac{\overline{m+n} \times \overline{2a-x}^{n} \times x^{m}}{mx^{m-1} \times \overline{2a-x}^{n} - n \times \overline{2a-x}^{n-1}\, x^{m}}$, and by dividing by x^{m-1}, $t = \dfrac{\overline{m+n} \times \overline{2a-x}^{n} \times x}{m \times \overline{2a-x}^{n} - n \times \overline{2a-x}^{n-1}\, x}$, and by dividing again by $\overline{2a-x}^{n-1}$, $t = \dfrac{\overline{m+n} \times \overline{2a-x} \times x}{m \times \overline{2a-x} - nx}$, and by multiplying $\overline{2a-x}$ by x, we shall have $BV = t = \dfrac{\overline{m+n} \times \overline{2ax-xx}}{m \times \overline{2a-x} - nx}$, and $AV = BV - BA, = \dfrac{\overline{m+n} \times \overline{2ax-xx}}{m \times \overline{2a-x} - nx}$ $- x = \dfrac{n \times \overline{2ax}}{m \times \overline{2a-x} - nx}$ For $BV = \dfrac{2max - mxx + 2nax - nxx}{2ma - mx - nx}$

and $AV = BV - BA = \dfrac{2max - mxx + 2nax - nxx}{2ma - mx - nx} - x$,

 whence

whence $AV = \frac{2max - mxx + 2nax - nxx - 2max + mxx + nxx}{2ma - mxx - nx}$

whence $AV = \frac{2nax}{2ma - mx - nx} = \frac{n \times \overline{2ax}}{m \times \overline{2a - x} - nx}$. Whence it follows, that all Ellipsis's, drawn about the same common Axis, will have the same Subtangent.

EXAMPLE III.

LET it be required to draw a Tangent to any Point C in the Parabola A C

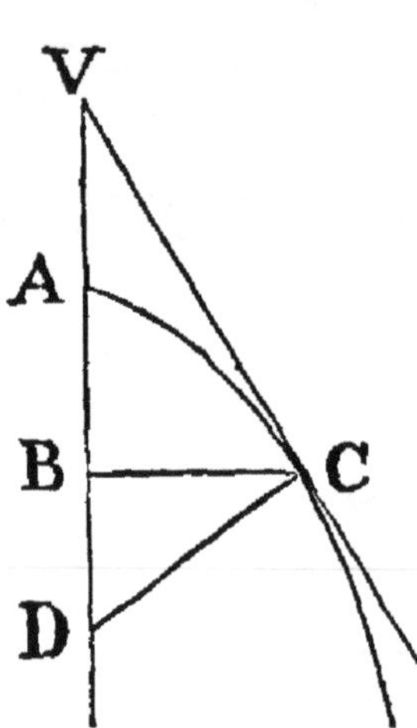

PUT, as before, $AB = x$ $BC = y$, and the Parameter $= 1$, and because, from the Nature of the Parabola $x = yy$, by taking the Fluxions of the Quantities on each Side of the Equation, we shall have $\dot{x} = 2y\dot{y}$, whence $t = 2yy$, and putting x in the room of yy, to which it is equal by Hypothesis, we shall have $t = 2x = VB$; wherefore making $AV = AB$, or $VB = 2AB$, we shall have the Point V in the Axis of the Parabola produced, to which if a Line, as V C, be drawn, it shall be a Tangent to the Curve in the Point C, which was the thing to be done

AND universally, if n represent the Exponent of the Power of B C, then $1x = y^n$, which expresses the Nature of all Parabolical Curves, whence $\dot{x} = ny^{n-1}\dot{y}$, and $t = \dot{x} \times \frac{y}{\dot{y}} = \frac{y}{\dot{y}} \times ny^{n-1}\dot{y} = ny^n$, and putting x in the room of y^n, to which it is supposed equal, we shall have $t = nx = BV$; wherefore universally as 1 n x t, that is, as Unity is to the Index of the Power of the Ordinate, so is the Abscisse to the Subtangent.

EXAM

EXAMPLE IV.

LET it be required to draw a Tangent to any Point C in the Hyperbola C c

LET A V and A D represent the Asymptotes of an Equilateral Hyperbola C c, and A the Centre of the opposite Hyperbolas. Suppose any Ordinate B C $= y$, and put A B $= x$; then because, from the Nature of the Curve, $aa = xy$, therefore $0 = x\dot{y} + y\dot{x}$, and $-y\dot{x} = x\dot{y}$, and $-\dot{x} = \frac{x\dot{y}}{y}$, and $t = \dot{x} \times \frac{y}{\dot{y}} = -x =$ A B

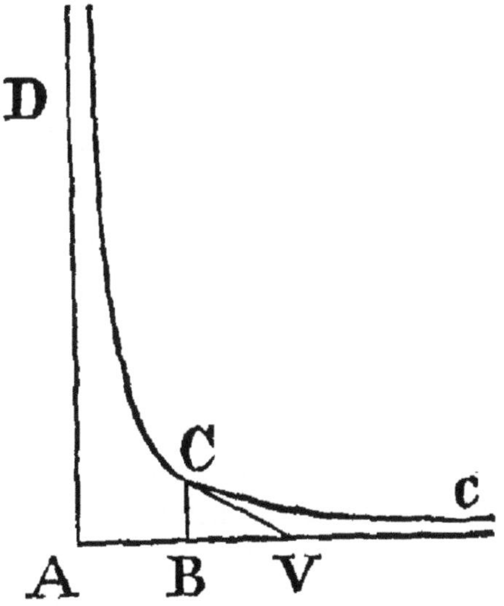

IF the Value of the Subtangent comes out positive, then V falls on the same Side of the Ordinate B C, with the Point A, the beginning of x, as in the Parabola, but if it comes out Negative, then it falls on the contrary Side of the Ordinate B C, in respect of A the beginning of the Axis, as in the Hyperbola.

LET the general Equation be $x = y^n$, which expresses the Nature of all Parabolas to Infinity, when the Exponent n is positive, whether it be a whole Number or a Fraction, but of all Kinds of Hyperbolas, when the Index n is negative; whence $\dot{x} = ny^{n-1}\dot{y}$, and consequently $t = \dot{x} \times \frac{y}{\dot{y}} = ny^n$, wherefore if $n = \frac{3}{2}$, the Equation will be $y^3 = axx$, which expresses the Nature of the Cubic Parabola, and the Subtangent B V will

will be $\frac{1}{2}x$; but if $n = -2$, the Equation will be $a^3 = xyy$ which expresses the Nature of one of the Cubic Hyperbolas, and the Subtangent B V, in this Case, will be $-2x$, and consequently the Point V will fall on the contrary Side of the Ordinate on which the Point A falls.

To draw a Tangent to the Point A, the Vertex of the Parabola, we must find what is the Ratio of $\dot{x}$ to $\dot{y}$ in this Point, since it is manifest, that if this Ratio be known, the Angle that the Tangent makes with the Axis, or Diameter, will be determined also Now $\dot{x}$ $\dot{y}$ $n y^{n-1}$ 1, whence it is manifest, that y being nothing, or vanishing in the Point A, the Ratio of $\dot{y}$ to $\dot{x}$ will be infinitely great, when n is greater than Unity, and infinitely less, when it is less than Unity; that is to say, the Tangent to the Point A will be parallel to the Ordinate B C in the first Case, but coincident with the Axis in the second Case.

If from C a Line, as C D, be drawn perpendicular to V C the Tangent, the Line B D is called the Subnormal, and because, in the Parabola, V B is equal to $2x$, $BC^2 = yy = ax$, and V B BC. B C B D, B D will be equal to $\frac{ax}{2x} = \frac{a}{2} = \frac{1}{2}a$, equal to half the Parameter, and consequently an invariable Quantity. [*See the Figure in Page* 100]

Again, if in the Hyperbola A B C we put $AB = x$. $BC = y$ $AD = a$ $VB = t$, and the Parameter A E equal to Unity, because, from the Nature of the Curve, $AB \times DB$ BC^2 $\overline{AD}$ AE, we shall have $x \times \overline{a - x}$ yy a 1, consequently $ax - xx = ayy$, and by taking the Fluxions of the Quantities on each Side of the Equation, we shall have $a\dot{x} + 2x\dot{x} = 2ay\dot{y}$, and

$\dot{x} =$

$\dot{x}=\frac{2ay\dot{y}}{a+2x}$, consequently V B $= t = \dot{x}\times\frac{y}{\dot{y}} = \frac{2ayy}{a+2x}\times\frac{y}{y}$ $= \frac{2ayy}{a+2x} = \frac{2\times\overline{ax+xx}}{a+2x}$ by putting $2\times\overline{ax+xx}$ in the room of $2ayy$, to which it is equal, and consequently B V $= t$ $= \frac{ax+xx}{\frac{1}{2}a+x}$. And universally,

If m be put for the Exponent of the Power of A B $= x$, and n for the Exponent of the Power of D B $= a+x$, we shall have this Equation $x^m\times\overline{a+x}^n = a\,y^{m+n}$, which expresses the Nature of all Kinds of Hyperbolas, whence taking the Fluxions on each Side of the Equation, we shall have $mx^{m-1}\dot{x}\times\overline{a+x}^n + n\times\overline{a+x}^{n-1}\dot{x}\times x^m = \overline{m+n}\times a y^{m+n-1}\dot{y}$, and consequently $\dot{x} = \frac{\overline{m+n}\,a\,y^{m+n-1}\dot{y}}{m\times x^{m-1}\times\overline{a+x}^n + n\times\overline{a+x}^{n-1}\times x^m}$, and $t = \dot{x}\times\frac{y}{\dot{y}} = \frac{\overline{m+n}\,a\,y^{m+n-1}\dot{y}}{mx^{m-1}\times\overline{a+x}^n + n\,\overline{a+x}^{n-1}\times x^m}\times\frac{y}{\dot{y}}$, whence $t = \frac{\overline{m+n}\times a\,y^{m+n}}{m\times x^{m-1}\times\overline{a+x}^n + n\times\overline{a+x}^{n-1}\times x^m}$, and putting $x^m\times\overline{a+x}^n$ in room of $a\,y^{m+n}$, to which it is equal, we shall have $t = \frac{\overline{m+n}\times x^m\times\overline{a+x}^n}{m\times x^{m-1}\times\overline{a+x}^n + n\times\overline{a+x}^{n-1}\,x^m}$, and by dividing by x^{m-1}, we shall have $t = \frac{\overline{m+n}\times x\times\overline{a+x}^n}{m\times\overline{a+x}^n + n\times\overline{a+x}^{n-1}\,x}$, and by dividing again by $\overline{a+x}^{n-1}$, we shall have $t = \frac{\overline{m+n}\times x\times\overline{a+x}}{m\times\overline{a+x}+nx}$, consequently B V $= \frac{\overline{m+n}\times\overline{ax+xx}}{ma+\overline{m+n}\,x}$, and

and $AV = BV - AB = \frac{\overline{m+n} \times \overline{ax+xx}}{ma + \overline{m+n}\,x} - x$, and consequently $AV = \frac{nax}{ma + \overline{m+n}\,x}$, which was the thing to be done.

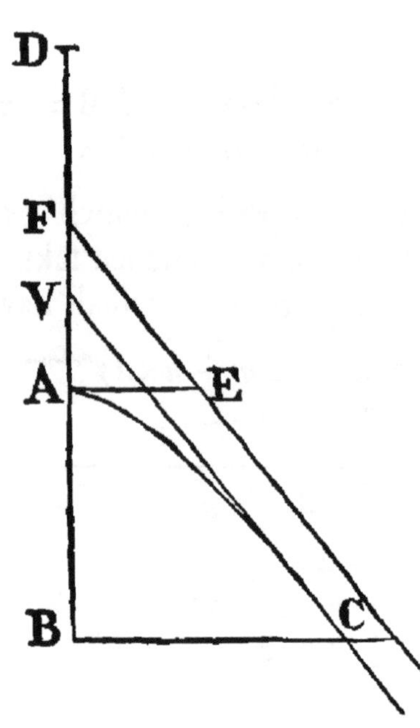

Now if we suppose the Abscisse AB to be infinitely produced, x will be infinitely great, and the Tangent VC will touch the Curve at an infinite Distance, and become the Asymptote FE, and in this Case $AV = \frac{nax}{ma + \overline{m+n}\,x}$ will be $= \frac{nax}{m+nx} = \frac{na}{m+n} = \frac{n}{m+n}\,a$, because ma vanishes Wherefore if, as in the common Hyperbola, where $m = 1$, and $n = 1$, $AF = \frac{1}{1+1}\,a = \frac{1}{2}\,a = \frac{1}{2}\,AD$, the Transverse Diameter; and this being the Centre of the opposite Hyperbolas, it follows, that the Asymptotes of the common opposite Hyperbolas intersect each other in one common Point the Centre.

And because the general Equation $\frac{ay^{m+n}}{b} = x^m \times \overline{a+x}^n$ (where b is put for the Parameter) when x becomes infinite and a vanishes, will be $\frac{ay^{m+n}}{b} = x^m \times x^n = x^{m+n}$, we shall have $ay^{m+n} = bx^{m+n}$, and consequently $y \times a^{\frac{1}{m+n}} = x \times b^{\frac{1}{m+n}}$; wherefore if the Asymptote be infinitely produced it it will be $\dot{x}$ $\dot{y}$. $a^{\frac{1}{m+n}}$ $b^{\frac{1}{m+n}}$. AF AE $\frac{n}{m+n}a$ $\frac{n}{m+n}$ $\dot{b}\, a\frac{m+n-1}{m+n}$, which determines the Position of the Asymptote, and because, in the common Hyperbola, $m = 1$, and $n = 1$, A E, equal to one half of the Conjugate Diameter, is a mean Proportional between the Parameter and the transverse Diameter A D.

If the Parameter be equal to the transverse Diameter, then is A E = A F = $\frac{1}{2}$ A D, and consequently the Angle A F E is a Semi right Angle, and therefore the Asymptotes stand at right Angles to each other, and the Curve, in this Case, is called an Equilateral Hyperbola.

EXAMPLE V.

Let it be required to draw a Tangent to the Point C of the Curve A C E, whose Abscisse A B is a Curve, from any Point of which Curve Line the Law of drawing Tangents is known.

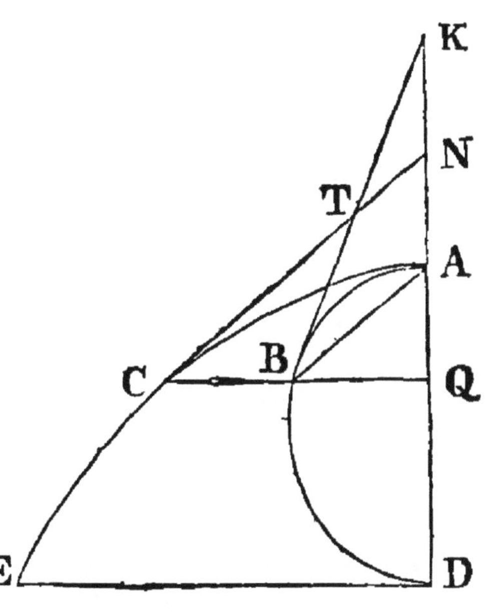

Put the Arch A B = x B C = y, then by *Proposition* I. $\dot{y}$ $\dot{x}$ y $\frac{y\dot{x}}{\dot{y}}$ = B T, for the Triangles C T B and C A B, in their evanescent Forms, will be similar.

Let us suppose the Curve A B D to be a Semicircle, then putting the Arch A B = x B C = y, the Arch of the Semicircle A B D = a, and D E = b, because from the Nature of

O the

the Curve $a\ b\ .\ x\ .\ y$, therefore $x = \frac{ay}{b}$, and $\dot{x} = \frac{a\dot{y}}{b}$,

whence $BT = \dot{x} \times \frac{y}{\dot{y}} = \frac{a\dot{y}}{b} \times \frac{y}{\dot{y}} = \frac{ay}{b} = x$.

If $a = b$, the Curve A C E will be the simple Cycloide.

If b be greater than a, it will be the protracted Cycloide.

If b be less than a, it will be the contracted Cycloide.

Therefore in the simple Cycloide, because $x = \frac{ay}{b} = y$, C B = A B = B T, whence the Point T, and consequently the Position of the Tangent C T, is determined.

But in the simple Cycloide, because C B = B T, the Angle B C T is equal to the Angle C T B, and the external Angle T B Q = 2 T C Q, but the Angle A B Q is equal to the Angle A B T, wherefore the Angle A B Q is equal to the Angle T C Q, and consequently C T is parallel to A B.

Whence to draw a Tangent to any Point C, in the common Cycloide, having drawn the Ordinate C B, join the Points B and A by the Chord Line B A, and draw the Line C T N parallel to A B, and the thing is done, and the Line C T N is the Tangent required to be drawn.

EXAMPLE VI.

Let there be a Curve Line I N, whose Diameter is I B, and A a given Point.

Let the Curve Line A M I be described, so that drawing any Diameter A B N, the Relation between A M, A B, A N, be expressed by any given Equation, 'tis required to draw the Tangent Line T M to touch the Curve in the Point M.

Having drawn K A H perpendicular to A N, meeting the Diameter I B in K, and the Tangent N H in H, on A as a Centre, with the Distances A N, A B, A M, describe the little Arches N Q, B o, M R, then A M R, A B o, and A N Q represent the nascent Triangles, putting therefore A R = s.

A H

AH $= t$, AB $= x$, AM $= y$, and AN $= z$; becauſe

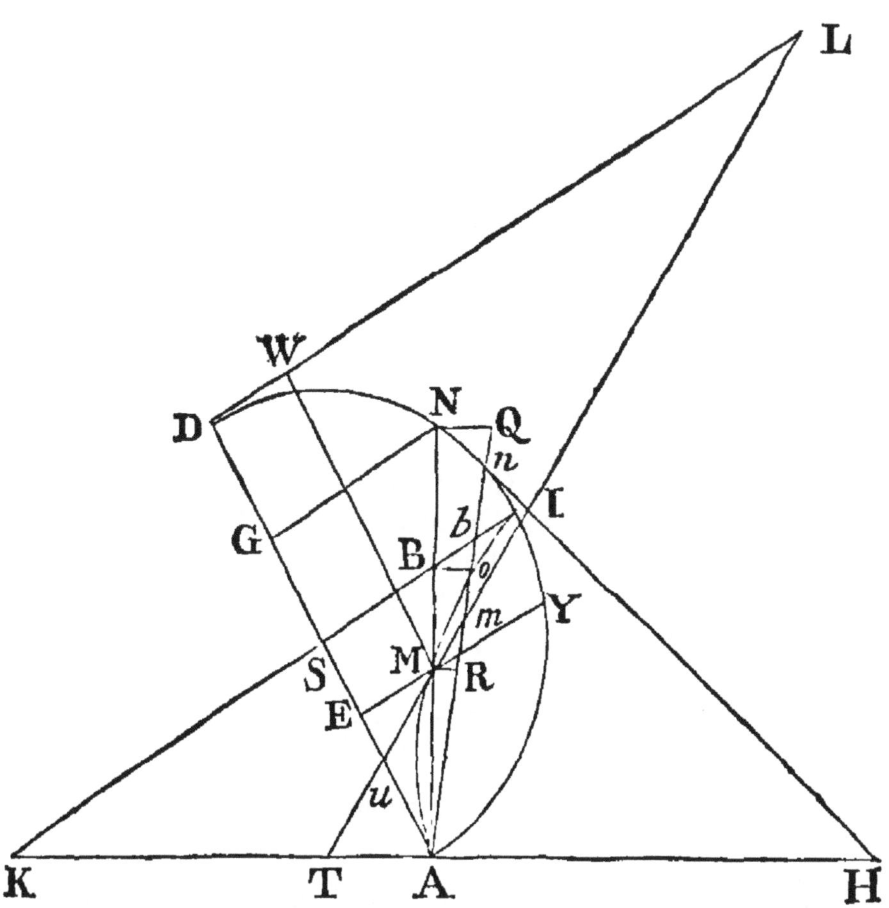

the Triangles BAK, $b\,o$B, alſo AMR, ABo, and ANQ are ſimilar, alſo HAN, NQn, MRm, and MAT, it will be as AB AK $b\,o$ oB, that is, $x \quad s \quad x \quad \frac{s x}{x}$, and as AB . AM · B$o$ · mR, that is, $x \quad y \cdot . \frac{s \dot{x}}{x} : \frac{s y \dot{x}}{x x}$, and as AB AN B$o$ NQ, that is, $x \quad z :. \frac{s x}{x} \quad \frac{s z x}{x x}$, and as

HA : AN :: NQ : Q*n*, that is, $t : z :: \frac{sz\dot{x}}{xx} : \frac{szz\dot{x}}{txx}$, and as MR : R*m* :: AM : AT, that is, $\dot{y} : \frac{sy\dot{x}}{xx} :: y : \frac{syy\dot{x}}{xx\dot{y}}$. Now having found the Values of y, m, x and z, and substituting for $\dot{z}$, its Value, $\frac{szz\dot{x}}{txx}$, all the Terms will then be affected with $\dot{x}$, whence the Value of AT, the Subtangent, will be expressed in known Terms.

If the Curve IN be a Circle passing through the Point A, situated so in regard to the Diameter IB, that AD is perpendicular to the Diameter, passing through S, the Centre of the Circle, and that BM = BN, the Curve AMI will be a Cyssoide, and its Equation $z + y = 2x$, whence $\dot{z} + \dot{y} = 2\dot{x}$, whence $\dot{y} = 2\dot{x} + \dot{z} = 2\dot{x} - \frac{szz\dot{x}}{txx} = \frac{2txx\dot{x} - szz\dot{x}}{txx}$ by substituting $\frac{szz\dot{x}}{txx}$ in the room of $\dot{z}$; therefore $\dot{y} = \frac{2txx\dot{x} - szz\dot{x}}{txx}$, but $\text{AT} = \frac{syy\dot{x}}{xx\dot{y}} = \frac{syy}{xx} \times \frac{\dot{x}}{\dot{y}}$; therefore $\text{AT} = \frac{styy}{2txx - szz}$; for $\frac{\dot{x}}{\dot{y}} = \frac{\dot{x}}{\frac{txx\dot{x} - szz\dot{x}}{txx}} = \frac{txx\dot{x}}{2txx\dot{x} - szz\dot{x}} = \frac{txx}{2txx - szz}$.

When the Point M falls in I, the Lines AN, AB, AM will become equal to each other, and to the Line AI; also the Line AK will become equal to AH, and consequently in this Case $\text{AI} = \frac{xxxx}{3xxx} = \frac{x}{3} = \frac{1}{3}x$, whence $\text{AT} = \frac{1}{3}\text{AI}$, whence the Tangent is easily had.

But the Tangent M T may be found after the following manner, for having drawn N G and M E perpendicular to A D, put A D $= 2a$. A E $=$ D G $= x$, and E M $= y$; then because the Triangles A E M and A G N are similar, it will be as $x \cdot y$ :: A G . G N, and as A G . G N :: G N $= \overline{2ax - xx}^{\frac{1}{2}} \cdot x$, wherefore $xx = y \times \overline{2ax - xx}^{\frac{1}{2}} = \overline{2axyy - xxyy}^{\frac{1}{2}}$, wherefore $x^4 = 2axyy - xxyy$, wherefore $x^3 = 2ayy - xyy$, and $yy = \frac{xxx}{2a - x}$, whence $2y\dot{y} = \frac{6axx\dot{x} - 3xxx\dot{x} + xxx\dot{x}}{\overline{2a - x}^2}$

$= \frac{6axx\dot{x} - 2xxx\dot{x}}{\overline{2a - x}^2}$, whence $\dot{y} = \frac{3axx\dot{x} - xxx\dot{x}}{\overline{2a - x}^2 \times y}$,

whence E $u = \frac{y\dot{x}}{\dot{y}} = \frac{\overline{2a - x}^2 \times yy}{3axx - xxx}$, whence E $u =$

$\frac{xxx \times \overline{2a - x}^2}{\overline{3axx - xxx} \times \overline{2a - x}} = \frac{xxx \times \overline{2a - x}}{3axx - xxx}$, putting $\frac{xxx}{2a - x}$ in the room of yy, whence E $u = \frac{2axxx - xxxx}{3axx - xxx} =$

$= \frac{2ax - xx}{3a - x}$

If D L be perpendicular to D A, and MW parallel to it, the Value of W L may be thus found

Put E Y $= z$, D E $= 2a - x$, and W L $= t$, then $t \cdot 2a - x$ :: $y \cdot x$, therefore $y = \frac{tx}{2a - x}$, but by the Property of the Curve $2ax - xx = zz$, therefore $2a\dot{x} - 2x\dot{x} = 2z\dot{z}$, wherefore $a\dot{x} - x\dot{x} = z\dot{z}$, and $\dot{z} = \frac{a\dot{x} - x\dot{x}}{z}$, and because in the Cyssoide D E, E Y, E A and E M are proportional;

onal; therefore $xx = yz$, and $2x\dot{x} = y\dot{z} + z\dot{y}$, therefore $z\dot{y} = 2x\dot{x} - y\dot{z}$, and $\dot{y} = \frac{2x\dot{x} - y\dot{z}}{z}$, and because $2ax - xx = zz$, and $yz = xx$, therefore $2ay - xy = xz$, but $\dot{y} = \frac{t\dot{x}}{2a - x} = \frac{2x\dot{x} - y\dot{z}}{z}$, therefore $tz\dot{x} = \overline{2a - x} \times \overline{2x\dot{x} - y\dot{z}} = 2zz\dot{x} - xx\dot{z}$, putting zz for $2ax - xx$, and zx for $2ay - yy$, therefore $\dot{z} = \frac{2z\dot{x} - t\dot{x}}{x} = \frac{a\dot{x} - x\dot{x}}{z} = \frac{2z - t}{x} = \frac{a - x}{z}$, wherefore $2zz - zt = ax - xx = zz - yz$, because $2ax - xx = \overline{2a - x} \times \overline{x} - xx$, therefore $2t = 3z + y$, wherefore $WL = t = \frac{1}{2}z + \frac{1}{2}y$, which is easily constructed, making $WL = \frac{1}{2}EY + \frac{1}{2}EM$.

EXAMPLE VII.

LET A B K be a Curve Line, whose Law of Tangents is known, and F a determinate Point. Suppose another Curve

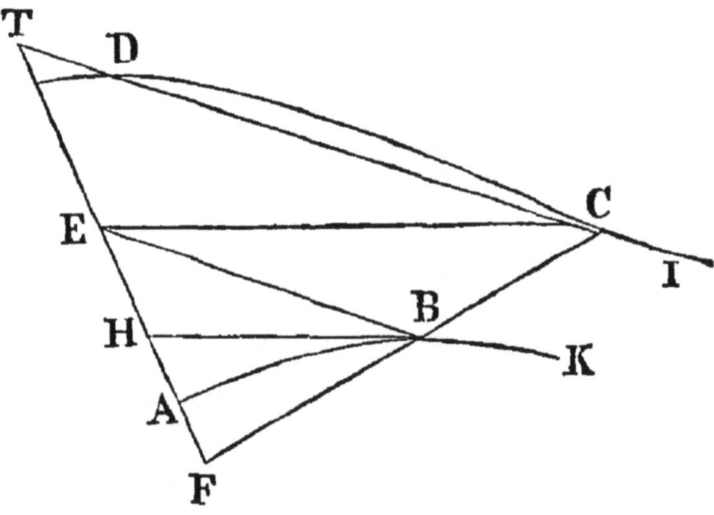

D C I, so that drawing any right Line F B C, the Ratio of F B to

to B C is always given, and let it be required to draw the Tangent T C.

HAVING drawn F H T perpendicular to F C, and put $FH = s$ $FB = x$, and $FC = y$, it will be as a s x $\frac{s\dot{x}}{x}$ and as x y $\frac{s\dot{x}}{x}$ $\frac{sy\dot{x}}{xx}$, and as y $\frac{sy\dot{x}}{xx}$ y $\frac{syy\dot{x}}{xxy} = TF$, whence the Tangent is had by the Help of the Equation given

SUPPOSE the Curve A B K becomes the Right Line H B, and the Equation, expressing the Nature of the Curve, *viz* of F B to F C, be $y - x = a$, that is, that B C be always equal to a right Line a, we shall have $\dot{y} - \dot{x} = 0$, and $\dot{y} = \dot{x}$, and consequently $FT = \frac{syy\dot{x}}{xxy} = \frac{syy}{xx}$, whence follows this Construction.

DRAW C E parallel to B H, and C T parallel to B E. I say C T is the Tangent required.

FOR F B FH F C F E, that is, x s y $\frac{sy}{x}$, and F B F E F C F T, that is, x $\frac{sy}{x}$ y $\frac{syy}{xx}$, whence it is evident, that the Curve D C I is the common Choncoid, whose Asymptote is B H, and Pole the Point F.

EXAMPLE VIII.

LET A R C be a Curve, the Method of drawing Tangents C H to it being known, and let the right Line D B A H V be a Diameter, without which let the Point F have a fixed Position, and from the same Point F let the indefinite Right Line F B E C be drawn cutting the Diameter in B, and Curve in C. Now if if you imagine the Line FBEC to revolve about the fixed

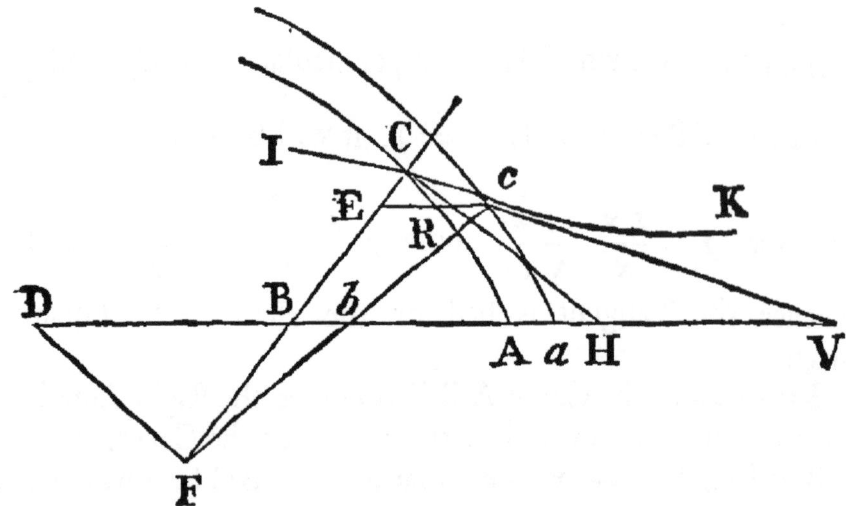

Point F, and at the same time the Plane BCA to move parallel to itself along the infinite immoveable Right Line DV, so that the Distance BA may be always the same, it is manifest that the continual Intersection C of the Curve Line AC, and the Right Line FC, by this Motion, will describe a Curve ICK, and let it be required to draw from the given Point C, in this Curve, a Right Line CV to touch the Curve in that Point.

IMAGINE the Plane BCA in a flowing State, and to move into the Place bca, and let the Line ERc be drawn parallel to BA, it is manifest, from the manner of Generation, that $Bb = Aa = Rc$, and consequently that $ER = Ec - Bb$, putting therefore $FB = x$. $FC = y$. $BH = s$. $CH = t$, because the Triangles FBb and FCc are similar, it will be as $Fb : Fc :: Bb : Ec$, that is, as $x : y :: (Bb =)\, \dot{z} : \frac{\dot{z}y}{x} = Ec$, whence $ER = Ec - Bb = \frac{y\dot{z}}{x} - \dot{z} = \frac{y\dot{z} - x\dot{z}}{x}$, and as $BH . HC :: ER . RC$; that is, as $s . t :: \frac{y\dot{z} - x\dot{z}}{x}$

ty

$\frac{ty\dot{z} - tx\dot{z}}{sx}$, and as R C : R c :: C H : H V, that is, as $\frac{ty\dot{z} - tx z}{sx} : \dot{z} :: t : \frac{sx}{y-x}$ = H V; whence, if F D be drawn parallel to C H, and H V be made equal to B D, the Line C V will be the Tangent required

If A C be a Right Line, the Curve I C K will be an Hyperbola, one of whose Asymptotes will be the right Line D V

If A C be a Circle, the Curve I C K will be the Chonoid of *Nicomedes*, the Line D V being its Asymptote, and the Point F its Pole

But if A C be a Parabola, the Curve I C K will be one of the Parabolick Kind, and at the same time would be described below the Right Line D V by the Intersection of F C with the other half of the Parabola

EXAMPLE IX.

Let A B O represent a given Curve, beginning at the Point A, and suppose the Method of drawing Tangents B V to it to be known.

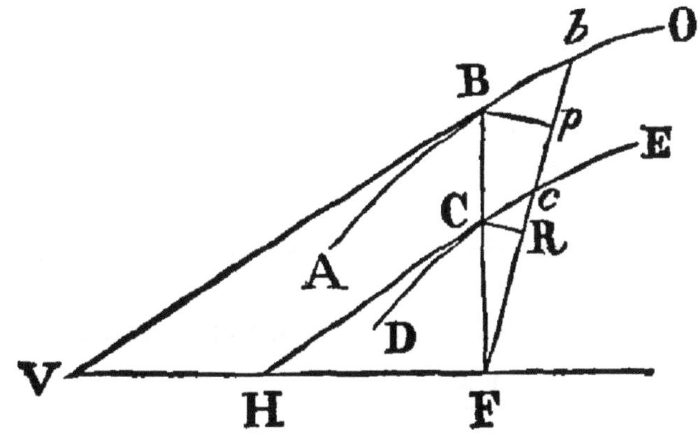

Let there be another Curve Line DCE, and an immoveable Point F, taken without the Curve, and having drawn any right Line as F C B, the Relation of F C to the Portion of the Curve A B being given, 'tis required to draw the Line C H to touch the Curve in the Point C.

P Let

LET FV be drawn perpendicular to FB, until it intersect the Tangent BV in V, and CH in H, and imagine the Line FB revolving about the fixed Point F to flow into the Place Fb, then will the Points B and C describe the nascent Increments Bp and CR in the same small Particle of Time, and the nascent Triangles Bbp and CcR will be similar to the Triangles FVB and FHC, put therefore BV $= t$, FV $= s$, FC $= y$, FB $= x$, and the Arch AB $= z$, and because as

BV : FV :: Bb : Bp, that is, as $t : s :: \dot{z} : \frac{s\dot{z}}{t} =$ Bp; and

because FB : FC :: Bp : CR; that is, as $x : y :: \frac{s\dot{z}}{t} : \frac{sy\dot{z}}{tx}$,

and because cR : CR :: FC : FH; that is, as $\dot{y} : \frac{sy\dot{z}}{tx} :: y :$

$\frac{syy\dot{z}}{tx\dot{y}} =$ FH; consequently FH may be found by substituting the Values of $\dot{z}$ and $\dot{y}$ deduced from the Equation expressing the Nature of the Curve in the general Equation $\frac{syy\dot{z}}{tx\dot{y}}$. For Example:

IF the Curve ABO be a Circle, and F its Centre, it is evident that the Tangent BV will become parallel and equal to the Subtangent FV, that is, t will become equal to s, since, in this Case, both FV and BV become Perpendiculars to FB, wherefore FH $= \frac{syy\dot{z}}{tx\dot{y}}$, will become $\frac{yy\dot{z}}{x\dot{y}}$, and putting a in the room of x, because FB becomes a constant Quantity, we shall have FH $= \frac{yy\dot{z}}{a\dot{y}}$.

NOW if we suppose the whole Circumference, or any determinate Portion of the Circle ABO to be equal to b, and if it be as $b : z :: a : y$, then the Curve Line DCE which now becomes FCE will

will be the Archimedian Spiral, and the Equation, expressing the Nature thereof, is $\frac{az}{b}=y$, whence $\frac{a\dot{z}}{b}=\dot{y}$; therefore F H = $\frac{yy\dot{z}}{a\dot{y}}$ is equal to $\frac{byy}{aa}=\frac{zy}{a}$, whence we have the following Construction.

JOIN the Points F and A, and on F as a Centre, with the Distance F C, describe the Arch Q C, and make F H = Q C, and draw the Line C H, which will touch the Spiral Line F C E in the Point C, for because the Sectors F B A and F C Q are similar, it will be as FB : F C :: A B : QC, that is, as $a : y :: z : \frac{zy}{a}$ = C Q. And universally,

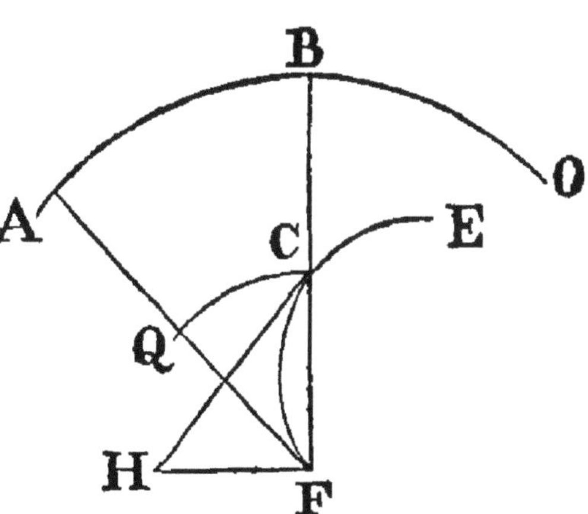

IF it be as $b^n : a^m :: z^n : y^m$, then $b^n y^m = a^m z^n$, and $m b^n y^{m-1}\dot{y} = n a^m z^{n-1}\dot{z}$, and dividing both Sides of the Equation by the Equation of the Curve, we shall have $my^{-1}\dot{y} = nz^{-1}\dot{z}$, that is, $mz\dot{y} = ny\dot{z}$, and $\dot{z} = \frac{mz\dot{y}}{ny}$, whence F H $= \frac{yy\dot{z}}{a\dot{y}} = \frac{myyz}{any} = \frac{myz}{na}$, whence by the Help of the Equation expressing the Nature of such Curve, z may be taken away, and the Subtangent express'd in straight Lines.

EXAMPLE X

LET D N and F Q represent two Curve Lines, D P and E I, their Axes cutting each other at right Angles in the Point A;

 and

and suppose the Method of drawing their Tangents N H, Q K

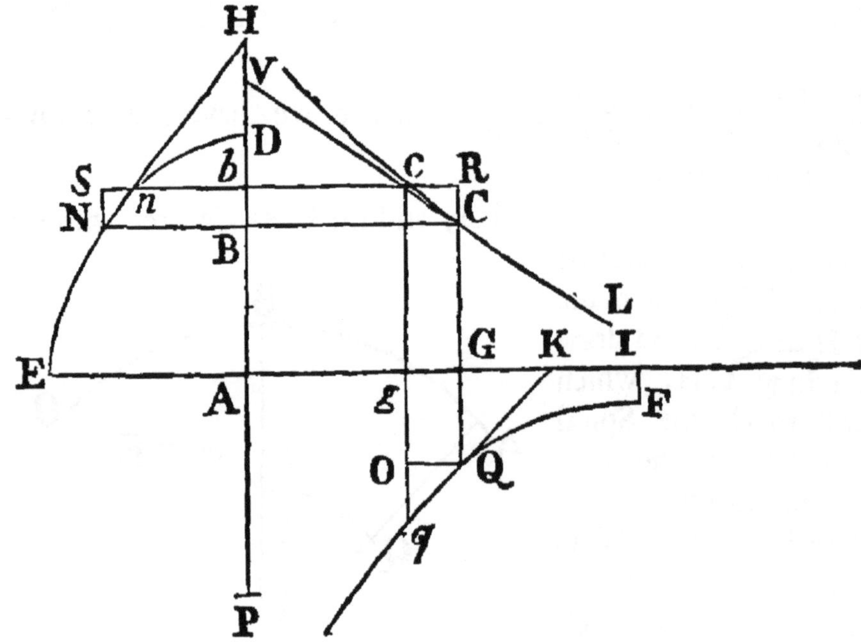

to be known; and supposing C L another Curve, such that the right Lines C G Q and C B N, drawn from any Point C taken in it parallel to their Axes P D and E I, the Relation of the Spaces I G Q F, and A B N E (the Point I being a fixed Point in E I, and I F being parallel to A P) be always the same, let it be required to draw from the Point C the right Line C V, a Tangent to the Curve C L in the Point C.

Put A B = G C = x, B C = A G = y, B N = v, G Q = z, the Space I G Q F = s, the Space A B N E = t, the Subtangent B H = a, G K = b, and imagine A B to flow into and become A b, then will the nascent Quantity B b = N S = C R be as $\dot{x}$, the nascent Quantity G g = R c = Q O, generated in the same small Particle of Time, be as $\dot{y}$, and S n = $-\dot{v}$ $= \frac{v\dot{x}}{a}$, for as $a : v :: \dot{x} :$ S n, because the nascent Triangle S N n is similar to the Triangle H B N, and because the Triangle

angle QGK is similar to the nascent Triangle $q\,o\,Q$, therefore as $b \, . \, z \;\; \dot{y} \;\; \frac{z\dot{y}}{b} = o\,q = \dot{x}$, and QG$g\,q$ will be as $\dot{s} = -z\dot{y}$, wherefore if in the fluxionary Equation arising from the Nature of the Curve you substitute $v\dot{x}$, $-z\dot{y}$, $\frac{-v\dot{x}}{a}$, $\frac{-z\dot{y}}{b}$ in the room of $\dot{t}$, $\dot{s}$, $\dot{v}$, $\dot{z}$, there will arise a new Equation, wherein the Relation of $\dot{y}$ to $\dot{x}$, or of C B to B V will be found.

Now if s be supposed equal to t, then $-z\dot{y} = v\dot{x}$, and $\frac{-z\dot{y}}{v}$ will be equal to $\dot{x}$, whence B V $= \frac{y\dot{x}}{\dot{y}}$ will be equal to $-\frac{zy}{v}$, wherefore because the Value of BV is negative, the Point V will fall on the contrary Side of B in respect of A, the beginning of A B or x, and if we suppose the Curve Line FQ to be an Hyperbola, AP and AI its Asymptotes, and that GQ $= z = \frac{cc}{y}$, and that the Curve DNE becomes a straight Line parallel to AD, so that B N $= v$ be always equal to a constant Quantity c, the Parameter of the Hyperbola, then it is manifest that AD will become an Asymptote to the Curve CL, and the Subtangent BV $= -\frac{zy}{v}$ will be $-\frac{cc}{v} = -c$ (by substituting z in the room of $\frac{cc}{y}$), that is, the Subtangent of the Curve CL will be a constant Quantity, and therefore the Curve, in this Case will be the Logarithmetick Line.

EXAMPLE XI.

Let BN, FQ represent two Curve Lines, whose common Axis is the right Line AB, in which take two Points A and E, and let LC be another Curve such, that drawing a right Line AN from

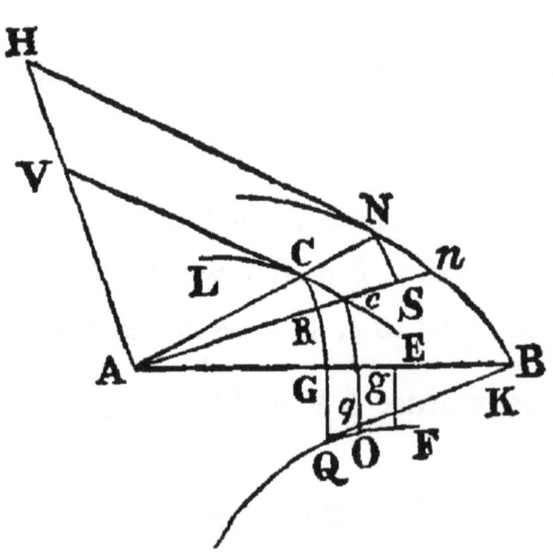

from any Point C taken in it, describing the Circular Arch CG from the Centre A, and drawing the Line GQ parallel to EF, and perpendicular to AB, the Relation of the Spaces EGQF, ANB, and the right Lines AC or AG, AN and GQ, be expressed by any given Equation. Let it be required to draw from the Point C the right Line CV, a Tangent to the Curve LC in the Point C.

Put $AC = AG = y$, $AN = z$, $QG = v$, the Space $EGQF = s$, the Space $NAB = t$, and having drawn the Line AVH perpendicular to ACN, let the Line ACN be imagined to flow into the Place Acn, then will the Points C and N describe the nascent Arches CR, NS, and conceive the Perpendicular cg to be drawn. Now supposing $AH = a$, $GK = b$, then will $Rc = Gg$ be as $\dot{y}$, Sn as $\dot{z}$; and because the nascent Triangle NSn is similar to the Triangle HAN, also the nascent Triangle QOq similar to the Triangle KGQ, therefore it will be as $z : a :: z : \frac{a\dot{z}}{z} = SN$, and as $b : v :: \dot{y} : \frac{v\dot{y}}{b} = Oq = -v$; and because $GQqg = -s = vy$, and ANn or $AN \times \frac{1}{2} NS = \dot{t} = \frac{1}{2} a\dot{z}$, if these several Values be substituted in the fluxionary Equation arising from the Equation expressing the Nature of the Curve, we shall have a new Equation, by which the Values of $\dot{z}$ in $\dot{y}$ will be easily found. Again, because the Triangles ANS and ACR, CRc and CAV are similar, it will be as $AN : AC :: NS : CR$; that is, as $z : y :: \frac{a\dot{z}}{z}$.

$\frac{ay\dot{z}}{zz} = CR$; and as cR CR $\cdot$ AC AV, that is, as $y\ \frac{ay\dot{z}}{zz} \cdot y \cdot \frac{ayy\dot{z}}{zz\dot{y}} = AV$, if instead of $\dot{z}$ you substitute its Value in $\dot{y}$, the Fluxions will vanish, and the Value of the Subtangent AV will be expressed in known Terms. For Example

IF $vy - s = zz - t$, then $v\dot{y} - y\dot{v} - \dot{s} = 2z\dot{z} - \dot{t}$, whence, by Substitution, we shall have $\dot{z} = \frac{4bv\dot{y} - 2vy\dot{y}}{4bz + ab}$, and substituting this Value in $\frac{ayy\dot{z}}{zz\dot{y}}$ in the room of $\dot{z}$, there will arise $\frac{4abvyy - 2avy^3}{4bz^3 + abzz}$ for the Value of AV.

AGAIN, if $s = 2t$, then $\dot{s} = 2\dot{t}$, that is, $-v\dot{y} = -a\dot{z}$, and $\dot{z} = \frac{v\dot{y}}{a}$, therefore $AV = \frac{ayy\dot{z}}{zz\dot{y}} = \frac{vyy}{zz}$.

IF the Line BN be a Circle, the Point A being the Centre, and the Radius be $AB = AN = c$, and if FQ be an Hyperbola, such that $GQ = v = \frac{ff}{y}$, then it is manifest, that the Curve LC makes an infinite Number of Revolutions about the Point A, before it arrives at the same, because the Spiral Space FEGQ becomes infinite when the Point G falls in A, and $AV = \frac{ffy}{cc}$; whence it follows, that the Ratio of AC to AV is a constant Quantity, and so the Curve LC is the Logarithmetical Spiral.

EXAMPLE XII.

LET it be required to draw Tangents to all Sorts of single Geometrical or Algebraic Curves.

ASSUME

ASSUME the general Equation $bx^m + cy^n + dx^p y^q + h = 0$, where x represents the Abſciſſe or intercepted Part of the Diameter, and y the Ordinate of the ſame Curve.

THEN $mbx^{m-1}\dot{x} + ncy^{n-1}\dot{y} + pdx^{p-1}\dot{x}y^q + qdx^p y^{q-1}\dot{y} = 0$, and $mbx^{m-1}\dot{x} + pdy^q x^{p-1}\dot{x} = -ncy^{n-1}\dot{y} - qdx^p y^{q-1}\dot{y}$, and $\dot{x} = \frac{-ncy^{n-1}\dot{y} - qdx^p y^{q-1}\dot{y}}{mbx^{m-1} + pdy^q x^{p-1}}$,

whence $t = \frac{y}{\dot{y}} \times \dot{x} = \frac{y}{\dot{y}} \times \frac{-ncy^{n-1}\dot{y} - qdx^p y^{q-1}\dot{y}}{mbx^{m-1} + pdy^q x^{p-1}}$,

and $t = \frac{-ncy^n - qdx^p y^q}{mbx^{m-1} + pdy^q x^{p-1}}$, the general Theorem expreſſing the Value of the Subtangent in all Curves, whoſe Terms may be found in the general Equation aſſumed. For Example

SUPPOSE it were required to find the Value of the Subtangent (by the former general Theorem) of the common Parabola, whoſe Equation is $ax = yy$, or $ax - yy = 0$.

Now becauſe $ax - yy = bx^m + cy^n$, therefore $b = a$ $m = 1$ $c = -1$. $n = 2$. $d = 0$. $p = 0$ $q = 0$. $h = 0$, and conſequently $t = \frac{2yy}{a} = \frac{2ax}{a}$ (becauſe $yy = ax$) equal to $2x$, inaſmuch as the Terms in the general Equation that are affected with the Quantities d, p, q and h vaniſh.

AGAIN, in the common Hyperbola (*See Page* 101.) where Cc repreſents the Curve, AD, AV the Aſymptotes, and VB the Subtangent required

LET the Equation expreſſing the Nature of the Curve $aa - xy$, be put equal to $bx^m + cy^n + dx^p y^q + h$, then $b = 0$. $m = 0$. $c = 0$. $n = 0$. $d = -1$. $p = 1$. $q = 1$, and conſequently $VB = \frac{-ncy^n - qdx^p y^q}{mbx^{m-1} + pdy^q x^{p-1}}$ will be equal $\frac{-1 \times -1 \times x^1 y^1}{+1 \times -1 \times y^1 \times x^{1-1}}$

$= \frac{+1 \times xy}{-1 \times yx^0} = \frac{xy}{-y} = -x$. After the ſame manner may the Value of any Subtangent be found by the former Theorem.

SECT

SECT. II.

Of the Use of FLUXIONS *in the Solution of Problems,* de Maximis & Minimis.

THE Method *de Maximis & Minimis,* is that Method whereby we arrive at the Knowledge of the greatest or least possible Quantity attainable in any Case.

THUS in Figure the First, if the Ordinate B C, flowing according to the Direction A F, continually increases 'till it arrive at a certain Place D E, after which it begins to diminish, the Ordinate D E in this Case is called the greatest Ordinate, or a *Maximum.*

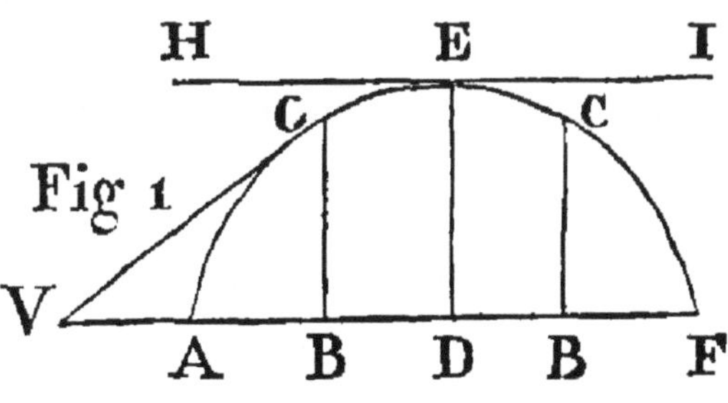

ON the Contrary, if, as in Figure 2, the Ordinate B C flowing according to the Direction A F, continually decreases 'till it come into the Place D E, and after that it begins to increase, the Ordinate D E in this Case is called the least Ordinate, or a *Minimum.*

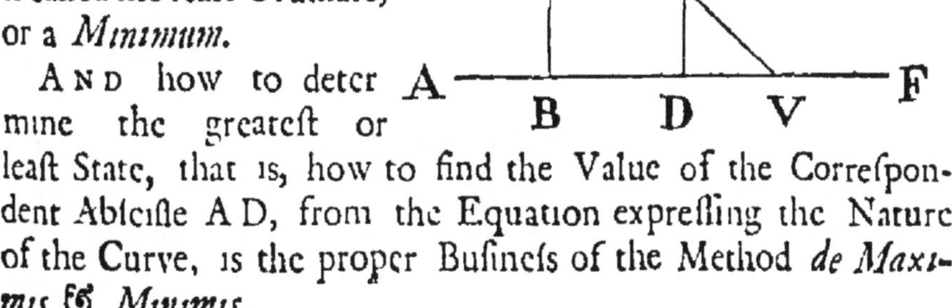

AND how to determine the greatest or least State, that is, how to find the Value of the Correspondent Abscisse A D, from the Equation expressing the Nature of the Curve, is the proper Business of the Method *de Maximis & Minimis.*

And to this End it has been demonstrated in the preceding Section, to which I refer the Reader, that the Fluxion of the Ordinate BC, is to the Fluxion of the Absciffe AB, as the Ordinate BC is to the Subtangent VB. Let us now suppose the Ordinate BC (*See Figure the First*) in a flowing State, moving according to the Direction AF, it is manifest that the nearer the Ordinate BC approaches the Ordinate DE, the greater will be the Subtangent BV, 'till when the Ordinate BC arrives at, or is coincident with the Ordinate DE, the Tangent HEI to the Point E, will be parallel to the Axis AF Consequently, the Subtangent BV will become infinite, in respect to the Ordinate DE, and the Fluxion of the Ordinate itself will vanish, or become equal to nothing

Whence to find the Value of the correspondent Absciffe, in this Case, let the Fluxionary Value of the Ordinate deduced from the Equation, expressing the Nature of the Curve, be put equal to o, or Nothing, by which means all those Members of the Equation in which it is found will vanish, and those that remain will determine the Place of the *Maximum.*

For Example, in Figure the First, where $AB = x$, $BC = y$, $AF = 2a$ Let us suppose the Equation of the Curve to be $2ax - xx = yy$, and let it be required to find the greatest Ordinate, or, which is the same Thing, the Length of its Correspondent Absciffe AB. Now because $2a\dot{x} - 2x\dot{x} = 2y\dot{y}$, whence $a\dot{x} - x\dot{x} = y\dot{y}$, we shall have $\dot{y} = \dfrac{a\dot{x} - x\dot{x}}{y}$ which being put equal to Nothing, we shall have $\dfrac{a\dot{x} - x\dot{x}}{y} = 0$, whence $a\dot{x} - x\dot{x} = 0$, and $a - x = 0$, consequently $a = x$; that is, AD will be equal to half AF

Again, Let us now suppose the Ordinate BC in the following Figure to move according to the Direction AD, it is likewise manifest that the nearer the Point B approaches to the Point D, that the lesser will be the Subtangent BV; 'till at last when the Point B arrives at, or is coincident with the Point

Point D, the Subtangent B V will vanish, and the Fluxion of the Ordinate will become infinite.

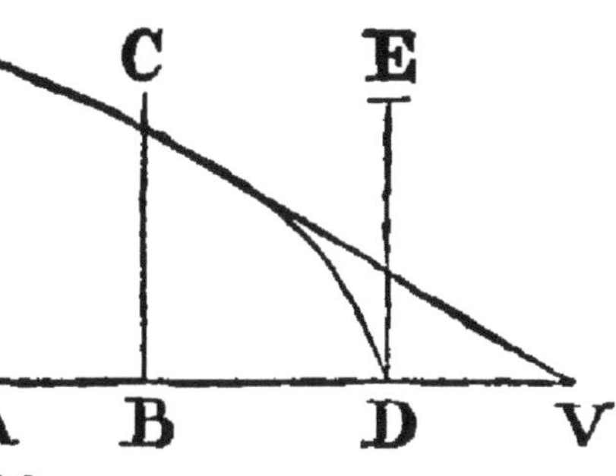

WHENCE to find the Value of the Abscisse in this Case, let the Fluxionary Value of the Ordinate be made equal to Infinite, then will the infinitely small Terms vanish, and the Remainder will determine the *Minimum.*

FOR Example; let us suppose $y - a = x^{\frac{2}{3}} \times \overline{a-x}^{\frac{1}{3}}$ to be the Equation of the Curve (having first supposed A B $= x$, and BC $= y$) then will $\dot{y} = - \frac{2\dot{x} \times \overline{a}^{\frac{1}{3}}}{3\overline{a-x}^{\frac{2}{3}}}$, which being put equal to an infinite Quantity, we shall have $3\,\overline{a-x}^{\frac{2}{3}} = 0$ (for the Numerator $- 2\dot{x} \times \overline{a}^{\frac{1}{3}}$ in this Case vanishes) whence $a - x = 0$, and $a = x$, that is, A B $= x$ becomes equal to A D, whence AD is the correspondent Abscisse.

AND hence we are taught a direct Method to determine the *Maximum* or *Minimum* in any Case whatsoever. Let it therefore be required in

EXAMPLE I

To find a Number, from which Number, if you take its Square, there shall remain the greatest Difference.

PUT x for the Number sought, then will $x - xx$ be the greatest Difference, or a *Maximum*; whence $\dot{x} - 2x\dot{x} = 0$, and $2x\dot{x} = \dot{x}$, consequently $2x = 1$, and $x = \frac{1}{2}$

Now if instead of $x - xx$ we put $x - x^{n+m}$, which is a general Equation for all Questions of this kind whatsoever, we shall have $x^n - x^{n+m} =$ a *Maximum*, whence $nx^{n-1}\dot{x} - \overline{n+m}\,x^{n+m-1}\dot{x} = 0$, consequently, $\overline{n+m}\,x^{n+m-1}\dot{x} =$

Qq 2 $n\dot{x}$

$n x^{n-1}\dot{x}$, and $\overline{n+m}\,x^m = n$, and $x^m = \frac{n}{n+m}$ whence $x = \overline{\frac{n}{n+m}}\Big|^{\frac{1}{m}}$

If $n = 1$, and $m = 1$, then the Question will be $x - xx$, whence $x = \frac{1}{1+1} = \frac{1}{2}$, as in the preceding Example.

If $n = 2$ and $m = 1$, then the Question will be thus expressed, $xx - xxx = Maximum$, and $x = \frac{2}{1+2} = \frac{2}{3}$.

If $n = 2$ and $m = 2$, then the Question will stand thus, $xx - xxxx$ = greatest Difference, and $x = \overline{\frac{2}{2+2}}\Big|^{\frac{1}{2}} = \overline{\frac{1}{2}}\Big|^{\frac{1}{2}}$ or $x = \sqrt{\frac{1}{2}}$, &c.

EXAMPLE II

To divide the Right Line AP in the Point D, so that the Product of the Square of one of its Parts AD, multiplied into the other Part DP, may be the greatest of all the Products made of the Square of any one part of the Line AP multiplied into the other Part.

Let a represent the whole Line AP, x the Part AD, then will $a - x$ be the other Part, then must $\overline{a-x} \times xx = axx - xxx$ be the greatest Rectangle that can be made of the Square of one of the Parts of the given Line multiplied into the other.

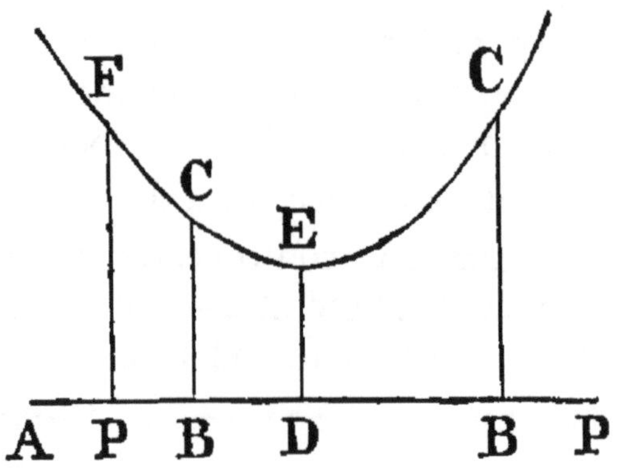

Let FCEC represent a Curve, whose Ordinate BC put equal to y, and the intercepted Part of the Diameter $AB = x$, and let

let the Relation of the Ordinate to the intercepted Diameter be expreſſed by this Equation $yaa = axx - xxx$, then will $y = \frac{axx - xxx}{aa}$, and $\dot{y} = \frac{2ax\dot{x} - 3xx\dot{x}}{aa} = 0$, whence $2ax\dot{x} - 3xx\dot{x} = 0$, and $2axx = 3xxx$, and $x = \frac{2a}{3}$ $= \frac{2}{3}a$

And univerſally, if we ſuppoſe $x^m \times \overline{a-x}$ which is a general Equation for all Problems of this kind, then $mx^{m-1}\dot{x} \times \overline{a-x}^n - nx^m \times \overline{a-x}^{n-1}\dot{x} = 0$; and dividing by $\overline{a-x}^{n-1}$ we ſhall have $mx^{m-1}\dot{x} \times \overline{a-x} - nx^m\dot{x} = 0$, and by dividing again by $x^{m-1}\dot{x}$, we ſhall have $ma - mx - nx = 0$, whence $mx + nx = ma$, and $x = \frac{ma}{m+n}$ equal to AD

If $m = 2$, and $n = 1$, then $\frac{m}{m+n}a$ will be equal to $\frac{2}{2+1}a = \frac{2}{3}a$, the ſame as in the preceding Example.

If $m = 2$, and $n = -1$, then $\frac{m}{m+n}a$ will become $\frac{2}{2-1}a = 2a$, and the Problem may be thus expreſſed, having produced AP to D, ſo that the Quantity $\frac{AD^2}{PD}$ may be the leaſt, that is poſſible, then the Equation of the Curve will be $\frac{xx}{a-x} = y$ wherein if we ſuppoſe $x = a$, then the Ordinate BC, which becomes equal to PF, will be equal to $\frac{aa}{0}$ or to Infinity, and ſuppoſing x infinite, we ſhall have $y = x$, that is, the Ordinate will be infinite alſo.

EXAM-

EXAMPLE III.

LET ACFDA represent a Semicircle, and let it be required to find the greatest Ordinate E F

PUT BC $= y$ AB $= x$ AD $= 2a$, then will BD $= 2a - x$, and because from the Nature of the Circle $2ax - xx = yy$, therefore $2a\dot{x} - 2x\dot{x} = 2y\dot{y}$, whence $a\dot{x} - x\dot{x} = y\dot{y}$, and $\dot{y} = \frac{a\dot{x} - x\dot{x}}{y} = 0$, wherefore $x\dot{x} = a\dot{x}$, and $x = a =$ A E, that is, when A B by flowing becomes equal to A E, B C will become equal to E F; so that E F is the greatest Ordinate

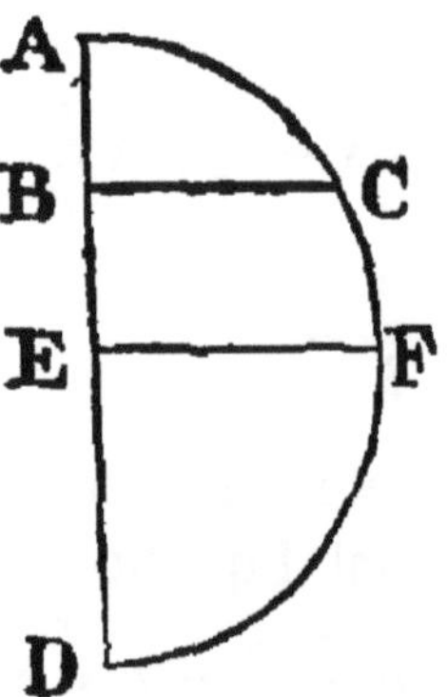

EXAMPLE IV.

LET ACFD represent a Semi-Ellipsis, and let it be required to find the greatest Ordinate, suppose E F

PUT EF $= b$. BC $= y$. AD $= 2a$ AB $= x$, then will BD $= 2a - x$, and because from the Nature of the Ellipsis

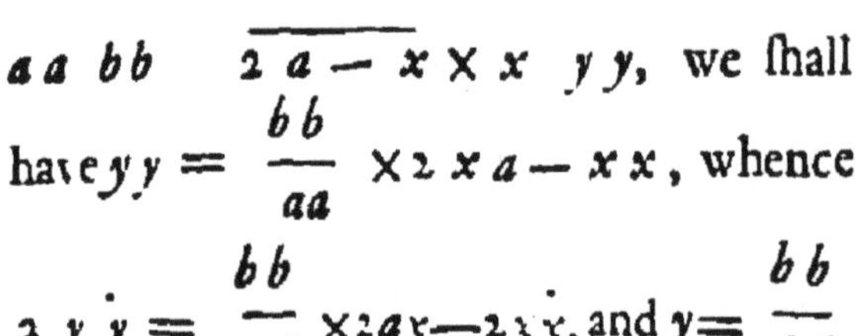

$aa \;\; bb \;\; \overline{2a - x} \times x \;\; yy$, we shall have $yy = \frac{bb}{aa} \times 2xa - xx$, whence $2y\dot{y} = \frac{bb}{aa} \times 2a\dot{x} - 2x\dot{x}$, and $\dot{y} = \frac{bb}{aa}$

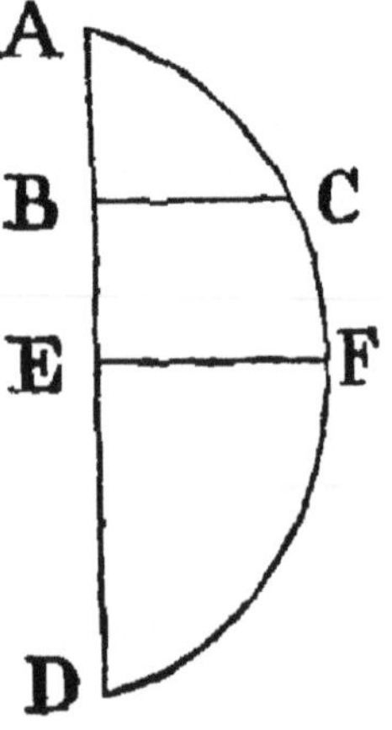

$\times \frac{2a\dot{x} - 2x\dot{x}}{2y} = 0$, and $a\dot{x} = x\dot{x}$, whence $x = a =$ EF, the Semi Conjugate Diameter will be the greatest Ordinate that can be applied to the same tranverse Diameter A D.

EXAM-

EXAMPLE V

LET ACEF be a contracted Semi Cycloid, whose Base FI is less than AOI the Semi-Circumference of the generating Circle, and whose Center is Q. Let it be required to find the Point D in the Diameter AI, so that DE shall be the greatest Ordinate that can be applied to the Axis AI.

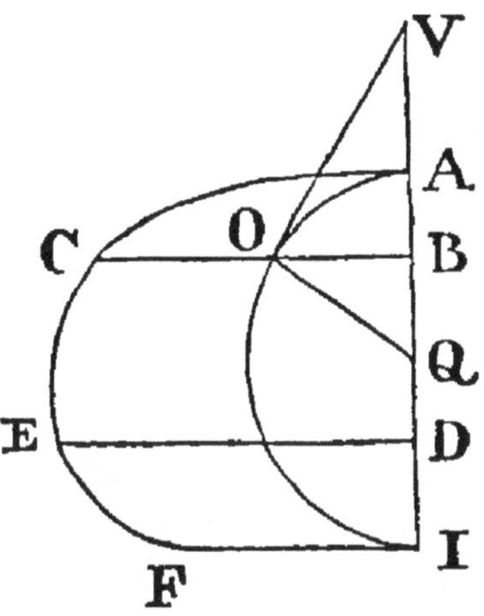

HAVING drawn the Ordinate BC intersecting the generating Circle in O, put AB $= x$, BO $= y$, the Arch AO $= z$, the Semi diameter AQ $= a$, the Semi circumference AOI $= c$, and the Base FI $= b$, and because from the Nature of the Cycloid AOI : IF :: AO : OC, that is, as $c : b :: z : \frac{bz}{c} =$ OC, whence $y + \frac{bz}{c} =$ BC, and $\dot{y} + \frac{b\dot{z}}{c}$ will be the Fluxion of the Ordinate BC.

AGAIN, because the Triangles QBO and OBV are similar, it will be as QO : QB :: VO : OB, but (by the 1st Proposition, of Sect. the 1st, of Part the 3d) as VO : OB :: $\dot{z} : \dot{y}$ therefore (OQ$=$) a : (QB$=$) $a - x :: \dot{z} : \dot{y}$, whence $\dot{y} = \frac{a\dot{z} - x\dot{z}}{a}$ and substituting this Value of $\dot{y}$ in the room of $\dot{y}$ in the former Value of the Ordinate BC, *viz.* $\dot{y} + \frac{b\dot{z}}{c}$ we shall have $\frac{a\dot{z} - x\dot{z}}{a} + \frac{b\dot{z}}{c} = \frac{ca\dot{z} - cx\dot{z} + ab\dot{z}}{ac}$, for the Fluxion of the Ordinate BC, but when the Point B flows in to the

Place

Place of D, then BC will become equal to DE the greateſt Ordinate Whence $\frac{ca\dot{z}-cx\dot{z}+ab\dot{z}}{ac}=0$. Conſequently, $ca-cx+ab=0$; and $cx=ca+ab$, whence $x=\frac{ca+ab}{c}=a+\frac{ab}{c}$ will be the Value of the Abſciſſe AD, whoſe Correſpondent and Ordinate DE will be the greateſt that can be applied to the Axis AI.

AGAIN, becauſe AD—AQ=QD, therefore $QD=a+\frac{ab}{c}-a=\frac{ab}{c}$, whence $QD\times c=ab$, conſequently it will be as $c \quad a \quad b$ QD, wherefore if QD be taken a fourth Proportional to the Circumference AOI, the Baſe FI, and the Radius OQ, then D will be the Point in the Axis, whoſe Ordinate Applicate will be the greateſt.

EXAMPLE VI.

LET ACE repreſent a Parabola, and P a given Point in the Axis AP, and let it be required to find the Point E in the Curve Line ACE, ſo that a right Line, as PE, drawn from the Point P to the Point E, may be the ſhorteſt Line that can be drawn from the ſame Point to the Curve Line ACE

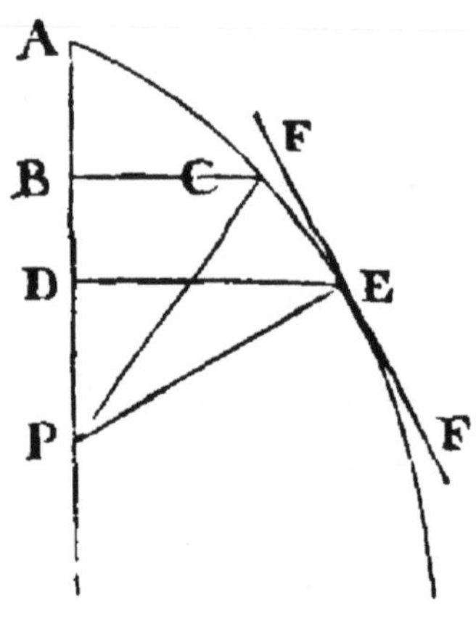

PUT $AB=x$. $BC=y$ $PC=z$. $AP=d$, then $BP=d-x$ and becauſe the Triangle BPC is Right angled at B, we ſhall have $PC^2=BC^2+PB^2$, that is, $zz=yy+dd-2dx+xx$, whence $2z\dot{z}=2y\dot{y}-2d\dot{x}+2x\dot{x}$, and $z\dot{z}=y\dot{y}-d\dot{x}+x\dot{x}$ and

and $z = \frac{yy - dx + xx}{z}$, but when AB by flowing becomes equal to AD, then the Points C and E will coincide, and PC will become equal to PE, and $\dot{z} = \frac{yy - d\dot{x} + x\dot{x}}{z} = 0$, whence

$yy - d\dot{x} + x\dot{x} = 0$, which is a general Equation for all Problems or Questions of this kind, wherein if we substitute in the room of $y\dot{y}$, its Value arising from the Nature of the Curve, we shall have an Expression whereby the Value of the Abscisse AD will be found.

Now because from the Nature of the Parabola $ax = yy$, therefore $a\dot{x} = 2y\dot{y}$ and $\frac{1}{2}a\dot{x} = y\dot{y}$ substituting therefore $\frac{1}{2}a\dot{x}$ in the room of $y\dot{y}$, in the former Equation, $y\dot{y} - d\dot{x} + x\dot{x}$, we shall have $\frac{1}{2}a\dot{x} - d\dot{x} + x\dot{x} = 0$, and $a\dot{x} - 2d\dot{x} + 2x\dot{x} = 0$ Whence $a - 2d + 2x = 0$, and $2x = 2d - a$ Consequently $x = d - \frac{1}{2}a$, will be the Value of the Abscisse AD But AP—AD = PD Whence PD $= d - d + \frac{1}{2}a = \frac{1}{2}a$ the Parameter, whence it follows,

That if from the given Point P you set off half the Parameter to D, and draw the correspondent Ordinate DE, the Line PE drawn from the given Point P, to the Point found E, will be the shortest Line that can be drawn from the same Point P, to the given Curve ACE.

Hence we are taught how to draw a Tangent to any Point E in the Parabola For since PE is the shortest Line that can be drawn from the Point P to the Curve Line ACE, it must be perpendicular to the Tangent to the Curve in the Point E, and consequently becomes the Subnormal, wherefore if half the Parameter be set off from D, the Place where the Ordinate drawn from the Point E cuts the Axis, and a Line, as PE be drawn, if another Line, as FE be drawn at Right Angles, to it, it will be a Tangent to the Curve in the Point E

Again, if PA be equal to $\frac{1}{2}a$, or the Parameter, then a Circle described on the Center P, with the Radius PA, will touch the Parabola in the Vertex A, and be altogether within the Parabola, for in this Case the Points E and A will coincide, and P E, which now becomes P A, will be the shortest Line that can be drawn from the given Point P to the Curve ACE.

EXAMPLE VII.

LET ACEF be an Ellipsis, and let it be required to find the Point E in the Curve Line ACEF, so that a Right Line PE drawn from a given Point P in the transverse Axis AF, may be the shortest of all Lines that can be drawn from the same Point P to the Curve Line ACEF.

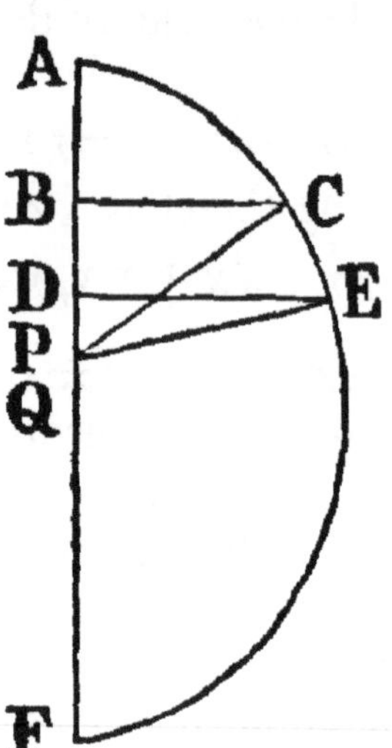

PUT $AB = x$. $BC = y$, the transverse Axis $AF = 2a$, and the Parameter equal to b, then because from the Nature of the Ellipses $2ayy = 2abx - bxx$, we shall have $4ayy = 2abx - 2bxx$ and $2ayy = abx - bxx$, whence $yy = \frac{abx - bxx}{2a}$, and substituting this in the room of $y\dot{y}$ in the general Equation, $y\dot{y} - d\dot{x} + x\dot{x} = 0$, there will arise $\frac{ab\dot{x} - bx\dot{x}}{2a} - d\dot{x} + x\dot{x} = \frac{ab\dot{x} - bx\dot{x} - 2ad\dot{x} + 2ax\dot{x}}{2a} = 0$ Whence $ab - bx - 2ad + 2ax = 0$, and $2ax - bx = 2ad - ab$, and $x = \frac{2ad - ab}{2a - b}$, and, consequently, $PD = d - x = \frac{ab - db}{2a - b}$.

IF we imagine ACEF to be a Semi-circle, and Q to be its Center, then because $2ax - xx = yy$ from the Nature of the Curve

Curve we shall have $2a\dot{x} - 2x\dot{x} = 2y\dot{y}$, and $y\dot{y} = a\dot{x} - x\dot{x}$ substituting this last Quantity in the general Equation $y\dot{y} - d\dot{x} + x\dot{x} = 0$ in the room of $y\dot{y}$, there will arise $a\dot{x} - x\dot{x} - d\dot{x} + x\dot{x} = 0$, whence $a\dot{x} = d\dot{x}$, and $a = d$, and, consequently, AD will become equal to AQ, the Semi-diameter, the Point P will fall in the Center, and E in any Part of the Circumference.

EXAMPLE VIII.

LET ACE be an Hyperbola, and let it be required to find the Point E in the Curve Line ACE, so that a right Line PE, drawn from a given Point P in the Axis AP, may be the shortest of all Lines that can be drawn from the same Point P to the Curve

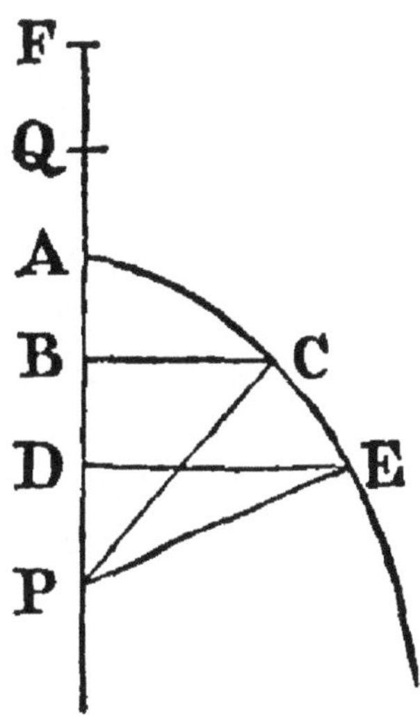

PUT $AB = x$. $BC = y$, the transverse Axis $AF = 2a$, and the Parameter $= b$, and because from the Nature of the Curve $2ayy = 2abx + bxx$, we shall have $4ay\dot{y} = 2ab\dot{x} + 2bx\dot{x}$, and $2ay\dot{y} = ab\dot{x} + bx\dot{x}$, whence $y\dot{y} = \frac{ab\dot{x} + bx\dot{x}}{2a}$, and substituting this last Quantity in the general Equation, $y\dot{y} + x\dot{x} - d\dot{x} = 0$, in the room of $y\dot{y}$, we shall have $\frac{ab\dot{x} + bx\dot{x}}{2a} + x\dot{x} - d\dot{x} = 0$ Whence $\frac{ab\dot{x} + bx\dot{x} + 2ax\dot{x} - 2ad\dot{x}}{2a} = 0$,

$=0$, and $ab+bx+2ax-2ad=0$, by dividing by x, and multiplying by $2a$, consequently $2ax+bx=2ad-ab$, and $x=\frac{2ad-ab}{2a+b}$, whence $DP=d-x=\frac{ab+db}{2a+b}$.

Now because $PD=\frac{ab+db}{2a+b}=\frac{a+d}{2a+b}\times b$, by reducing the Equation to a Proportion, we shall have $2a+b$: b :: $a+d$: PD, and by Division it will be $2a$: b :: $a+d-$PD : PD, wherefore (if Q be the Center of the Hyperbola, because $a+d=$QP) it will be as $2a$: b :: (QP$-$PD$=$) QD : PD, that is, as the transverse Diameter AF is to the Parameter, so is QD to DP, whence PD may be had by Construction.

Again (by the preceding Example) because in the Ellipsis DP is equal to $\frac{ab-db}{2a-b}=\frac{a-d}{2a-b}\times b$, reducing the Equation to an Analogy; it will be as $2a-b$: b :: $a-d$: DP, wherefore by Composition $2a$: b :: $a-d+$DP : DP (now if Q be the Center of the Ellipsis, then $a-d=$QP) whence $2a$: b :: (QP$+$DP$=$) QD : DP, that is, as the transverse Diameter to the Parameter, so is QD to DP, whence DP may be had by Construction.

Now if we suppose AP$=d$ equal to half the Parameter, then PD in the Hyperbola equal to $\frac{ab+db}{2a+b}$ will become $\frac{2ab+bd}{4a+2b}=\frac{1}{2}b$, and in the Ellipsis $\frac{ab-db}{2a-b}$ will become $\frac{2ab-bd}{4a-2b}=\frac{1}{2}b$, whence PD will be equal to AP. Consequently the Points E and A will coincide, and a Circle described on the Center P, with the Radius PA, or PE, will touch the Hyperbola or Ellipses in the Vertex A, and be altogether within them.

And hence we have a general Method for drawing Tangents to Curves; for inasmuch as PE is the Subnormal, as being

ing the shortest Line that can be drawn from the given Point P to the Curve, if the Value of P D from the Equation expressing the Nature of the Curve be determined, the Point P will be determined also, whence a Line drawn through E, the Extremity of the Ordinate D E at right Angles to P E, will be a Tangent to the Curve in the Point E.

EXAMPLE IX.

LET it be required to find the Point P in the right Line M D, lying in the same Plane with the Points R and A, that a Particle of Light, in going from R to P, with a given Velocity v, and from P to A, with a given Velocity c, shall travel from R by P to A in the shortest Time.

LET P be the Point required, and from the Points R and A having drawn the Lines R S, A E perpendicular to M P D, put $RS=a$, $AE=b$, $SE=d$, $SP=x$, then will $PE=d-x$, $RP=\overline{aa+xx}|^{\frac{1}{2}}$ and $AP=\overline{bb+dd-2dx+xx}|^{\frac{1}{2}}$.

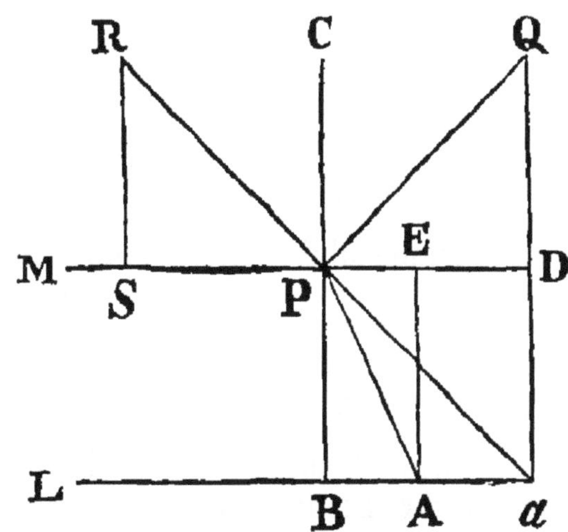

NOW by the known Laws of Motion, if a Body move from R to P with the Velocity v, and from P to A with the Velocity c, if the Velocities are equal, then the Times will be as the Spaces described P R and P A, and if the Spaces R P and P A are equal, and the Velocities unequal, the Times will be reciprocally as the Velocities. Wherefore if the Spaces described, and the Velocities are both unequal, then the Times will be in a Ratio compounded of the direct Ratio of the Spaces, and the reciprocal Ratio of the Velocities, and consequently

consequently the Time that a Particle of Light will take to move from R to P, with the Velocity v, will be represented by $\frac{\overline{aa+xx}|^{\frac{1}{2}}}{v}$; and the Time that the same Particle will take in moving from P to A with the Velocity c, will be represented by $\frac{\overline{bb+dd-2dx+xx}|^{\frac{1}{2}}}{c}$, and consequently their Sum $\frac{\overline{aa+xx}|^{\frac{1}{2}}}{v}$ $+\frac{\overline{bb+dd-2dx+xx}|^{\frac{1}{2}}}{c}$ or $c\times\overline{aa+xx}|^{\frac{1}{2}}+v\times\overline{bb+dd-2dx+xx}|^{\frac{1}{2}}$ will be the shortest Time that a Particle of Light will require to move from R by P to A, with the respective Velocities v and c, wherefore $\frac{2c\dot{x}x}{2\overline{aa+xx}|^{\frac{1}{2}}}+\frac{2v\dot{x}x-2dv\dot{x}}{2\overline{bb+dd-2dx+xx}|^{\frac{1}{2}}}=0$, and (by dividing by 2, expunging $\dot{x}$, and substituting PR in the room of $\overline{aa+xx}|^{\frac{1}{2}}$, and PA in the room of $\overline{bb+dd-2dx+xx}|^{\frac{1}{2}}$) we shall have $\frac{cx}{PR}=\frac{dv-vx}{PA}$.

LET us now suppose PR = PA, for the Refraction is the same in the Point P, whether the Ray PA be longer or shorter, then will $cx=dv-vx$. Consequently by reducing the Equation to an Analogy, we shall have $v:c::x:d-x$, that is, $v:c::$ SP : PE.

NOW if PR equal to PA be considered as the Radius of a Circle, SP will be the Sine of the Angle SRP equal to the Angle RPC, the Angle of Incidence, and PE equal to BA the Sine of the Angle of Refraction BPA. Whence it follows that the Sines of the Angles of Incidence and Refraction are directly as the Velocities v and c of the Particle of Light, in its Passage through the different Mediums.

AND because the Velocities of Bodies moving through different Mediums are reciprocally proportional to the Densities of the respective Mediums, it follows, that the Sines of the Angles of Incidence and Refraction of a Particle of Light passing through different Mediums, are reciprocally proportional to the Densities of those Mediums; and this is the fundamental Law upon which the Science of Dioptricks is founded

NOW if the Particle of Light in moving from R to A by P, when it arrives at P, instead of being refracted towards A, it be reflected towards Q in the right Line PQ, in this Case the Medium being still the same, the Velocities v and c will be equal Wherefore putting RS $= a$, QD $= b$, SD $= d$ SP $= x$, whence PD $= d - x$, we shall have PR $= \overline{aa+xx}|^{\frac{1}{2}}$, and PQ $= \overline{bb+dd-2dx+xx}|^{\frac{1}{2}}$ Wherefore $\overline{aa+xx}|^{\frac{1}{2}}$ $\overline{+bb+dd-2dx+xx}|^{\frac{1}{2}}$, will give the shortest Time, consequently

$$\frac{x\dot{x}}{\overline{aa+xx}|^{\frac{1}{2}}} + \frac{x\dot{x}-d\dot{x}}{\overline{bb+dd-2dx+xx}|^{\frac{1}{2}}} = \frac{x\dot{x}}{PR} + \frac{x\dot{x}-d\dot{x}}{PQ} = 0,$$

and supposing PR and PQ to be equal (for the Reflexion is the same in whatsoever part of the Line PQ, the Point Q be taken, we shall have $x\dot{x} + x\dot{x} - d\dot{x} = 0$, whence $2x = d$, and $x = \frac{1}{2}d$, that is, SP will be equal to PD, and because PR is equal to PQ, by the Hypotheses, and the Angles at S and D right Angles, therefore the Triangles RSP and PDQ will be mutually equal Wherefore the Angle SRP will be equal to PQD, and because CP is perpendicular to the Line SD, in the Point of Incidence, P, therefore the Angles CPR, SRP, PQD and CPQ are equal to each other, whence the Angle CPR the Angle of Incidence is equal to CPQ the Angle of Reflexion, and this is the fundamental Law upon which the Science of Catoptricks is founded.

EXAM-

EXAMPLE X.

LET it be required to find the Curve of *swiftest Descent*, or the Nature of a Curve in which a heavy Body, descending by the Force of its own Gravity, shall move from one given Point to another given Point in the *shortest Time*, or in less Time than in any other Line passing between those Points.

LET ADEFP represent the Curve, AK the Axis, D and F two Points given by Position, and let it be required to find the Nature of the same Curve ADEFP, so that a heavy

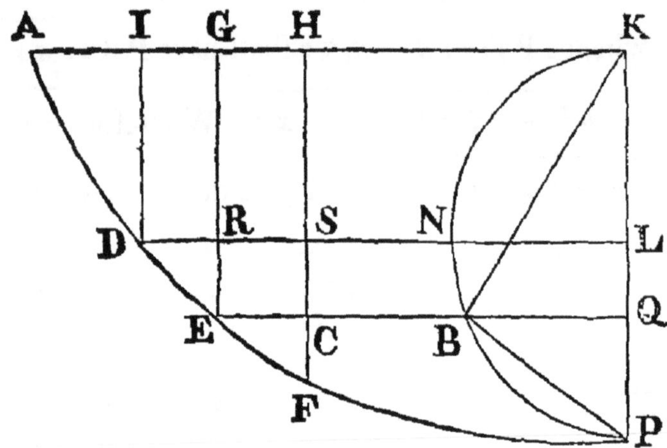

Body moving therein, when it arrives at the Point D, shall pass from that Point to any other Point, suppose F, in the shortest Time possible, or in less Time than through any other Curve whatever

FROM the Points D and F, let the Ordinates DI, FH, be drawn perpendicular, and the Line DL parallel to the Axis AK, and imagine the Ordinate DI in a flowing State to move till it come into the Place GE, which is situated in such a Position that the Segment RE may be equal to the Segment FC of the Ordinate FH, cut off by the Line EQ, drawn from the Point E, parallel to the Axis AK.

FOR

FORASMUCH as the Points D and F are fixed Points, the Ordinates FH, DI, in this Case, are constant Quantities, and so is the Ordinate GE, inasmuch as there can be but one Situation of the intermediate Point E, that will answer the Condition, and because RE is supposed to be always equal to FC, these will also be fixed or constant Quantities, as will be the Line DS, consequently the Arches DE, FE, and the Lines DR, EC, will be variable, or flowing Quantities. Put therefore $EG = a$, $FH = b$, $DS = c$, $RE = FC = CS = d$, $DR = z$, $EC = v$, then will $DS = c = z + v$, and the Arch DE, in its nascent or arising Form, will be equal to $\overline{zz + dd}|^{\frac{1}{2}}$, as will the Arch EF at the same time be equal to $\overline{vv + dd}|^{\frac{1}{2}}$.

NOW since the Velocities that heavy Bodies acquire in their Descent, are in a Subduplicate Ratio of the Altitudes they fell from, the Velocity of the heavy Body in the Point E will be $\sqrt{a}$, and the Velocity of the same Body in the Point F, will be $\sqrt{b}$, and because the Times are reciprocally as the Velocities, the Time in which the Body will descend from D to E, will be as $\frac{\overline{zz+dd}|^{\frac{1}{2}}}{\sqrt{a}}$, as will the Time of the Descent through EF, as $\frac{\overline{vv+dd}|^{\frac{1}{2}}}{\sqrt{b}}$, and since these Velocities, in their arising State, are as the Arches DE and EF, described in the same infinitely small Particle of Time, and since the Time of the Descent from D to F is the shortest possible (by Hypothesis) therefore $\frac{\overline{zz+dd}|^{\frac{1}{2}}}{\sqrt{a}} + \frac{\overline{vv+dd}|^{\frac{1}{2}}}{\sqrt{b}}$ must be a *Minimum*, and consequently $\frac{z\dot{z}}{\sqrt{a} \times \overline{zz+dd}|^{\frac{1}{2}}} + \frac{v\dot{v}}{\sqrt{b} \times \overline{vv+dd}}$ $= 0$, and because $z + v = c$, a fixed or constant Quantity,

S therefore $\dot{z} + \dot{v} = 0$; whence $z = -v$, and $\frac{z}{\sqrt{a} \times \overline{zz+dd}|^{\frac{1}{2}}} - \frac{v}{\sqrt{b} \times \overline{vv+dd}|^{\frac{1}{2}}} = 0$; whence $\frac{z}{\sqrt{a} \times \overline{zz+dd}|^{\frac{1}{2}}} = \frac{v}{\sqrt{b} \times \overline{vv+dd}|^{\frac{1}{2}}}$, and $z \times \sqrt{b} \times \overline{vv+dd}|^{\frac{1}{2}} = v \times \sqrt{a} \times \overline{zz+dd}|^{\frac{1}{2}}$ whence $\overline{vv+dd}|^{\frac{1}{2}} : \overline{zz+dd}|^{\frac{1}{2}} :: v \times \sqrt{a} : z \times \sqrt{b}$, that is, as EF : ED :: $\sqrt{EG} \times EC$: $\sqrt{HF} \times DR$, so that supposing the Curve to commence at the Point A, AG, AH will be Abscisses, GE, HF Ordinates rightly applied, and DR, EC, will be as the Fluxions of the Abscisses AG, AH, as will the Lines RE, CF, be as the Fluxions of the Ordinates GE, HF, and the Arches DE, EF, as the Fluxions of the Curve Lines AD, AF, generated in the same very small Particle of Time, whence it follows, that the Property of the Curve of swiftest Descent is, that the Fluxions of the Curve are in the Ratio compounded of the direct Ratio of the Fluxions of the Abscisses, and the reciprocal Subduplicate Ratio of the Ordinates, and this being the Property of the common Cycloid, it follows, that the Curve of swiftest Descent is an inverted Cycloid

SCHOLIUM

IF a Ray of Light fall upon a Medium, whose Rarity increases in a Subduplicate Ratio of its Depth, the Ray in its Passage through such a Medium, will describe the same Track as a heavy Body does in its swiftest Descent, for since, in the Descent of a heavy Body, the Velocities are in the Subduplicate Ratio of the perpendicular Depths or Descents, and likewise the Velocity of a Particle of Light is ever proportional to the Rarity of the Medium it passes through, it follows that the Velocity of a Ray of Light, in such a Medium as is here supposed, will be increased in a Subduplicate Ratio of its per-

pendicular

pendicular Descent, and consequently the Curve of Refraction, in this Case, will be the same with the Curve of the swiftest Descent, that is, a Cycloid.

EXAMPLE XI.

LET it be required to investigate the Nature of the Curve D K, which being revolved about its Axis A M, shall describe

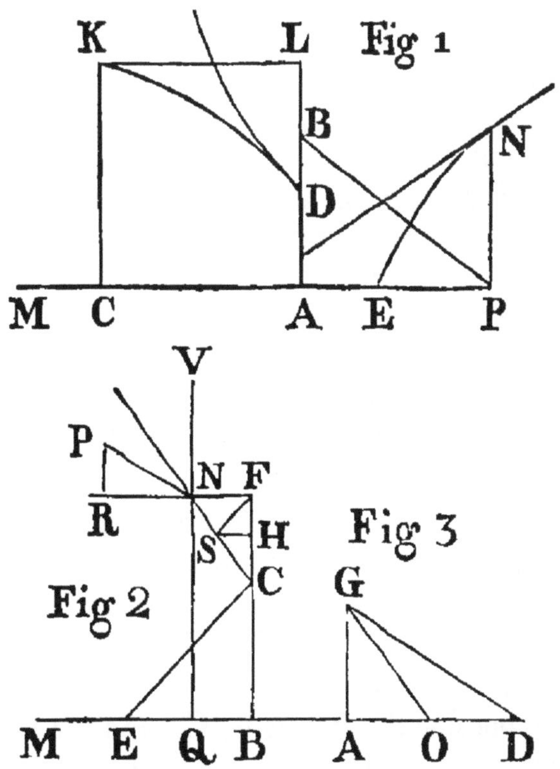

the Surface of a Solid, which moving in a Fluid whose Particles are at rest, according to the Direction M A, from M towards A, shall be less resisted by the Fluid than any other Solid generated by a Curve having the same Axis A M, (*Fig* 1) and passing through the same Points D and K, given by Position

LET (*Fig.* 2) C N P represent a small Portion of a Curve Line, N Q, C B, Ordinates rightly applied to the Axis A M, and let R N F be drawn parallel to the Axis, cutting the Curve C N P in the Point N, and perpendicular to it draw the Lines P R and C F, as also C E perpendicular to the Curve in the Point C.

NOW if the right Line C F, and the Portion of the Curve C N, be supposed to move in the Direction of the Axis M A, from M towards A, it is evident, that the Force of Resistance of the Fluid, in this Case, is equal to the Action of the Fluid moving with the same Velocity, and in a direct contrary Direction from A towards M, on the Line C F, and the small Portion of the Curve Line C N supposed at rest. Wherefore draw F S perpendicular to N C, and S H parallel to R F, or M A.

NOW if F N represent the Force of a Particle of the Fluid, against Q N V, in the Direction A M, or from A towards M, then F S will represent the Force of the same Particle of the Fluid against C N, according to the Direction C E, or from C towards E. And again, if F S represent the Force of the same Particle of the Fluid against C N, in the Direction C E, or from C towards E, then S H will represent the Force of the same Particle of the Fluid against C N, in the Direction A M, or from A towards M. Wherefore because the Triangles E B C, C F N, F N S, and F S H are similar, it will be as F N : F S :: F S : S H, consequently from the Nature of continued Proportionals, as F N : F S :: FN^2 : SH^2, and so is CE^2 to EB^2, or as F N : F S :: C E : E B.

NOW supposing the Points P, C, and the Line R F, given by Position, to lye in the same Plane with the Axis B M, we are to find the Point N in the Curve Line C P, so that the Surface generated by the Revolution of the nascent Augment of the Curve C N P, may generate the nascent Augment of a Surface that shall meet with a lesser Resistance than any other Surface generated from the same Data.

AND forasmuch as the Quantities C F, C B, N Q, P R, in the present Case, are fixed or constant Quantities, and F N, N R

N R, variable or flowing Quantities, put C F = a, C B = b, P R = c, N Q = d, F N = v, N R = z; whence C N = $\overline{aa+vv}^{\frac{1}{2}}$, and P N = $\overline{cc+zz}^{\frac{1}{2}}$ Now ſuppoſing r to repreſent the Reſiſtance of a Particle of the Fluid againſt the Body moving in the Direction M A or from M towards A, or, which is the ſame, the Velocity of a Particle of the Fluid moving in a contrary Direction, or from A to M, and ſtriking againſt the Body ſuppoſed at reſt, then will the Force of the ſame Fluid, upon the Plane deſcribed by the Line C F, revolving about the Axis B M at the Diſtance of B C, oppoſed to the Motion of the Fluid, be as the Surface deſcribed multiplied into the Velocity, that is, $\bar{r} \times \bar{a} \times \bar{b}$ Whence to find the Force of the Fluid moving in the Direction A M, or from A towards M, againſt the Surface generated by the Part of the Curve C N, it will be $\overline{vv+aa}^{\frac{1}{2}}\ aa\ \ r\,ab\ \ \frac{ra^3b}{\overline{vv+aa}^{\frac{1}{2}}}$, and conſequently by the ſame way of Reaſoning, the Force which the Surface, generated by the Part N P, revolved about the Axis A M, will be impelled with, will be $\frac{rcccd}{\overline{cc+zz}^{\frac{1}{2}}}$, conſequently $\frac{raaab}{\overline{aa+vv}^{\frac{1}{2}}} + \frac{rcccd}{\overline{cc+zz}^{\frac{1}{2}}}$ will be a *Minimum*, whence $\frac{2aaabv\dot{v}}{\overline{aa+vv}^{\frac{1}{2}}} + \frac{2cccdz\dot{z}}{\overline{cc+zz}^{\frac{1}{2}}} = 0$, and $\frac{aaabv\dot{v}}{\overline{aa+vv}^{\frac{1}{2}}} = \frac{-c^3dz\dot{z}}{\overline{cc+zz}^{\frac{1}{2}}}$, but becauſe $v + z$ = R F, a conſtant Quantity, therefore $\dot{v} + \dot{z} = 0$, whence $\dot{v} = -\dot{z}$, and conſequently $\frac{aaabv}{aa+vv} = \frac{cccdz}{\overline{cc+zz}^{\frac{1}{2}}}$ Wherefore if the right Line AG, (*Fig* 3) drawn perpendicular to the Axis A M, be made equal to r, and from the Point G the Line G O be drawn parallel to the Tangent to the Curve in the Point N, it will be as 4 AG × A O $\overline{GO}^3$

G

: GO :: BC; for because the Triangles CFN and GAO are similar, it will be as CF : FN :: GA · AO; that is, as $a : v :: r : \frac{vr}{a} = AO$, and as FC : CN : GA . GO, that is, as $a : \overline{aa+vv}^{\frac{1}{2}} :: r . \frac{r \times \overline{aa+vv}^{\frac{1}{2}}}{a} = GO$; whence $\frac{4r^3 v}{a} : \frac{r^3 \times \overline{aa+vv}^{\frac{3}{2}}}{a^3} :: \frac{r \times \overline{aa+vv}^{\frac{1}{2}}}{a} \cdot b$; consequently $\frac{4br^3 v}{a} = \frac{r^4 \times \overline{aa+vv}^2}{a^4}$, and $4a^3bv = r \times \overline{aa+vv}^2$, whence $\frac{1}{4}r = \frac{a^3bv}{\overline{aa+vv}^2}$

AGAIN, if from the same Point G the right Line GD be drawn parallel to the Tangent to the Curve in the Point P, it will be as $\overline{GA}^2 \times AD \cdot \overline{GD}^3 :: GD, NQ$; for because the Triangles PRN and GAD are similar, it will be as PR : RN :: AG : AD, that is, as $c : z :: r : \frac{zr}{c} = AD$; and again, as PR : PN :: AG : GD, that is, as $c : \overline{cc+zz}^{\frac{1}{2}} :: r : \frac{r \times \overline{cc+zz}^{\frac{1}{2}}}{c} = GD$, whence $\frac{4r^3 z}{c} : \frac{r^3 \times \overline{cc+zz}^{\frac{3}{2}}}{c^3} :: \frac{r \times \overline{cc+zz}^{\frac{1}{2}}}{c} : d$ Wherefore $\frac{4dzr^3}{c} = \frac{r^4 \times \overline{cc+zz}^2}{c^4}$, and $4dz = \frac{r \times \overline{cc+zz}^2}{c^3}$, whence $dc^3 z = \frac{r \times \overline{cc+zz}^2}{4}$, and $\frac{1}{4}r = \frac{dc^3 z}{\overline{cc+zz}^2}$, and consequently $\frac{a^3bv}{\overline{aa+vv}^2} = \frac{c^3dz}{\overline{cc+zz}^2}$, which is the same with the general Equation before found.

WHENCE it is evident, that the Nature of the Curve DK, (*Fig* 1) which being revolved about its Axis AM, generates the Solid

Solid of least Resistance, is such that drawing A L perpendicular to the Axis A M, and taking $AB = r$, and drawing B P parallel to the Tangent to the Curve in the Point K, then it will always be as $\overline{4\,AB}^2 \times AP \quad BP^3 \quad BP \quad AD$, the Ordinate passing through the Point D

Now in order to construct the Curve, let A L be drawn perpendicular to the Axis A M, and make A B equal to r, and $AE = \overline{\tfrac{1}{3} r r}^{\frac{1}{2}}$, and through the Point E let the Logarithmetical Curve E N be drawn, and let A L be the Asymptote, and the Subtangent equal to $\frac{1}{4} r$, then taking A P of any Length, draw P N parallel to A L, till it meet the Logarithmetical Curve in N, then putting $AP = z$, make A L equal to $\frac{rr}{4z} + \frac{z}{2} + \frac{zzz}{4rr}$, and $AC = \frac{zz}{4r} + \frac{3z^4}{16r^3} - \frac{\pm r}{48} + PN$, if A P be greater than A E, but $- PN$, if A P be less than A E, and compleat the Parallelogram A C K L I say, the Point K, wherein C K and L K intersect, will be a Point in the Curve.

For A P being equal to z, if A C be put equal to x, and C K equal to y, then, by the Property of the Curve, A L or $CK = y = \frac{r^4 + 2r^2z^2 + z^4}{4rrz}$, and consequently $\dot{y} = \frac{\dot{z}}{2} + \frac{3zz\dot{z}}{4rr} - \frac{rr\dot{z}}{4zz}$, and because B P is parallel to the Tangent in the Point K, therefore the Triangle A B P is similar to the nascent Triangle at the Point K; and consequently as $r \; z : \dot{y} \cdot \frac{z\dot{y}}{r} = \dot{x} = \frac{z\dot{z}}{2r} + \frac{3zzz\dot{z}}{4r^3} - \frac{r\dot{z}}{4z}$, whence the Fluent $AC = x = \frac{zz}{4r} + \frac{3z^4}{16r^3} - \frac{r\dot{z}}{4z}$, but by the Property of the Logarithmetical Curve, as $z \; \frac{1}{4}r \; . \; \dot{z} \; \frac{r\dot{z}}{4z}$, whence

1 ±

$\pm \frac{rz}{4z} = PN$ Therefore $AC = x = \frac{zz}{4r} + \frac{3z^4}{16r^3} - PN \pm$ a constant Quantity $\frac{\pm r}{48}$, and consequently when PN vanishes, then AC will vanish also, therefore DK is the required Curve.

WHENCE it is evident, that the Curve DK cannot approach nearer the Axis AM then in the Point D, where it intersects the Perpendicular AL, and that afterwards, when AP is less than AE, the Portion of the Curve DK will be described Convex towards the Axis AM So that the Surface of the Solid of least Resistance may be Convex as well as Concave towards the Axis

---

SECT. III.

Of the Use of FLUXIONS *in the Invention of Points of* Inflexion *and* Retrogression.

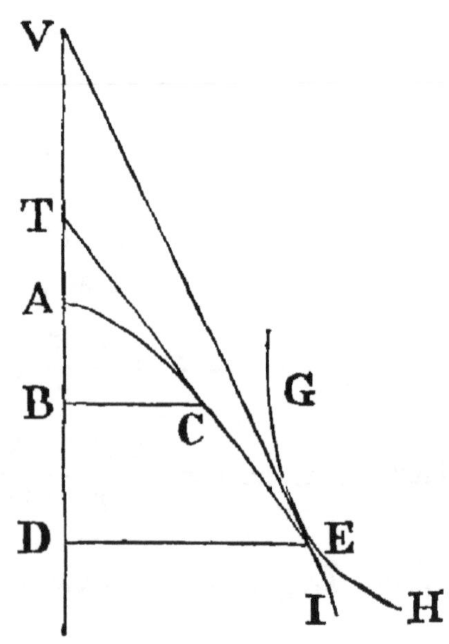

IN the Formation of a Curve Line ACEH, if the generating Point, after it has described a Portion of it AC Concave towards the Axis AD, shall begin to move by a Law different from what it first set out with, so as to describe the Part EH Convex towards the same right Line AD, the Point E, where the generating Point received the new Direction, which divides the Concave from the Convex Part, and consequently is at the End of one, and at the Beginning of the other, is called the Point of *Inflexion*, as long as long as the Curve, being continued in F, keeps its Direction the ſame But it is called the Point of *Retrogreſſion*, when it inflects back again towards that Part or Side from whence it took its Original

THESE Things being premiſed, from E, the ſuppoſed Point of Inflexion, let the Ordinate D F be drawn, and the Tangent F V to meet the Diameter A D produced in V Again, from C, ſome other Point of the Curve, ſituated between E, the Point of Inflexion, and the Vertex of the Curve A, let another Ordinate B C, be drawn parallel to the former Ordinate D E, and T C a Tangent to the Point C, to cut the ſame Diameter A D produced in T This being done, it is evident (ſuppoſing the Ordinate B C in a flowing State) that the nearer it approaches the Ordinate D E, the greater will be the Diſtance A T, intercepted between the Vertex of the Curve A, and the Interſection T of the Tangent, with the Diameter prolonged, 'till at laſt, when the Ordinate B C arrives at, and coincides with the Ordinate D E, the Point T will coincide with the Point V, and conſequently the Diſtance V A, between A the Vertex, and the Interſection V of the Tangent V E with the Diameter A D produced, will, in this Caſe, become a *Maximum*

WHEREFORE putting A D $= x$, D E $= y$, it will be (by *Propoſition* I. of *Part* II *Sect* I) as y x y $\frac{yx}{y} =$ D V, from whence taking $x =$ A D, we ſhall A V $= \frac{yx}{y} - x$ a *Maximum*, conſequently (ſuppoſing x a conſtant Quantity) its Fluxion $\frac{yyx - yyx}{yy} - x = 0$, or Nothing, by the preceding *Section* · whence $\frac{yyx - yyx - yyx}{yy} = 0$, conſequently, $\frac{-yyx}{yy} = 0$. Whence $-y\ddot{y}x = 0$, and $y = 0$.

And hence we have a general Rule to find the Point of Inflexion or Retrogression in any Curve, for the Equation of the Curve being given, if we find the Value of $\dot{y}$ in $\dot{x}$, and again, find the Fluxion of that Value (supposing $\dot{x}$ to be a constant Quantity) we shall have the Value of $\ddot{y}$ in $\dot{x}\dot{x}$, which being put equal to Nothing, or Infinity, as the Case requires, we shall have such a Value of A D, that its correspondent Ordinate D E shall intersect the Curve A C E in the Point of Inflexion or Retrogression, as will more evidently appear from the following Examples.

EXAMPLE I.

LET A E F be a protracted Semi-cycloid, whose Base is longer than the Circumference of the generating Circle A H B, whose Centre is C, 'tis required to find the Point D in the Diameter A B, so that the Ordinate Applicate D E shall cut the Semi cycloid in E, the Point of contrary Flexion.

PUT B F $= b$, A B $= 2r$, the Arch of the generating Semi circle, A H B $= c$, A D $= x$, D H $= z$, the Arch A H $= v$, and D E $= y$, because, from the Nature of the Curve $y = z + \frac{bv}{c}$, we shall have $\dot{y} = \dot{z} + \frac{b\dot{v}}{c}$, but from the Nature of the Circle, we shall have $z = \overline{2rx - xx}^{\frac{1}{2}}$

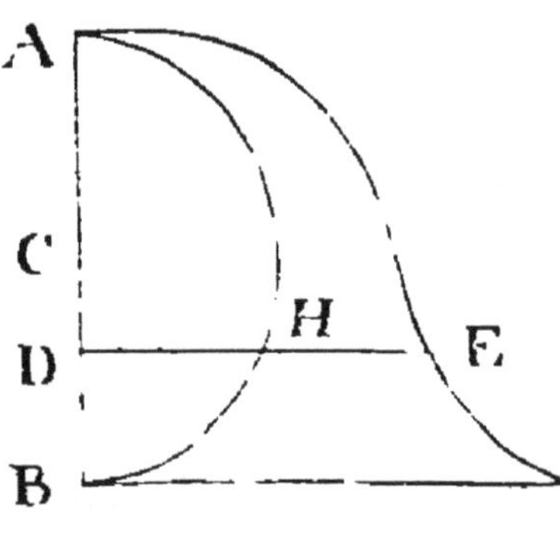

consequently $\dot{z} = \frac{r\dot{x} - x\dot{x}}{\overline{2rx - xx}^{\frac{1}{2}}}$, and $\dot{v} = \overline{\dot{x}\dot{x} + \dot{z}\dot{z}}^{\frac{1}{2}} = \frac{r\dot{x}}{\overline{2rx - xx}^{\frac{1}{2}}}$. Wherefore substituting in the room of $\dot{y}$ and $\dot{v}$

in

in the Equation $y = z + \frac{bv}{c}$, their respective Values, and we shall have $\dot{y} = \frac{r\dot{x} - x\dot{x}}{\overline{2rx - xx}|^{\frac{1}{2}}} + \frac{br\dot{x}}{c \times \overline{2rx - xx}} = \frac{cr\dot{x} - cx\dot{x} + br\dot{x}}{c \times \overline{2rx - xx}|^{\frac{1}{2}}}$, whose Fluxion (supposing $\dot{x}$ a constant Quantity) is $\ddot{y} = \frac{\overline{brx - crr - brr} \times \dot{x}\dot{x}}{\overline{2rx - xx} \times \overline{2rx - xx}|^{\frac{1}{2}}} = 0$, whence $\overline{brx - crr - brr} \times \dot{x}\dot{x} = 0$, and $bx - cr - br = 0$ (by dividing by $r\dot{x}\dot{x}$) whence $bx = br + cr$, and $AD = x = r + \frac{cr}{b}$, whence $AD - AC = CD = \frac{cr}{b}$. Whence it is manifest, that to have a Point of contrary Flexion, the Base BF must be greater than the Semi-circumference AHB of the generating Circle, for if it be less, then CD would be greater than CB.

EXAMPLE II.

LET it be required to find the Point B of contrary Flexion in the Conchoid ABΓ of *Nichomedes*.

LET C be the Pole of the Choncoid, DE the Asymptote, and since, from the Nature of the Curve, the Segments AD, BN, of the Lines CA, CB, drawn from the Pole C to the Points A and B in the Curve Line, cut off by the Asymptote DE, are equal amongst themselves, and to a given right Line. Having drawn CDA perpendicular to the Asymptote, and BH parallel to it, and NP parallel to DH, put $DA = NB = a$, $CD = b$, $DH = x$, $HB = y$, then will $PB = \overline{aa - xx}|^{\frac{1}{2}}$, and $CH = b + x$, and because the Triangles CHB and NPB are similar, it will be as NP . PB :: CH . HB, that is, as $x \; \overline{aa - xx}^{\frac{1}{2}} \quad b + x \quad \frac{\overline{b + x} \times \overline{aa - xx}^{\frac{1}{2}}}{x} = HB$ $= y$, and consequently $\dot{y} = \frac{x^3 \dot{x} + aab\dot{x}}{xx \times \overline{aa - xx}^{\frac{1}{2}}}$, and $\ddot{y}$ $= \frac{\overline{2a^4 b - aax^3 - 3aabxx} \times \dot{x}\dot{x}}{aaxxx - x^5 \times \overline{aa - xx}^{\frac{1}{2}}} = 0$, supposing $\dot{x}$ to be a constant Quantity Whence $2a^4 b - aax^3 - 3aabxx = 0$, and dividing by aa, we shall have $2aab - xxx - 3bxx = 0 = x^3 + 3bxx - 2aab = 0$, and one of the Values of the Root x will be equal to DH

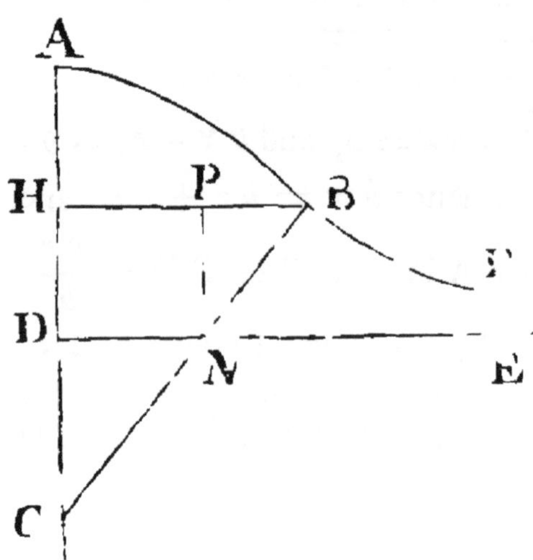

If CD = DA, then $b = a$, and the Equation will be $xxx + 3axx - 2aaa = 0$, which being divided by $x + a$, the Quotient $xx + 2ax - 2aa = 0$, and consequently $x = -a + \overline{3aa}^{\frac{1}{2}}$

EXAMPLE III.

Suppose the Property of the Conchoid ABF (*See the preceding Figure*) to be such, that if a right Line, as CB, be drawn from the Pole C to any Point B in the Curve, intersecting the Asymptote DE in N, that the Rectangle CN × NB may be always equal to a constant Rectangle CD × DA, and let it be required to find the Point of Inflexion B.

Put CD $= b$, DA $= a$, DH $= x$, HB $= y$, then will CN × NB $= ab$, and because the Lines DN and HE are parallel as CN × NB . CD × DH .. CB^2 . CH^2, that is, as as $ab : bx :: bb+2bx+xx+yy : bb+2bx+xx$, whence $bbx+2bxx+xxx+yyx=abb+2abx+axx$, and

$$yy=\frac{abb+2abx+axx-bbx-2bxx-xxx}{x},$$

and $y=\overline{b+x}\times\frac{\overline{a-x}^{\frac{1}{2}}}{x}=\frac{x}{\overline{ax-xx}^{\frac{1}{2}}}+\frac{b\times\overline{a-x}^{\frac{1}{2}}}{x}$,

whose Fluxion will be $\dot{y}=\frac{ax\dot{x}+2xx\dot{x}+ab\dot{x}}{2x\times\overline{ax-xx}^{\frac{1}{2}}}$, and consequently its second Fluxion $\ddot{y}=\frac{\overline{3aab-aax-4abx}\times\dot{x}\dot{x}}{4axx-4xxx\times\overline{ax-xx}^{\frac{1}{2}}}$

$=0$ (supposing $\dot{x}$ a constant Quantity), whence $3aab-aax-4abx=0$, and $ax+4bx=3ab$, whence

$x=\frac{3ab}{a+4b}=DH$.

EXAMPLE IV.

Let AEK be a given Curve Line, AB its Diameter, and supposing the Relation of the Ordinate y, to its Abscisse x, be expressed by this Equation $axx=xxy+aay$, let it be required to find the Value of AD, so that its correspondent Ordinate DE may intersect the Curve AEK in the Point of contrary Flexion.

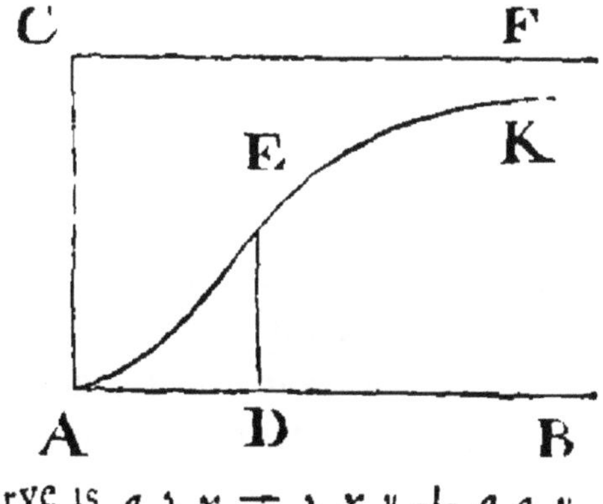

The Equation of the Curve is $axx=xxy+aay$, whence $y=\frac{axx}{xx+aa}$, and $\dot{y}=\frac{2aaax\dot{x}}{\overline{xx+aa}^{2}}$, and (supposing $\dot{x}$ a standing Quantity) $\ddot{y}=2a^{3}\dot{x}\dot{x}\times\overline{xx+aa}^{-2}-8a^{3}$

$-\frac{8a^3 x\dot{x}\dot{x}x \times \overline{xx+aa}}{\overline{xx+aa}^4} = 0$, whence $2a^3\dot{x}\dot{x} \times \overline{xx+aa}^{-1}$ $-8a^3 x\dot{x}\dot{x}x \times \overline{xx+aa} = 0$, and dividing by $2a^3\dot{x}\dot{x} \times \overline{xx+aa}^2$, and multiplying by $\overline{xx+aa}^4$, we ſhall have $xx+aa-4xx=0$, whence $3xx=aa$, and $AD = x = a \times \sqrt{\frac{1}{3}}$

If we ſubſtitute $\frac{1}{3}aa$ in the room of xx, in the Equation of the Curve $y = \frac{axx}{aa+xx}$, then $y = \frac{\frac{1}{3}a^3}{\frac{4}{3}a^2} = \frac{1}{4}a = CD$ So that we may determine the Point of Inflexion E, without ſuppoſing the Curve to be deſcribed

If AC be drawn parallel to the Ordinate DE, and equal to the given Line a, and if CF be drawn parallel to AB, it will be an Aſymptote to the Curve AEK; for if x be ſuppoſed to be infinite, than the Equation of the Curve $y = \frac{axx}{aa+xx}$ will become $y = \frac{axx}{xx} = a$ So that the Ordinate DE of the Curve cannot be equal to AC, before the Abſciſſe AD be infinite.

EXAMPLE V.

Let AEK be a Curve, whoſe Axis is the right Line AB, and let the Nature of it be ſuch, that any Tangent, EB, being drawn, meeting AB in the Point B, the intercepted Part AB will be always to the Tangent BE, in a given Ratio, as m to n, it is required to determine the Point of Retrogreſſion E. Put $AD = x$, $DE = y$, then DB will be equal $-\frac{y\dot{x}}{\dot{y}}$, and $EB = \frac{y \times \overline{\dot{x}\dot{x}+\dot{y}\dot{y}}^{\frac{1}{2}}}{\dot{y}}$ Now from the Nature of the Curve

AD

as AD + DB = AB : BE :: $m : n$, that is, as $\frac{x\dot y - y\dot x}{\dot y}$: $\frac{y\times\overline{\dot x\dot x+\dot y\dot y}^{\frac{1}{2}}}{\dot y}$ :: $m : n$.

Therefore $m\times\overline{\dot x\dot x+\dot y\dot y}^{\frac{1}{2}} = \frac{nx\dot y}{y} - n\dot x$, and the Fluxion of this last Quantity (supposing $\dot x$ a constant Quantity) will be $\frac{m\dot y\ddot y}{\overline{\dot x\dot x+\dot y\dot y}^{\frac{1}{2}}} = \frac{-ny\dot x\dot y + nxy\ddot y - nx\dot y\dot y}{yy}$, whence we shall have $\ddot y = \frac{ny\dot x\dot y - nx\dot y\dot y\times\overline{\dot x\dot x+\dot y\dot y}^{\frac{1}{2}}}{m\dot y yy - nxy\times\overline{\dot x\dot x+\dot y\dot y}^{\frac{1}{2}}}$, which being equal to Infinity, the Numerator will vanish, consequently $m\dot y yy - nxy\times\overline{\dot x\dot x+\dot y\dot y}^{\frac{1}{2}} = 0$, and $my\dot y = nx\times\overline{\dot x\dot x+\dot y\dot y}^{\frac{1}{2}}$ and $\overline{\dot x\dot x+\dot y\dot y}^{\frac{1}{2}} = \frac{my\dot y}{nx} = \frac{nx\dot y - ny\dot x}{my}$ from the Equation of the Curve: wherefore $\dot x = nnxx\dot y - mmyy\dot y$ and squaring both Sides of the Equation $my\dot y = nx\times\overline{\dot x\dot x+\dot y\dot y}^{\frac{1}{2}}$, we shall have $\dot x = \frac{\dot y\times\overline{mmyy - nnxx}^{\frac{1}{2}}}{nx} = \frac{nnxx\dot y - mmyy\dot y}{nnxy}$, and consequently $y\times\overline{mm-nn}^{\frac{1}{2}} = nx$, from whence we have the following Construction.

On the Diameter AC = m describe a Semi-circle AHC, and take the Chord AH = n, and draw the Line AH. This produced, will intersect the Curve AEK in E, the Point of Retrogression.

For if HP be drawn perpendicular to AB, because of the similar Triangles CHA, HPA, EDA, CH : HA :: HP : PA

E D : D A, that is, as $n : \overline{mm-nn}^{\frac{1}{2}} :: y : x$, therefore $y \times \overline{mm-nn}^{\frac{1}{2}} = nx$.

It is manifest, that B E is parallel to C H, because as A B : B E :: A C : C H, whence the Angle A E B will be a right Angle, and so the Lines A B, B E and B D are continual Proportionals.

EXAMPLE VI.

Let A B C be an Arch of a Circle, and A its Centre, and let the Property of the Curve Line A E K be such, that drawing any Ray D E B, at Pleasure, the Square of BE be equal to the Rectangle comprehended under the Arch A B, and a given Line a, 'tis required to find the Point E of contrary Flexion.

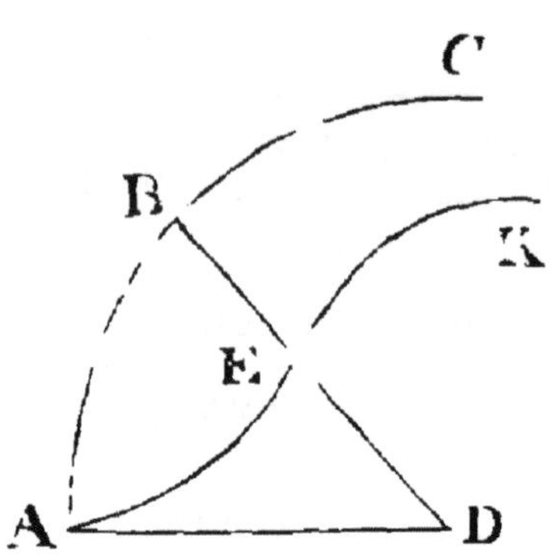

Put the Radius A D = r, the Ordinate DE = y, the Arch of the Circle A B = z, and the Portion of the Curve Line A E = x, then will B E = $r - y$, and because, by the Property of the Curve A B $\times a$ = B E², we shall have $az = rr - 2ry + yy$, and $\dot{z} = \frac{2y\dot{y} - 2r\dot{y}}{a}$, and forasmuch as the Triangles D A B and D A E, in their nascent Form, are similar, it will be as $r : y :: \frac{2y\dot{y} - 2r\dot{y}}{a} : \dot{x}$, whence $r\dot{x} = \frac{2y^2\dot{y} - 2ry\dot{y}}{a}$, and $\dot{x} = \frac{2yy\dot{y} - 2ry\dot{y}}{ar}$, and (supposing $\dot{x}$ a constant Quantity) we shall have $4y\dot{y}\dot{y} - 2a\dot{y}\dot{y} + 2yy\ddot{y} - 2ay\ddot{y} = 0$, consequently $y\ddot{y} = \frac{a\dot{y}\dot{y} - 2y\dot{y}\dot{y}}{y - a}$. Now

if

if we substitute these Values of xx and yy, in the general Theorem $yy = xx + yy$, there will arise this Equation

$$\frac{ryy - 2yyy}{y - a} = \frac{4y^4yy - 8ry^3yy}{aarr} + \frac{4rryyyy + rraayy}{aarr},$$

which, by the Reduction, will give $4y^5 - 12ry^4 + 12rry^3 - 4rrryy + 3rraay - 2r^3aa = 0$, and one of the Values of the Root y will be equal to D E.

It is manifest that the Curve A E K, which may be called a Parabolical Spiral, must have a Point of Inflexion E, for because the Circumference of the Circle A B C does not at first sensibly differ from the Tangent in A, it follows, from the Nature of the Parabola, that it must at first be Concave towards the Tangent, and afterwards, when the Curvature of the Circumference becomes sensible about that Centre, it must become Concave towards the said Curve.

SECT. IV.

Of the Use of FLUXIONS *in finding the* Evoluta *of a given Curve.*

DEFINITION.

LET A B C D represent a given Curve, and supposing the Point D fixed, let the Curve be imagined to unbend itself uniformly, beginning at the Point A, and conceive the Point A, at the same time to move according to the Direction A G, in such a manner, that the several Distances E B, F C, G D of the Point A from the Curve A B C D may be always equal to the respective Portions A B, A C, A D of the same Curve intercepted between the Points B, C, D, and the Point A, then the Curve Line A E F G is called the Involute Curve, or Curve of Evolution, as is the Curve

A B C D, first given, called the *Evoluta*, or Evolute of the Curve A E F G

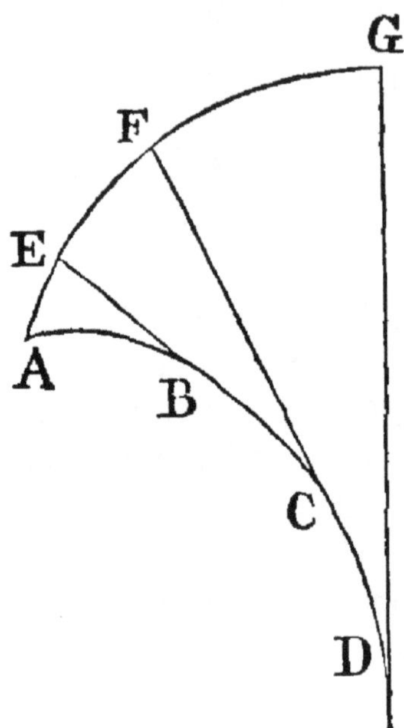

The Lines B E, C F, which are always equal to the intercepted Portions B A, C E of the *Evoluta*, are call'd the Radii of the Curvature of the Involute Curve in the Points E, F, and consequently every Ray of the *Evoluta*, as C F, is equal to C B A, the Portion of the Curve evolved; whence it follows *First*, That these Radii B E, C F, D G, become Tangents to the *Evoluta* in the several Points B, C, D, and Perpendiculars to the several Points E, F, G, in the involute Curve A E F G, where they intersect it, as is evident from the Generation of the Curve of Evolution.

Secondly, That the Ray D G, the Tangent to the *Evoluta* in the Extreme Point of it, D is equal to the whole Curve Line A B C D.

Thirdly, And because the Curvature of Circles are in a reciprocal Ratio of their respective Rays, it follows, that the Curvature of the involute Curve A E F G, in the Point E, is to the Curvature of the same Curve in the Point F reciprocally as the Ray B E to the Ray C F, or as the Ray C F is to the Ray B E whence it is evident, that the nearer the Point F (supposing it in a State of flowing) approaches the Point G, the lesser will be the Curvature of the Curve A F E G, 'till at last, when the Point F coincides with the Point G, it will be least of all, and consequently a *Minimum* Again, the nearer the Point F (supposing it still in a State of flowing) approaches to the Point A, the greater will be the Curvature, 'till at last, when the Point F arrives at or coincides with the Point A, the Curvature

vature of the involute Curve A E F G will be the greatest, or a *Maximum*

How from any Curve A E F G, considered as an involute Curve supposed to be known or given, to find its *Evoluta* A B C D, shall be fully exemplified in the Course of this *Section.*

PROBLEM I

THE Nature of the Curve A C F being given, together with the Position of a Perpendicular C H in the Point C, to find the Length of the Ray C H of the Evolute Curve

LET A D be the Axis of the Curve A C F, C B an Ordinate at right Angles to it, from H, the Extremity of the Ray CH, draw H E parallel to the Axis A B D, to meet the Ordinate C B produced in E, then will the Triangles V B C and C E H be similar (for the Angles at B and E are right Angles, and the Angles E C H and C V B are equal to each other) wherefore putting A B $= x$, B C $= y$, the Arch A C $= v$, and C F $= z$, it will be (by *Prop* II of *Sect.* I. *Part* II) as

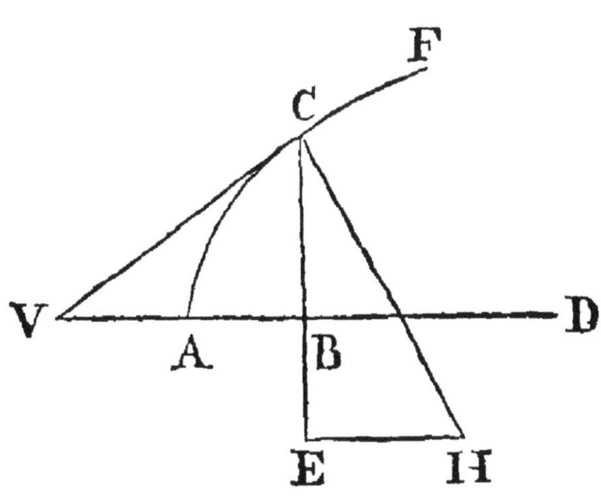

$x \quad v \quad$ BV VC CE CH, but $\dot{v} = \overline{x x + y y}^{\frac{1}{2}}$ (by *Prop* III. of *Sect* I of *Part* III) wherefore $x \quad \overline{x x + y y}^{\frac{1}{2}}$

$$z \quad \frac{z \times \overline{x x + y y}^{\frac{1}{2}}}{x} = \text{C H},$$ whence supposing $\dot{x}$ a constant

Quantity) $\dot{z} \times \overline{x x + y y}^{\frac{1}{2}} + z \times \frac{1}{2} \overline{x x + y y}^{-\frac{1}{2}} \; 2 \; y \; y$ divided by $\dot{x}$, or $\dot{z} \times \overline{xx+yy} + \frac{zy\dot{y}}{\overline{xx+yy}|^{\frac{1}{2}}}$ divided by $\dot{x}$, that is $\frac{\dot{z}xx+\dot{z}yy+zy\dot{y}}{\dot{x}\times\overline{xx+yy}|^{\frac{1}{2}}} = 0$, whence $z = \frac{\dot{z}xx+\dot{z}yy}{-\dot{y}y}$ $= \frac{x\dot{x}+yy}{-y} =$ C E (by putting y in the room of z), but because as $x : v :: $ C E : C H (by the preceding Part of the Demonstration) if we substitute $\overline{xx+yy}|^{\frac{1}{2}}$ in the room of z, and $\frac{xx+yy}{-y}$ in the room of C E (to which it has been proved to be equal) we shall have $x : \overline{xx+yy}|^{\frac{1}{2}} :: \frac{xx+yy}{-y} :$ $\frac{\overline{xx+yy}\times\overline{xx+yy}|^{\frac{1}{2}}}{-xy} = \frac{\overline{xx+yy}|^{\frac{3}{2}}}{-xy} =$ C H, for the Ray of the *Evoluta* of the Curve A C F

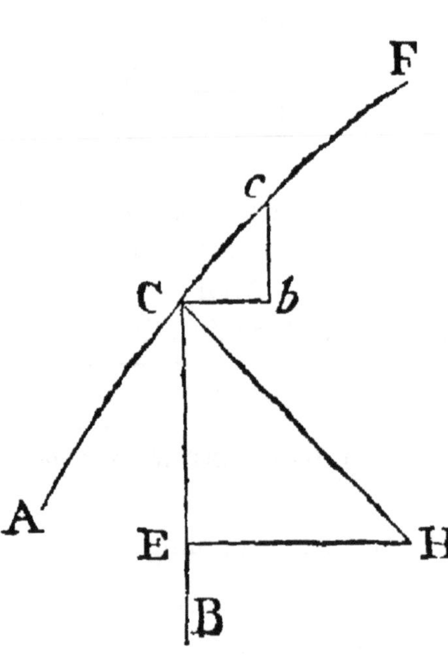

BUT if the Ordinates B C issue from the same Point H, draw H E perpendicular to C B, and let C$b$$c$ represent the nascent or fluxionary Triangle, which, because of the Equality of the Angles cCb, and E C H, cbC and C E H, will be similar to the Triangle CEH, and putting C E $= z$, C B $= y$, then will Cc be equal to $\overline{\dot{x}\dot{x}+\dot{y}\dot{y}}|^{\frac{1}{2}}$, and H E $= \frac{z\dot{y}}{\dot{x}}$, for as C$b$: bc :: C E : E H

EH, and because as Cb : Cc :: EC : CH, it will be as $\dot{x} : \overline{\dot{x}\dot{x}+\dot{y}\dot{y}}^{\frac{1}{2}} :: z : CH$, whence $CH = \frac{z \times \overline{\dot{x}\dot{x}+\dot{y}\dot{y}}^{\frac{1}{2}}}{\dot{x}}$, whence $\dot{z} \times \overline{\dot{x}\dot{x}+\dot{y}\dot{y}}^{\frac{1}{2}} + z \times \frac{1}{2}\overline{\dot{x}\dot{x}+\dot{y}\dot{y}}^{-\frac{1}{2}} 2\dot{y}\ddot{y} = \dot{z} \times \overline{\dot{x}\dot{x}+\dot{y}\dot{y}}^{\frac{1}{2}} + \frac{z\dot{y}\ddot{y}}{\overline{\dot{x}\dot{x}+\dot{y}\dot{y}}^{\frac{1}{2}}}$ divided by $\dot{x}$, supposed to be a constant Quantity, will give $\frac{\dot{z}\dot{x}^2+\dot{z}\dot{y}^2+z\dot{y}\ddot{y}}{\dot{x}\times\overline{\dot{x}\dot{x}+\dot{y}\dot{y}}^{\frac{1}{2}}} = 0$, whence $z = \frac{\dot{z}\dot{x}\dot{x}+\dot{z}\dot{y}\dot{y}}{-\dot{y}\ddot{y}}$, but $y : \frac{z\dot{y}}{\dot{x}} :: \dot{x} : \frac{z\dot{y}}{y}$, and $\dot{z} = \frac{y\dot{y}-z\dot{y}}{y}$, wherefore $z = \frac{\dot{z}\dot{x}\dot{x}+\dot{z}\dot{y}\dot{y}}{-\dot{y}\ddot{y}} = \frac{y\dot{x}\dot{x}+y\dot{y}\dot{y}-z\dot{x}\dot{x}-z\dot{y}\dot{y}}{-y\ddot{y}}$; consequently $-zy\ddot{y}+z\dot{x}\dot{x}+z\dot{y}\dot{y} = y\dot{x}\dot{x}+y\dot{y}\dot{y}$, and $z = \frac{y\dot{x}\dot{x}+y\dot{y}\dot{y}}{\dot{x}\dot{x}+\dot{y}\dot{y}-y\ddot{y}}$. Now if we suppose the Ordinate y to be infinite, the Terms $\dot{x}\dot{x}$ and $\dot{y}\dot{y}$ will vanish, and this last Form will coincide with the preceding Form.

AGAIN, because of the Similitude of the Triangles Cbc, CEH, we shall have as Cb : Cc :: CE : CH, that is, it will be $\dot{x} : \overline{\dot{x}\dot{x}+\dot{y}\dot{y}}^{\frac{1}{2}} :: \frac{y\dot{x}\dot{x}+y\dot{y}\dot{y}}{\dot{x}\dot{x}+\dot{y}\dot{y}-y\ddot{y}} : \frac{y\dot{x}\dot{x}+y\dot{y}\dot{y}\times\overline{\dot{x}\dot{x}+\dot{y}\dot{y}}^{\frac{1}{2}}}{\dot{x}\dot{x}\dot{x}+\dot{y}\dot{y}\dot{x}-\dot{x}y\ddot{y}}$ the Value of the Ray CH: whence it follows, That one Curve can have but one *Evoluta*, because the Value of CE or CH is but one and the same.

If the Value of CE $= \frac{\dot{x}\dot{x}+\dot{y}\dot{y}}{-\ddot{y}}$ (in the first Case where the Ordinates are supposed parallel) or $\frac{y\dot{x}\dot{x}+y\dot{y}\dot{y}}{\dot{x}^2+\dot{y}^2-y\ddot{y}}$ (in the

second

ſecond Caſe, where they are ſuppoſed to iſſue from a Point) be poſitive, we muſt take the Point E on the ſame Side with the Axis A D, or the Point B, as has been ſuppoſed in the preceding Inveſtigation. Whence it is alſo evident, that the Curve will be Concave toward the ſame Point or Axis, but if the Value of C E be negative, the Point E muſt be taken on the Side of the Curve oppoſite to the Axis A D, and then the Curve will be Convex towards the Axis A D, or Point B.

Now if the Nature of the Curve be given, we may get the Values of $y y$ and y in $\dot{x} x$, or of $x x$ and y in $\dot{y} y$, which being ſubſtituted in the preceding Forms, there will ariſe an Expreſſion for C E freed from Fluxions; and then drawing E H perpendicular to C E, it will cut C H, the Perpendicular to the Curve, in the Point H; whence the Length of the Ray of Evolution will be determined.

Now if we ſuppoſe A C K (*See the following Figure*) to be a Curve of Evolution, whoſe Axis A D is at right Angles to the Tangent in the Point A, and it be required to find the Point R, wherein the ſaid Axis touches the *Evoluta* R H.

If the Point C be ſuppoſed to be infinitely near the Vertex A, it is manifeſt, that the Perpendicular C Q will interſect the Axis in the required Point R, whence if you would find the Value in general of $B R = \frac{y y}{x}$ in x or y, and afterwards you make x or $y = 0$, we may determine the Point B, which is to coincide with A, and the Point Q, which coincides with the Point R required, that is, B Q will then become equal to A R, as will be more fully explained in the Sequel of this *Section*.

EXAM-

EXAMPLE I.

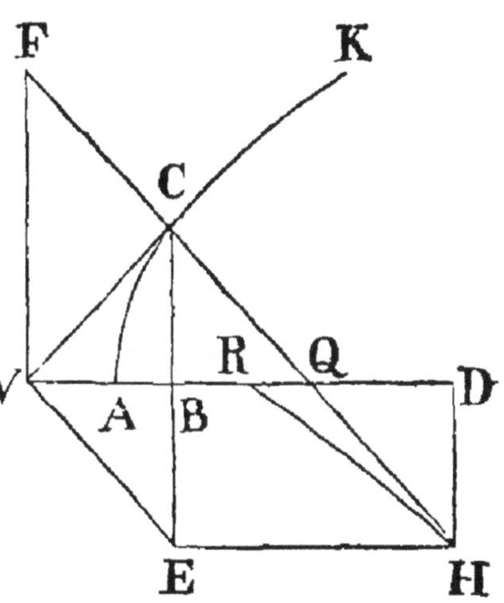

Let ACK be a Parabola, AD its Axis, and supposing the Line CQH to be drawn perpendicular to the Curve in the Point C, let it be required to determine the Point H in the *Evoluta* of the Parabola. Put AB $= x$, BC $= y$, the Parameter $= a$, then will $ax = yy$, from the Nature of the Curve, and $a\dot{x} = 2y\dot{y}$, and $\dot{y} = \frac{a\dot{x}}{2y} = \frac{a\dot{x}}{2\times\overline{ax}^{\frac{1}{2}}}$ (by putting $\overline{ax}^{\frac{1}{2}}$ in the room of y, to which it is equal) and taking again the Fluxion of this last Expression, we shall have (supposing $\dot{x}$ a constant Quantity) $\ddot{y} = \frac{a\dot{x}\times -\frac{1}{2}\overline{ax}^{-\frac{3}{2}}\times a\dot{x}}{2} = \frac{-a\dot{x}\dot{x}}{4x\times\overline{ax}^{\frac{1}{2}}}$, and substituting these Values in the room of $\dot{y}$ and $\ddot{y}$, in the general Equation $\frac{\dot{x}\dot{x}+\dot{y}\dot{y}}{-\ddot{y}}$, we shall have CE $= \frac{\overline{a+4x\times\overline{ax}^{\frac{1}{2}}}}{a} = \overline{ax}^{\frac{1}{2}} + \frac{4x\times\overline{ax}^{\frac{1}{2}}}{a}$ Whence we have the following Construction.

From the Point V, in which the Tangent CV cuts the Axis, draw VE parallel to CH, I say, it will intersect the Line CB produced in E, the Point required for the Angles CBV

C B V and C V E, being right Angles, as C B B V V B. B E, that is, as $\overline{4x}^{\frac{1}{2}}$ $2x$ $2x$ $\frac{4xx}{\overline{ax}^{\frac{1}{2}}}$ = B E = $\frac{4x\times\overline{ax}^{\frac{1}{2}}}{a}$ (for $\frac{ax}{\overline{ax}^{\frac{1}{2}}}=\overline{ax}^{\frac{1}{2}}$, and $\frac{x}{\overline{ax}^{\frac{1}{2}}}=\frac{\overline{ax}^{\frac{1}{2}}}{a}$) and consequently C B + B E = C E = $\overline{ax}^{\frac{1}{2}}+\frac{\overline{4x}\times\overline{ax}^{\frac{1}{2}}}{a}$

Again, because the Triangles C B Q and C E H are similar, as B C B Q C E E H, that is, as $\overline{ax}^{\frac{1}{2}}$ $\frac{1}{2}a$ $\overline{ax}^{\frac{1}{2}}+\frac{\overline{4x}\times\overline{ax}^{\frac{1}{2}}}{a}$ E H = B D = $\frac{1}{2}a+2x$, and consequently Q D is equal to $2x$ From whence we get this new Construction; Take Q D, the Double of A B, or (which is the same) take B D = V Q, and draw D H parallel to C E, this will meet the Perpendicular C H in the Point H, which will be in the *Evoluta* R H

Now to find the Point R, where the Axis A D touches the Evolute R H, we have B Q = $\frac{yy}{x}=\frac{1}{2}a$; and since this Quantity is invariable, the Subnormal R Q will always be the same, whatever Point of the Curve C is in; and consequently when C coincides with A, then B will coincide with A, and Q will coincide with R, and A R will be equal to $\frac{1}{2}a$ = B Q, that is, the Vertex of the *Evoluta* R H is distant from the Vertex of the Parabola $\frac{1}{2}$ of the Parameter of the Parabola

And to investigate the Nature of the *Evoluta* R H, put the intercepted Diameter R D = z, the Ordinate B E or D H = v, whence D H = $v=\frac{\overline{4x}\times\overline{ax}^{\frac{1}{2}}}{a}$, and A B + B D — A R = $z=3x$, and consequently $\frac{1}{3}z=x$, and substituting $\frac{1}{3}z$ in the room of x, in the Equation, $v=\frac{\overline{4x}\times\overline{ax}^{\frac{1}{2}}}{a}$, we

shall

shall have $27avv = 16z$, which expresses the Relation of RD to DH, and shews that RH, the *Evoluta* of the Parabola, is a Cubical Paraboloid, whose Parameter is $\frac{27}{16}$ of the Parameter of the Parabola.

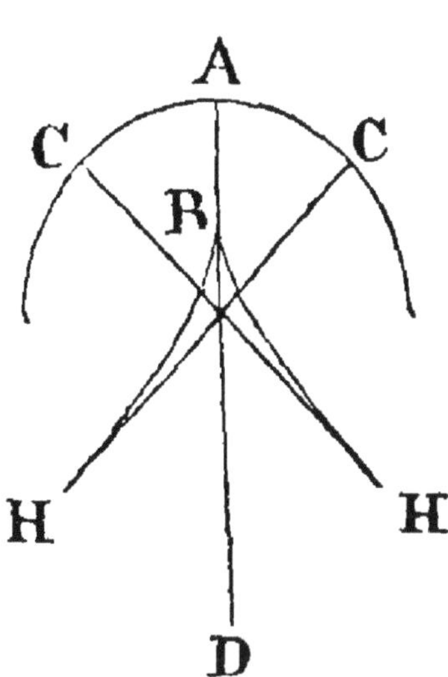

IT is evident, that if the Curve of Evolution CAC be a whole Parabola, as in the adjacent Figure, the *Evoluta* HRH will consist of two Parts HR, HR, having contrary Convexities, so that R will be the Point of Retrogression.

EXAMPLE II.

LET the Curve of Evolution be an Hyperbola within its Asymptotes, and let it be required to determine the Point H in the *Evoluta*. (*See the following Figure.*)

LET CAC represent an Hyperbola AD, AM its Asymptotes, CH the Ray of the *Evoluta*.

PUT $AB = x$, $BC = y$, and the Parameter $= a$, and because, from the Nature of the Curve $aa = xy$, we shall have $x = \frac{aa}{y}$, and $x = \frac{-aay}{yy}$, and supposing x a constant Quantity, the Fluxion of this last Quantity $\frac{-aayyy + 2aayyy}{y^4} = 0$. Whence $-aay^2y + 2aayy^2 = 0$, and $2aayy = aay^2y$, and dividing each Part by aay, we shall have

$2y^2 = yy$, and $y = \frac{2yy}{y}$, and putting this Value in the

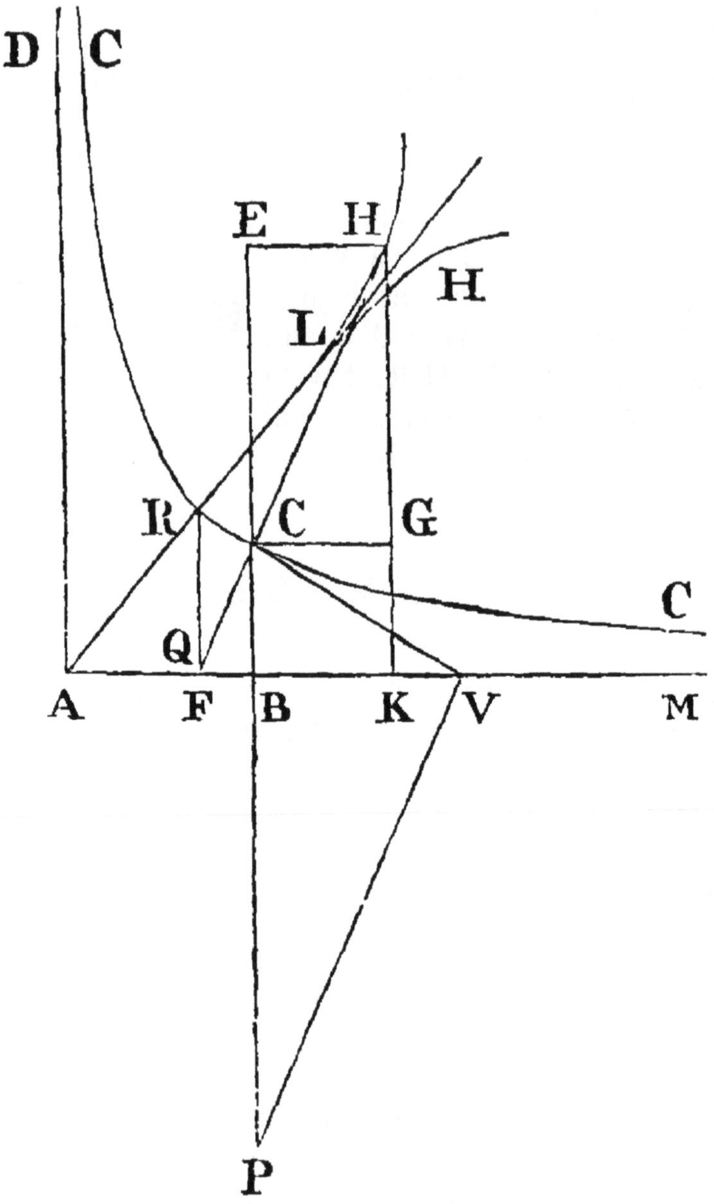

room of y in the general Equation $\frac{xx + yy}{-y}$, we shall have

— 2

$\frac{y}{-2yy} \times \frac{xx+yy}{1} = \frac{yxx+yyy}{-2yy} =$ C E And because the Triangles C B Q and E C H are similar, it will be as C B B Q C E E H, that is, as x y $\frac{yxx+yy\dot{y}}{-2yy}$ $\frac{-yy}{2x}$ $-\frac{yx}{2y} =$ E H or B K, and hence arises the following Construction.

THROUGH the Point V, where the Tangent C V cuts the Asymptote A M, draw V P parallel to C H, until it intersect C B produced in P, take C E equal to half C P, on the opposite Side of the Curve, in respect of the Asymptote A M, which is instead of an Axis, because the Value of C E is negative, or take B K = ½ Q V on the same Side of the Ordinate with V I say, if E H be drawn parallel to A M, or K H be drawn perpendicular to A M, either of them will intersect the Ray CH in H, the Point required, for it is evident, that V Q $= \frac{yy}{x} + \frac{yx}{y}$, because as y x y $\frac{yx}{y} =$ B V, and x y y $\frac{yy}{x} =$ B Q, and C P $= \frac{yxx+yyy}{yy}$, because C B $= y$; and as y $\dot{x}$ C B B V $= \left(\frac{yx}{y}\right)$ C V V P $= \frac{yx\dot{x}}{yy}$, whence C B + B P $= \frac{yxx+yyy}{yy} =$ 2 C E.

FROM an Inspection of the Figure of the Hyperbola C R C it will appear that the *Evoluta* H L H will have a Point of Retrogression L, in like manner as the *Evoluta* of the Parabola.

Now to determine the Point L, the Vertex of the *Evoluta*, or the Point of Retrogression, it must be observed that the Ray of the *Evoluta* R L is the shortest; whence it follows, that the Fluxion of $\frac{\overline{\dot x\dot x+\dot y\dot y}\times\overline{\dot x\dot x+\dot y\dot y}^{\frac{1}{2}}}{-\dot x\ddot y}=\frac{\overline{\dot x\dot x+\dot y\dot y}^{\frac{3}{2}}}{-\dot x\ddot y}$ will be equal to o, and consequently supposing $\dot x$ a constant Quantity $\frac{-3\,\overline{\dot x\dot x+\dot y\dot y}^{\frac{1}{2}}\times\dot x\dot y\ddot y\ddot y}{\dot x\dot x\ddot y^{2}}+\frac{\dot x\dddot y\times\overline{\dot x\dot x+\dot y\dot y}^{\frac{3}{2}}}{\dot x\dot x\ddot y^{2}}=0$, whence $-3\,\overline{\dot x\dot x+\dot y\dot y}^{\frac{1}{2}}\times\dot x\dot y\ddot y^{2}+\dot x\dddot y\times\overline{\dot x\dot x+\dot y\dot y}^{\frac{3}{2}}=0$, and dividing by $\overline{\dot x\dot x+\dot y\dot y}^{\frac{1}{2}}$, we shall have $\frac{-3\dot x\dot y\ddot y^{2}+\dot x\dddot y\times\overline{\dot x\dot x+\dot y\dot y}}{\dot x}=0$, and dividing again by $\dot x$, there will arise $-3\dot y\ddot y^{2}+\dddot y\times\overline{\dot x\dot x+\dot y\dot y}=0$, which Equation will serve to find A F, the Value of the Absciss. So that drawing the Ordinate R F, and the Ray of the *Evoluta* R L, the Point L will be the Point of Retrogression.

Thus in the present Example $y=\frac{aa}{x}$, and $\dot y=\frac{-aa\dot x}{xx}$, and $\ddot y=\frac{-2aa\dot x^{2}}{xxx}$, and $\dddot y=\frac{-6aa\dot x^{3}}{x^{4}}$, and substituting these Quantities in the Equation $\dot x\dot x\dddot y+\dot y^{2}\dddot y-3\dot y\ddot y^{2}=0$, we shall have $\frac{-6aa\dot x^{5}}{x^{4}}-\frac{6a^{6}\dot x^{5}}{x^{8}}+\frac{12a^{6}\dot x^{5}}{x^{8}}=0$, and multiplying by x^{8}, and dividing by $aa\dot x^{5}$, we shall have $-6x^{4}-6a^{4}+12a^{4}=0$, that is, $6x^{4}=6a^{4}$, that is, $a^{4}=x^{4}$, consequently $a=x=$ AF, whence it follows, that the Point R is the Vertex of the Hyperbola, and that the Lines A R, R L, make but one straight Line A L, which is the Axis of the Hyperbola, and the Point of Retrogression L is in the said Axis, and may be determined by the foregoing general Construction.

EXAM

EXAMPLE III

LET the general Equation $x = y^m$ express the Nature of all sorts of Paraboloids, when the Exponent m is a positive Number, whole or broken, and all sorts of Hyperboloides, when m represents a negative Number; and let it be required to find a general Theorem expressing the Value of the Ray of the Curvature of all such Curves.

BECAUSE $x = y^m$, therefore $\dot{x} = my^{m-1}\dot{y}$, and finding again the Fluxion of this Fluxion (supposing $\dot{x}$ a constant Quantity), we shall have $\overline{mm - m}\,y^{m-2}\dot{y}^2 + my^{m-1}\ddot{y} = 0$, and dividing by my^{m-1}, there will arise $-\ddot{y} - \overline{m-1}\,y^{-1}\dot{y}^2 = 0$, whence $-\ddot{y} = \overline{m-1}\,y^{-1}\dot{y}^2$, and $\ddot{y} = \frac{\overline{m-1}\,\dot{y}^2}{y}$, and substituting this Value in the general Equation $\frac{\dot{x}\dot{x} + \dot{y}\dot{y}}{-\ddot{y}}$, we shall have $\frac{y}{\overline{m-1} \times \dot{y}\dot{y}} \times \frac{\dot{x}\dot{x} + \dot{y}\dot{y}}{1} = \frac{y\dot{x}\dot{x} + y\dot{y}\dot{y}}{\overline{m-1} \times \dot{y}\dot{y}} = CE$, and consequently $LH = \frac{y\dot{y}}{\overline{m-1}\,\dot{x}} + \frac{y\dot{x}}{\overline{m-1}\,\dot{y}}$, whence arises this general Construction.

THROUGH the Point V (*See the Figure to Example* I) in which the Tangent CV cuts the Axis, draw VE parallel to CH until it intersect CB produced in E, and then take $CI = \frac{1}{m-1}$ of the Distance between this Intersection and the Point C (which, if m be negative, or a Fraction, will be negative) or take $BD = \frac{1}{m-1}$ VQ, then it is evident, that if through the Point E we draw a Line parallel to the Axis AD, or through the Point D we draw a Perpendicular to the same Axis AD, they will intersect the Ray CH in the Point

Point H, the required Point in the *Evoluta*, for C S is equal to $\frac{y x x - y y y}{y y}$, therefore $\frac{1}{m-1}$ C S is equal to $\frac{y x x + y y y}{\overline{m-1}\, y y}$ and Q V is equal to $\frac{y x}{y} + \frac{y y}{x}$, therefore Q V is equal to $\frac{y x}{\overline{m-1}\, y} + \frac{y y}{\overline{m-1}\, x}$.

EXAMPLE IV.

LET the Curve A C be an Hyperbola, or an Ellipsis whose Axis, or transverse Diameter A E, is equal to a, and Parameter equal to b, and let it be required to find the Ray C H of the *Evoluta* R H

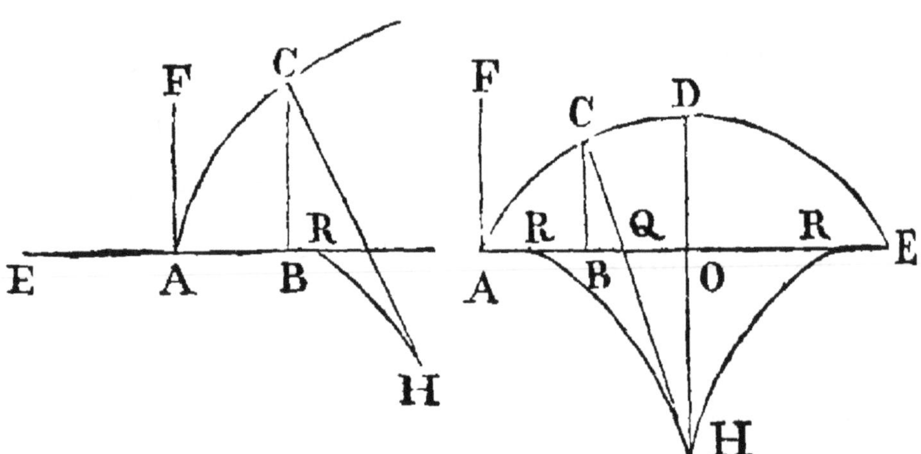

BECAUSE the Equation, expressing the Nature of the Curve, is $y = \frac{\overline{a b x \mp b x x}^{\frac{1}{2}}}{a^{\frac{1}{2}}}$, we shall have y equal to $\frac{a b x \mp 2 b x x}{\overline{2 a a b x \mp a b x x}^{\frac{1}{2}}}$, and putting p equal to the Numerator,

and

and q equal to the Denominator $y = \frac{p}{q}$, and $\dot{y} = \frac{q\dot{p} - p\dot{q}}{qq}$
$= \frac{-aaabbx\dot{x}}{\overline{4aabx \mp 4abxx} \times \overline{aabx}^{\frac{1}{2}} \mp abxx}$ (by putting for p and q their Values) and substituting this last Quantity in the general Equation $\frac{\overline{\dot{x}\dot{x}+\dot{y}\dot{y}} \times \overline{\dot{x}\dot{x}+\dot{y}\dot{y}}^{\frac{1}{2}}}{-\dot{x}\ddot{y}} = \frac{\overline{\dot{x}\dot{x}+\dot{y}\dot{y}}^{\frac{3}{2}}}{-\dot{x}\ddot{y}} = CH$,
we shall have $CH = \frac{\overline{aabb \mp 4abbx + 4bbxx + 4aabx \mp 4abxx}}{2aaabb}$
$\times \frac{\overline{aabb \mp 4aabx + 4bbxx + 4aabx \mp 4abxx}^{\frac{1}{2}}}{2aaabb}$ equal
(because $CQ = \frac{y \times \overline{\dot{x}\dot{x}+\dot{y}\dot{y}}^{\frac{1}{2}}}{\dot{x}} = \frac{\overline{aabb \mp 4abbx + 4bbxx}}{2a}$
$\frac{\overline{+4aabx + 4abxx}^{\frac{1}{2}}}{2a}$) $\frac{4CQ^3}{bb}$, whence arises the following Construction.

FIND a fourth continual Proportional to the Parameter b, and the Perpendicular CQ, by making b, CQ, $\frac{CQ^2}{b}$, $\frac{CQ^3}{bb}$ continued Proportionals, and multiplying the last Proportional $\frac{CQ^3}{bb}$ by 4, we shall have $\frac{4CQ^3}{bb} = CH$, for the Ray of the *Evoluta*, whence H is a Point in the *Evoluta* to be found. Whence it follows.

First, If x be put equal to 0, then the Radius of the Curvature AR will be $\frac{1}{2}b$, or the Parameter: and in the Ellipsis, if we suppose $x = \frac{1}{2}a$, the Transverse Axis, then the Radius of the Curvature DH will be $\frac{a \times \overline{ab}^{\frac{1}{2}}}{2b}$ equal to half the Parameter of the ſhorteſt, or Conjugate Diameter, whence it is evident in the Ellipſis, that the *Evoluta* R H terminates in the Point H in the ſhorteſt Axis D O, but in the Parabola and Hyperbola, it runs out infinitely

Secondly, In the Ellipſis, if $a = b$, then C H $= \frac{1}{2} a$ is a conſtant Quantity, whence it follows, that all the Rays of the *Evoluta* are equal between themſelves, which conſequently can be but a ſingle Point, that is, the Ellipſis, in ſuch a Caſe, degenerates into a Circle, whoſe *Evoluta* is its Centre.

EXAMPLE V.

LET A C D be the common Logarithmetick Curve, the Nature whereof is ſuch, that drawing (from any Point in the Curve C) the Line C B perpendicular to the Aſymptote KQ and CV, touching the Curve in the Point C, and interſecting the Aſymptote in V, the Subtangent B V will be always equal to a conſtant Quantity a.

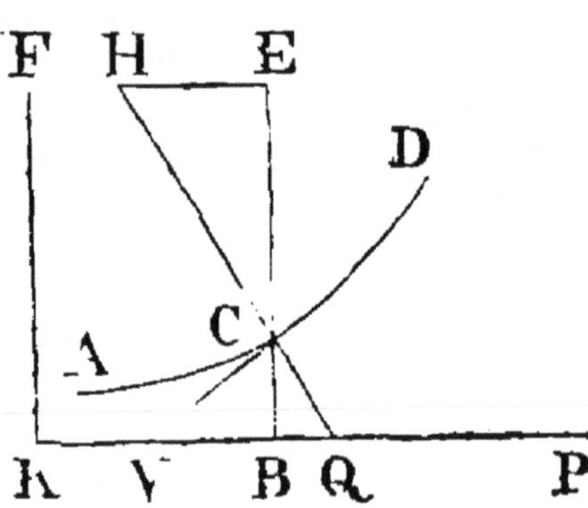

Now becauſe as y x y a, (putting the Ordinate BC $= y$ (by *Prop* I *Sect* I. *Part* II) therefore B V $= a = \frac{y x}{y}$, whence $y = \frac{y x}{a}$, and $y = \frac{y x^2}{a} = \frac{y x^2}{a a}$, by ſubſtituting $\frac{y x}{a}$ in the room of y, and ſuppoſing x a conſtant Quantity, but C E is equal to $\frac{\overline{x x + y y}}{-y}$ by the general Equation,

whence

whence $CE = \frac{-aa-yy}{y}$, by substituting $\frac{yyxx}{aa}$ in the room of yy, and $\frac{yxx}{aa}$ in the room of y, and consequently, because as $VB : BC :: BC : BQ$; that is, as $a : y :: y : \frac{yy}{a} = BQ$, and as $CB : BQ :: CE : EH$, that is, as $y : \frac{yy}{a} :: \frac{-aa-yy}{y} : \frac{aa-yy}{a} = \frac{-aa-yy}{a}$ will be equal to EH, whence we have the following Construction.

TAKE $BK = QV$, on the same Side of the Ordinate with the Point V (because its Value is negative) and draw KF parallel to BC, until it intersect the Perpendicular to the Curve CH in H, a Point in the *Evoluta*. For VB $= a$, and $BQ = \frac{yy}{a}$, and consequently VQ is equal to $\frac{aa+yy}{a}$.

EXAMPLE VI.

LET ACK be the Logarithmetick Spiral Line, and let it be required to investigate the Value of the Ray CH of the *Evoluta*.

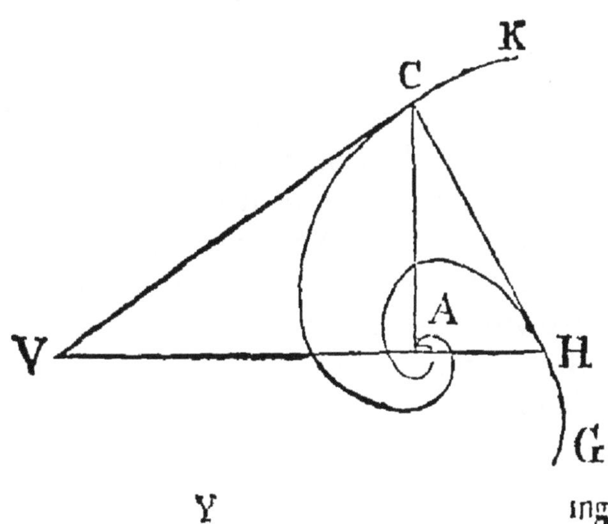

INASMUCH as the Nature of the said Curve is such, that drawing from any Point of the Curve, as C, the right Line C A to the Centre A, and the Tangent C V, the Angle A C V will always be the ſame.

AND becauſe the Angle A C V is a conſtant Quantity, the Ratio of the Fluxion of the Ordinate, to the Fluxion of the Abſciſs, will be a conſtant Ratio (*Prop* I. *Sect.* I *of Part* II) and conſequently $\frac{\dot{\dot{y}}}{\dot{x}} = 0$, whence $\ddot{y}$ (ſuppoſing $\dot{x}$ a conſtant Quantity) will be equal to nothing, and conſequently the general Equation $\frac{y\dot{x}\dot{x}+y\dot{y}\dot{y}}{\dot{x}\dot{x}+\dot{y}\dot{y}-y\ddot{y}}=$ C E will become $\frac{y\dot{x}\dot{x}+y\dot{y}\dot{y}}{\dot{x}\dot{x}+\dot{y}\dot{y}}$ (ſince the Quantity $y\ddot{y}$ will vaniſh) and this being divided by $\dot{x}\dot{x}+\dot{y}\dot{y}$, the Quotient y will be the Value of C E, that is, C E will be equal to C A, from whence we have the following Conſtruction

DRAW A H perpendicular to A C, and C H perpendicular to the Curve in the Point C, then the mutual Interſection of theſe two Lines will give the Point H a Point in the *Evoluta*, whence it follows

Firſt, THAT the Angles A C V and A H C are equal, for each is the Complement of the Angle A C H Therefore the *Evoluta* A H G is alſo a Logarithmic Spiral Line, and the Curves A C K and A H G differ only in Poſition.

Secondly, IF a Point H in the *Evoluta* A H G be given, and it be required to find the Length of the Ray C H equal to the Portion of the Curve A H (which makes an infinite Number of Revolutions before it terminates in the Centre) draw A C perpendicular to A H, until it interſect the Tangent H C in C, then is H C equal to A H, the Portion of the Spiral evolved; and if A V be drawn perpendicular to A C, then is the Tangent C V equal to the Portion A C of the given Spiral Line.

EXAM

EXAMPLE VII

LET ACD be one of the infinite Sort of Spiral Lines formed in the Sector of a Circle PAD, and let it be required to find the Length of the Ray of the *Evoluta* CH.

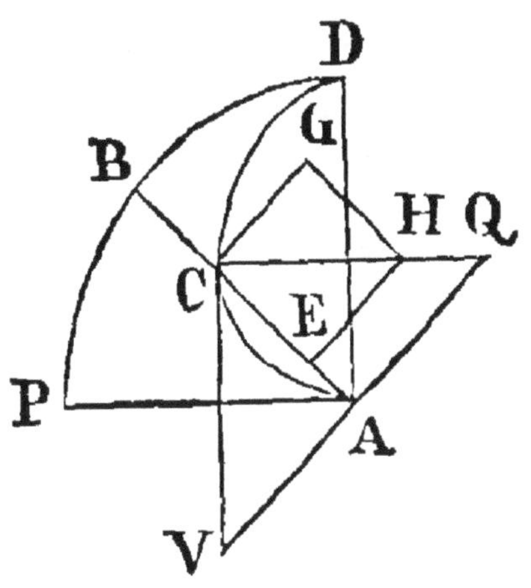

PUT the whole Arch PBD $= b$, $PB = z$, $AP = AB = a$, and $AC = y$, and let the Equation, expressing the Nature of the Spiral Line ACD, be $y^m = \frac{a^m z}{b}$, then is $m y^{m-1} y = \frac{a^m z}{b}$, but as AC AB x z, because the Arches are in the same Ratio with their respective Rays, wherefore as y a x z, consequently $z = \frac{a x}{y}$, which being substituted in the room of z in the preceding Equation, we shall have $m y^m \dot{y} = \frac{a^{m+1} x}{b}$, and the Fluxion of the Equation (supposing x a constant Quantity) is $m m y^{m-1} y y + m y^m y = 0$, whence $m y y + y y = 0$, by dividing by $m y^{m-1}$, whence $-y y = m y y$, and consequently $CE = \frac{y \overline{x x + y y}}{x x + y y - y y}$ is equal to $\frac{y \overline{x x + y y}}{x x + \overline{m+1} y y}$ (by substituting $m y y$ in the room of $y y$, to which it is equal) the Value of CE, whence we have the following Construction.

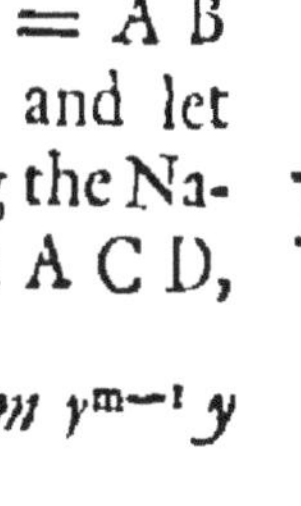

 THROUGH

THROUGH the Centre A draw the right Line V A Q perpendicular to A C, and intersecting the Tangent C V in V, and the Perpendicular to the Curve Q C in Q, then say, as $VA+\overline{m+1}\,AQ$ VQ CA CE. I say, E H drawn parallel to V Q, will intersect the Perpendicular C Q in H, the Point in the *Evoluta* required.

FOR (because the Line C G is parallel to A Q) C Q $=\frac{\overline{m+1}\,yy}{x}+x$, and as x y $\frac{yy}{x}$ $\frac{yy}{x}+x$ V A $+\overline{m+1}\,AQ$ VQ· (AC=) y CE $=\frac{yyxx+yy}{xx+\overline{m+1}\,yy}$

EXAMPLE VIII.

IF the Curve ACD be a simple Cycloid, whose Base D P is equal to the Semi-circumference of the generating Circle A E P, let it be required to find the Value of the Ray of the *Evoluta* H C.

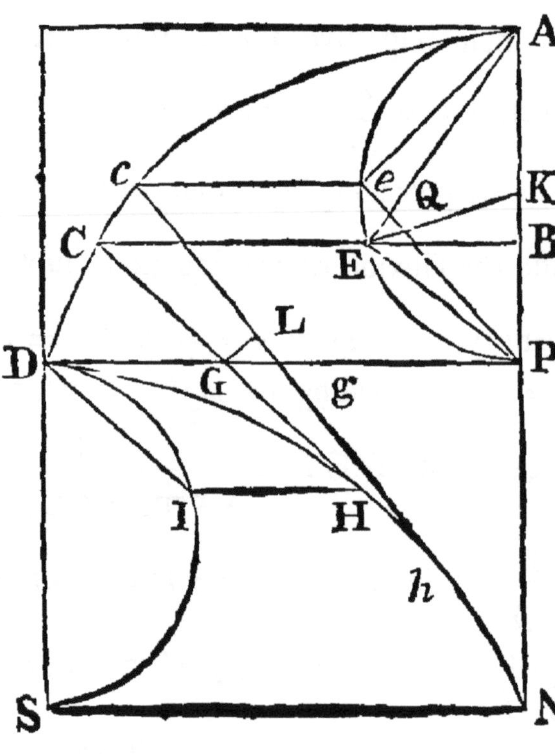

PUT A B $=x$, B C $=y$, the Arch A E $=z$, and A P $=2a$, and because, from the Nature of the Circle, B E is equal to $\overline{2ax-xx}|^{\frac{1}{2}}$ and, from the Nature of the Cycloid, B C $=y=z+$ $+\overline{2ax-xx}|^{\frac{1}{2}}$, there-

therefore $\dot y = \dot z + \frac{a\dot x - x\dot x}{\overline{2ax - xx}^{\frac{1}{2}}}$, but $\dot z = \frac{a\dot x}{\overline{2ax-xx}^{\frac{1}{2}}}$, therefore $\dot y = \frac{2a\dot x - x\dot x}{\overline{2ax-xx}^{\frac{1}{2}}} = \dot x \times \frac{2a - x}{\overline{2ax-xx}^{\frac{1}{2}}} = \dot x \times \frac{2a-x}{x^{\frac{1}{2}} \times \overline{2a-x}^{\frac{1}{2}}}$ $= \dot x \times \frac{\overline{2a-x}^{\frac{1}{2}}}{x}$ (by dividing by $\overline{2a-x}^{\frac{1}{2}}$), whence (supposing $\dot x$ a constant Quantity) $\ddot y = \frac{-a\dot x\dot x \times x^{-\frac{1}{2}}}{xx \times \overline{2a-x}^{\frac{1}{2}}} = \frac{-a\dot x\dot x}{x \times \overline{2ax-xx}^{\frac{1}{2}}}$, and substituting this Value in the general Equation, $\frac{\overline{\dot x\dot x + \dot y\dot y} \times \overline{\dot x\dot x + \dot y\dot y}^{\frac{1}{2}}}{-\dot x\ddot y} = \frac{\overline{\dot x\dot x + \dot y\dot y}^{\frac{3}{2}}}{-\dot x\ddot y}$, we shall have (because $\dot y = \dot x \times \frac{\overline{2a-x}^{\frac{1}{2}}}{x^{\frac{1}{2}}}$)

$$\frac{\overline{\frac{2a\dot x\dot x}{x}}\Big|^{\frac{3}{2}}}{-\dot x\ddot y} = \frac{\overline{\frac{8a^3\dot x^6}{x^3}}\Big|^{\frac{1}{2}}}{-\dot x\ddot y} = \frac{\overline{\frac{8a^3\dot x^6}{x^3}}\Big|^{\frac{1}{2}} \times x \times \overline{2ax-xx}^{\frac{1}{2}}}{a\dot x^3}$$

$$= \frac{\overline{\frac{8a^3}{x^3}}\Big|^{\frac{1}{2}} \times x \times \overline{2ax-xx}^{\frac{1}{2}}}{a} = \frac{\overline{\frac{16a^4x^3 - 8a^3x^4}{x^3}}\Big|^{\frac{1}{2}}}{a} =$$

$= 2 \times \overline{4aa - 2ax}^{\frac{1}{2}} = CH = (2 \times \overline{EP^2 + BP^2} = 2\,EP)$ $= 2\,CG$, because CH, perpendicular to the Curve in the Point C, is parallel to the Chord PE. From whence it follows

First, If x be supposed equal to Nothing, then is AN $= 2 \times \overline{4aa}^{\frac{1}{2}} = 4a$ equal to the Ray of the *Evoluta* on the Vertex. And if we suppose $x = 2a$, then CH is equal to $2 \times \overline{4aa - 4aa}^{\frac{1}{2}} = 0$; that is, the Ray of the *Evoluta* in D is equal to Nothing, and in A it is equal to twice the Diameter of the generating Semicircle; and hence it is evident, that

that the *Evoluta* begins in D, and ends in N; so that P N is equal to P A

Secondly, THE *Evoluta* D H N is a Semicyclod, equal to the Semicycloid A C D Compleat the Parallelogram P S, and on the Diameter D S describe the Semicircle D I S, and draw the Lines D I, C H, E P parallel to each other, then is the Angle P D I equal to the Angle E P D, and consequently the Arches D I and P E are equal, but F P = C G = G H, therefore G H = D I; and if I H be drawn, it will be equal and parallel to D G Now, by the Nature of the Cycloid, D G is equal to the Arch E P, equal to the Arch D I, and consequently the *Evoluta* D H N is a Semicycloid, whose Base is S N, equal to half the Circumference of the generating Circle D I S, that is, the *Evoluta* is equal to the given Cycloid, and the same with it, only placed in a contrary Position

Thirdly, THE Length of the Curve of the Cyclod D H N is equal to twice A P, equal to twice the Diameter of the generating Circle, and any Portion of the Cycloid, as D H is equal to twice H G, equal to twice D I, equal to twice the corresponding Chord in the generating Circle.

BUT the Length of the Ray of the *Evoluta* C H may be determined, without any Calculation, after this manner

IMAGINE the Perpendicular C H, to the Curve A C D, in the Point C, to be in a flowing State, and move into the Place C *h*, in which Time the Line C E will become *c e*, and the Chords P E and A E will become P *e* and A *e*, then will the nascent Triangles G L *g* and E Q *e* be similar and equal, for the nascent Augments G *g* and E *e* are equal (because P G = E C is equal to the Arch A E) and L *g* = *c g* − C G = E *e*, or P *e* − P E, and G L = E Q Now the Angle

Angle C h c = E P, because the Perpendiculars C H, c h, are parallel to the Chords P E, P e, and the Arches G I, E Q, the Measures of those equal Angles are also equal, inasmuch as they are generated in the same small Particle of Time, therefore their Rays H G and P E are also equal, and consequently the Ray of the *Evoluta* C H is equal to twice the Chord P E, equal to twice C G

PROPOSITION.

To find any Number of Involutes A C, B N, K F O, to a given Evolute B F H.

It is manifest, that while the given Line H F B A revolves about the fixed Point H, that the Points A, B, F will describe the Curves A C, B N, F O, to which the given Curve B F H is the common *Evoluta*; but because the Curve F O is described by the Evolution of the Part H F, it does not begin in the Point F, and in order to find where it does begin, the Part B F must be taken as the Evolute, the Point B being the fixed Centre, and beginning at F, the Part K F of the Involute K F O must be described, which begins in K, and is the Involute to the whole Curve B F H. Whence it follows

First, That the Involute Curves A C, B N, F O differ very much from each other as to their Nature, since in the Vertex A of the Curve A C, the Radius of the Evolution is equal to A B, whereas that of the Curve B N is nothing It is likewise evident, from the Figure of the Curve K F O, that it differs very much from the Curves A C, B N.

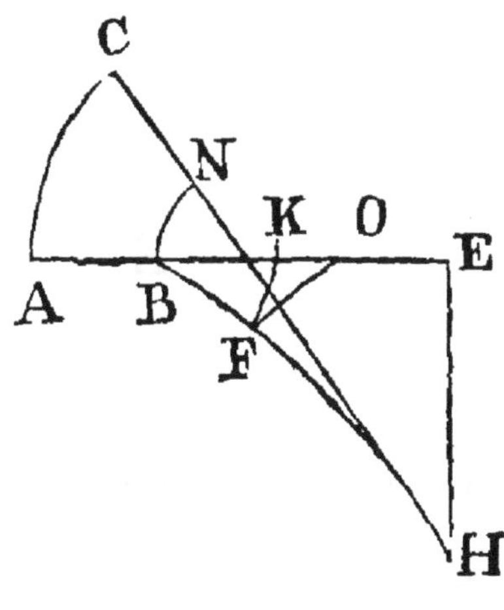

Secondly,

Secondly, THAT the Curves A C, B N, K F O, are Geometrical Curves only, when the given *Evoluta* B F H is a Geometrical Curve, and rectifiable: For if the Curve B F H be not a Geometrical Curve, when B E is assumed for an Abscis, the Ordinate E H cannot be determined Geometrically, and if it be not rectifiable, when the Tangent H C is drawn, the Points C, N, O, cannot be determined in the Curves A C, B N, K F O, because straight Lines cannot be found equal to the Curve B F H, and its Parts B F, F H.

IF the Evolute B A N M has a Point of Inflexion in A, then from the Evolution of the Part B A D, beginning at the Point D, there will be formed the Part D E F of the Invo

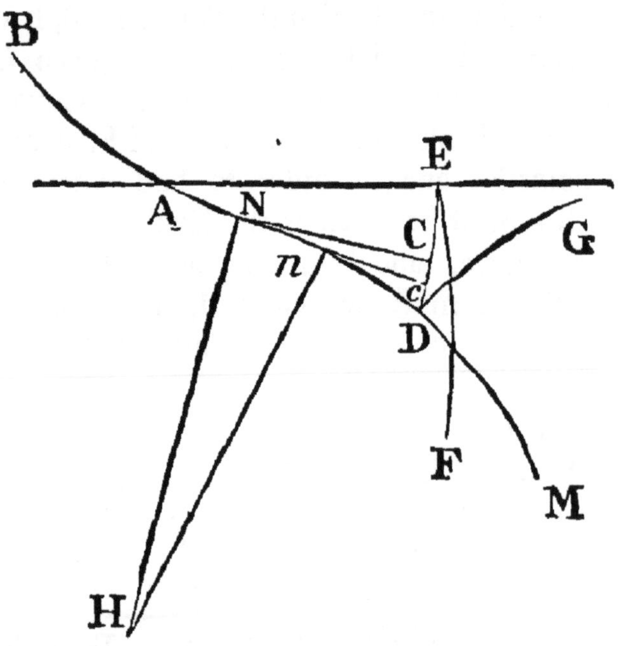

lute, and from the Evolution of the Part D M will be generated the remaining Part D G of the Involute. So that the whole Involute Curve, formed from the Evolution of the Curve B A M, will be F E D G, whence it is apparent, that this Curve has two Points, D and E, of Retrogression, with this Difference, that at D the Parts D E, D G have opposite Convexities,

vexities, and at E the Concavities of D E and E F lie in the same way. And in order to find the Point of Retrogression F which may be called a Point of Retrogression of the second Kind

FROM any Point C, in the Curve D E, draw C N a Perpendicular to it in the Point C, and from the Point N, where the Ray touches the Evolute D A B, draw a Perpendicular N H, and imagine the Lines H N and N C to flow into the Places H *n* and *n c*, then will the nascent Sectors C N *c* and N H *n* be similar, because the Angles C N *c* and N H *n* are equal, therefore as N *n* C *c* N H N C Now in the Point A of Inflexion the Ray H N becomes infinite, or vanishes, and the Ray C N, which becomes A E, continues finite, therefore in the Point E of Retrogression of the second Kind, the Ratio of the Fluxions of the Ray of Evolution C N, and of the Curve D E, which are as the nascent Augments N *n*, C *c*, will vanish, or become infinite And because the Fluxion of the Ray C N is equal to $\frac{-3xyy^2 \times \overline{x^2+y^2}^{\frac{1}{2}} + xy \times \overline{x^2+y^2}^{\frac{3}{2}}}{x^2 y^2}$, and the Fluxion of the Curve D E is $\overline{x^2+y^2}^{\frac{1}{2}}$, therefore $\frac{x^2y + y^2y - 3yy^2}{xy^2} = 0$, whence $x^2y + y^2y - 3yy^2 = 0$ Which is a general Expression for determining the Point of Retrogression of the second Kind.

NOW if an Involute D E F, or H D F F G, (*See the following Figure*) has a Point of Retrogression of the second Kind, the Evolute B A C may have a Point of Retrogression of the second Kind also, so that the second Point A of Retrogression answers to the second Point E, that is, both lie in the Ray of Evolution issuing from the Point E. Now in this Supposition it is evident, that the Ray of Evolution E A will always be a *Maximum* or a *Minimum*, and therefore the Fluxion

Z of

of $\frac{\overline{\dot{x}\dot{x}+\dot{y}\dot{y}}^{\frac{3}{2}}}{-\dot{x}\ddot{y}}$, the general Expreſſion for the Rays of Evo-

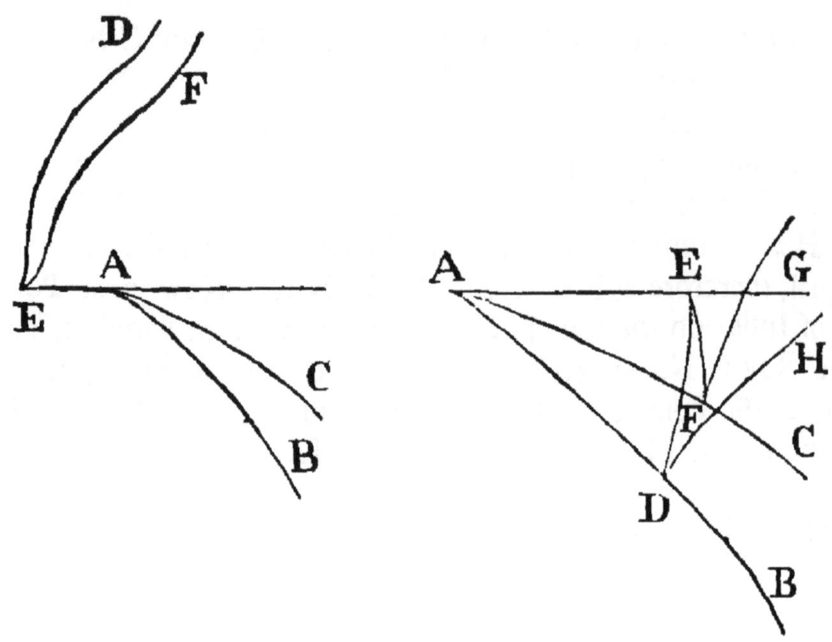

lution will vaniſh, or become infinite, whence the ſame general Expreſſion is obtained, as before, and which muſt be uſed to inveſtigate the Points of Retrogreſſion of the ſecond Kind

---

SECT. V.

Containing the Uſe of FLUXIONS *in finding the* Cauſtick Curves *by Reflection.*

LET ACD repreſent a Curve, KC a Perpendicular to the Tangent to the Point C, BC an Incident Ray iſſuing from the luminous Body B, CF the ſame Ray reflected from th-

the Point C, and F the Focal Point Now if the extreme Point C of the Ray B C be carried along the Curve A C D, and the Angle F C K, formed by the reflected Ray F C, and the Line K C, the Perpendicular to the Curve in the Point C, be in every Point of the Curve A C D equal to the Angle B C K, formed by the same Perpendicular K C, and the Incident Ray BC, the Point F will, by this means, generate the Curve Line F H, which is called the Catacaustick Curve, or Caustick Curve by Reflection.

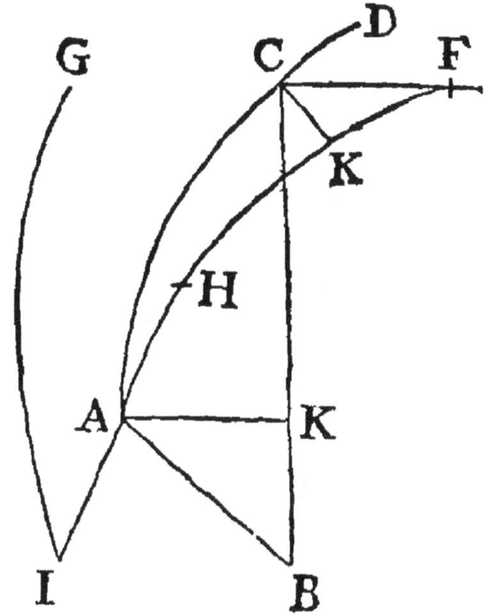

In the following *Figure* let H A be produced to I, so that A I = A B ; and if the Caustick H F N be evolved, and the Curve, described by such Evolution, begin in the Point I, the Curve I L G will be described, and the Tangent F L will always be equal to the Portion of the Caustick F H, encreased by the right Line H I.

IMAGINE the Incident Ray B C, and the reflected Ray C F in a flowing State, then will the nascent Triangles C O P and C E P be similar, for the Angle O C P is equal to the Angle E C D, equal to the Angle E C P, and the Hypothenuse C P is common to both, therefore the Sides O C, E P, are equal between themselves. Now O P and C L are as the Fluxions of L C and B C generated in the same very small Particle of Time, and consequently their Fluent will be equal amongst themselves. Wherefore C L − I A = A H + H F − C F (equal to the Fluent) = B C − B A ; and consequently

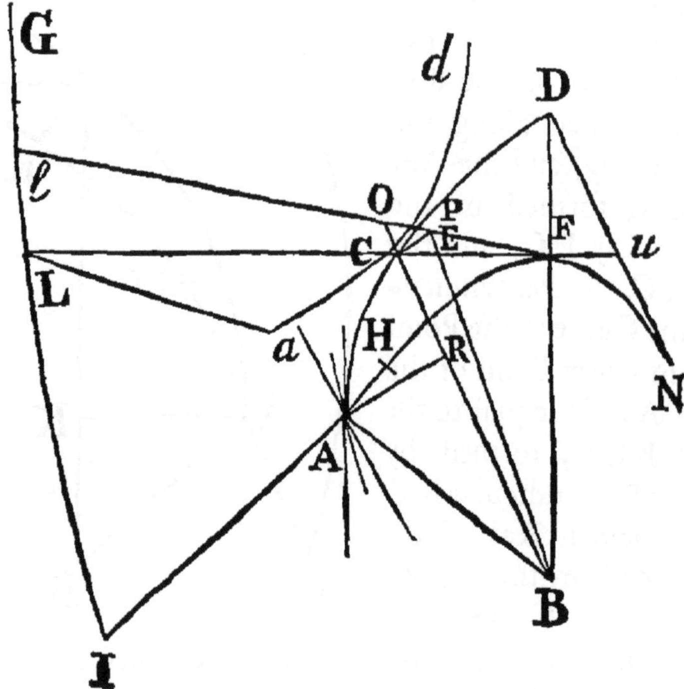

H F (the Portion of the Caustick H F N is equal to B C — B A + C F — A H. Whence it follows,

First, If on the Centre B the Arch A R be described, it is evident that R C is equal to C B — A B, and if we suppose the luminous Point B to be at an infinite Distance from the Curve A C D, the Rays of Incidence B A, B C, will become parallel, and the Arch A R will become a straight Line, cutting the said Rays at right Angles.

Secondly, If we imagine the Figure B A C D to be reverted on the same Plane, so that the Point B falls on the Point I, and that the Line touching the Curve A C D in A, touch the same in the reverted Position in the same Point, and if we imagine the Curve A C D immoveable, and that the reverted Curve *a* C *d* revolves on the same, so that the Portions A C, *a* C, be always equal between themselves I say, the Point B or I, by such a Motion, will describe a sort of a Cycloid I L G, whose *Evoluta* is the Caustick H F N.

FOR

FOR, from the Genisis of the Curve, it is evident, *First*, that the Line L C, drawn from the describing Point L to the Point of Contact C, is perpendicular to the Curve I L G. *Secondly*, L a = I A = B A, and L C equal to B C *Thirdly*, the Angles made by the right Lines C L, B C, and the Tangent in C (common to both Curves) are equal, and consequently if C L be perpendicular to F, the Ray C F will be the reflected Ray of the Ray of Incidence B C, whence it is evident, that the Perpendicular L F touches the Caustick H F N, and because this holds good in whatever Point of the Curve I G, the Point L be taken, it follows, that the Curve I L G is generated by the Evolution of the Caustick H F N + H I

Thirdly, AND hence it appears, that the Portion F H, or F L − H I, is equal to B C + C F − B A − A H, as has already been demonstrated

Fourthly, IF the Tangent D N be drawn infinitely near the Tangent C F, the Points of Contact N, F, and the Point of Intersection V, will coincide, so that to find the Point F, where the Ray C F touches the Caustick H F N, is the same thing as to find the Point V, in which the reflected Rays O F, C F, infinitely near each other, concur.

PROPOSITION I

THE Nature of the Curve A C K, the luminous Point B, and the Ray of Incidence B C being given, to find in the reflected Ray C F, given by Position, the Point F where it touches the Caustick.

HAVING found the Length of the Ray C H of the *Evoluta* to the Point C, suppose the same Ray C H to flow uniformly into the Place H c, and draw the right Lines B c, H c, c F, on the Centres B and F describe the small Arches C D, C O, and draw the Perpendicular H E, H e, H G, H g, to the Rays of Incidence and Reflection, and put B C = y, and C F or C G = a

THEN

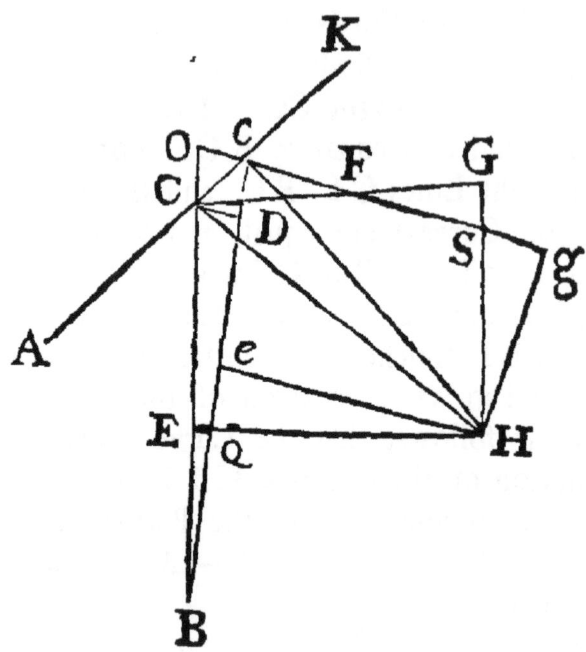

THEN it is evident that the Triangles CDc, COc, are similar and equal, and consequently CD is equal to CO, and because the Angles of Incidence and Reflection are equal, and, consequently, therefore HE is equal to HG, and $He = Hg$, and consequently $HE - He = EQ$ is equal to $HG - Hg = GS$, and because the Triangles BCD, BEQ, FCO, FGS are similar, it will be as $BC + BE$ BC. $CD + EQ = CO + GS$ $CD = CO$ CG cF. Wherefore $BC + BE$ BC CG CF, that is, as $2y - a$ y a $\frac{ay}{2y-a} = CF$ Whence it follows

First, IF the luminous Point B fall on the other Side of the Point E, in respect of C, or (which is the same thing) if the Curve Line ACK be convex towards the luminous Point B, then y, instead of being positive, will become negative, consequently CF will be equal to $\frac{-ay}{-2y-a} = \frac{ay}{2y+a}$

Secondly, IF we suppose y to become infinite, that is to say, if the luminous Point B be at an infinite Distance from the Curve ACK, the Rays of Incidence will be parallel amongst themselves, and CF equal to $\frac{ay}{2y \mp a}$, will become $\frac{1}{2}a$, because a is equal to nothing in respect of y.

Thirdly,

Thirdly, THE Curve A C K can have but one Cauſtick by Reflection H F N; for one and the ſame Curve can have but one *Evoluta*, and the Ray or Tangent thereof enters into the Value C F, ſo that there can be but one Value of C F.

Fourthly, WHEN A C K is a Geometrical Curve, it is evident that its *Evoluta* is a Geometrical Curve alſo (becauſe in that Caſe we can find the Relation between the Abſciſſa and Ordinate of the *Evoluta*) that is, all the Points H may be determined Geometrically; whence it is manifeſt, that all the Points F of its Cauſtick may alſo be determined Geometrically; that is, the Cauſtick H F N will be a Geometrical Curve.

Fifthly, IF the Curve A C K be convex towards the luminous Point B, the Value of C F $= \frac{ay}{2y - a}$ will be always poſitive, and conſequently we muſt take the Point F on the ſame Side of the Curve with the Point H, in reſpect of C, as has been ſuppoſed in the preceding Calculation, whence it is evident, that the Rays of Reflection, infinitely near one another, diverge.

Sixthly, IF the Curve A C K be convex towards the luminous Point B, the Value of C F $= \frac{ay}{2y - a}$ will be poſitive when $y = \frac{1}{2} a$ whence it is manifeſt, that if a Circle be deſcribed, whoſe Diameter is $\frac{1}{2}$ C H, the Ray of the *Evoluta*, then, if the luminous Point B be without the Circumference of the ſaid Circle, the reflecting Rays will converge, if within, they will diverge, and if the ſaid Point happen to be in the Circumference, they will be all parallel one to the other.

Seventhly, IF the Ray of Incidence B C touch the Curve A C K in the Point C, then is C E $= a = 0$, and conſequently C F $= 0$, becauſe the refracted Ray is in the ſame Direction with the Ray of Incidence, and the Nature of the Cauſtick being ſuch, that it touches all the reflected Rays, it follows, that it muſt alſo touch the Ray of Incidence B C in C, that is, B C will be a Tangent to both Curves in the Point C.

Eighthly,

Eighthly, If the Ray of the *Evoluta* CH be equal to nothing, then is C E equal to nothing, and consequently C F is equal to nothing, whence it is manifest, that the given Curve, and the Caustick, make an Angle in the Point C, which is common to both, equal to the Angle of Incidence.

Ninthly, If the Ray of the *Evoluta* be infinite, the fluxionary Arch C c will be a straight Line, and C F $= \frac{ay}{2y \mp a}$ (because C E, or a, being infinite, y will vanish) will be equal to $\mp y$, and if the luminous Point B be on the same Side with the Point H, then the Value of C F will be negative, and consequently the reflected Rays will diverge, and if the luminous Point B be on the contrary Side of the Curve, with respect to H, the Value of C F will be positive, that is, the Point F will be on the same Side of the Curve with the Point H, and consequently the reflected Rays will also, in this Case, diverge, whence it is manifest, that Rays issuing from any luminous Point, and reflected by any plain Surface, will, after Reflection, diverge

Tenthly, If any two of the three Points B, H, F, be given, the third may be found For Example, if the Curve A C K be a Parabola, and the luminous Point B in the Focus, it is evident, that all the reflected Rays will be parallel to the Axis, and consequently, because the Point F, where two Rays of Reflection intersect each other, is at an infinite Distance, C F will be infinite, where ever C be taken; but C F $= \frac{ay}{2y - a}$ equal to Infinity, therefore $2y - a = 0$, and $2y = a$ whence if C E be taken equal to 2 C B, and the Perpendicular E H be drawn, it will cut C H, the Perpendicular

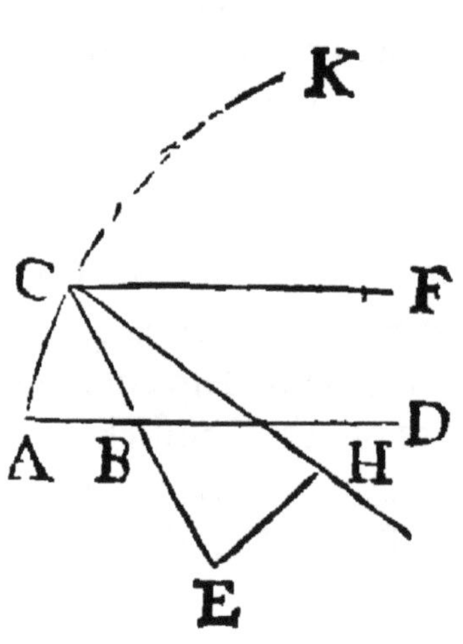

pendicular to the Curve in H, which will be in the *Evoluta* of the Parabola.

AGAIN, if the Curve ACK be an Ellipsis, and the luminous Point be in one of the *Foci*, it is manifest, that all the reflected Rays will meet in the other Focus F, whence if CF be supposed equal to z, then is $z = \frac{ay}{2y - a}$, and consequently CE equal to a, is equal to $\frac{2yz}{y + z}$, but if the Curve ACK be an Hyperbola, then the Focus F will be in the opposite Section, or on the other Side of the Curve, the reflected Rays themselves will diverge, but being produced, they will unite in the Focus of the opposite Section, therefore EC will be negative, and $-z = \frac{ay}{2y - a}$, that is, $CE = a = \frac{-2yz}{y - z} = \frac{2yz}{z - y}$ which gives the following Construction for the Ellipsis.

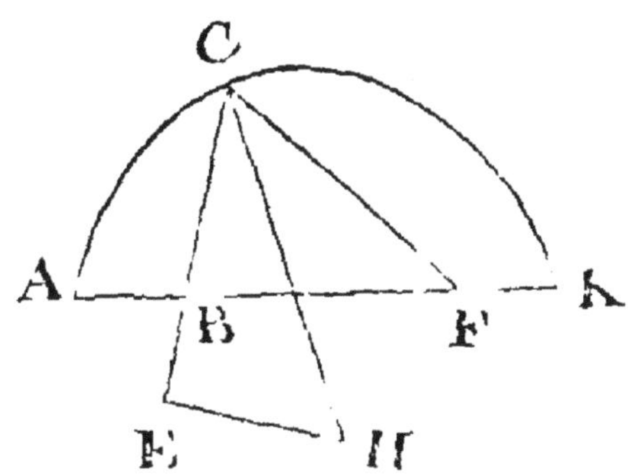

IF CE be taken a fourth Proportional to half the transverse Axis, the Ray of Incidence, and the reflected Ray, and the Perpendicular EH be drawn, it will cut CH, the Perpendicular to the Curve in C, in H, the Point in the *Evoluta*

EXAMPLE I.

LET ADCE be a plain Surface, or right Line, (*See the following Figure*) and let B be a luminous Point, and let it be required to find the Caustick by Reflection.

IF the right Line AE be imagined to be a Curve Line concave towards the luminous Body B, whose Centre E is removed at an infinite Distance, then a will vanish, and CF equal to $\frac{ay}{2y - a}$, will become $\frac{ay}{-a} = -y$, equal to BC,

 where-

wherefore having drawn B D perpendicular to A E in B D produced, take D F equal to BD, then will the reflected Ray C G, produced towards F, converge to the Point F, for the Triangles B C D and F C D are similar and equal, wherefore C B is equal to CF Whence it follows.

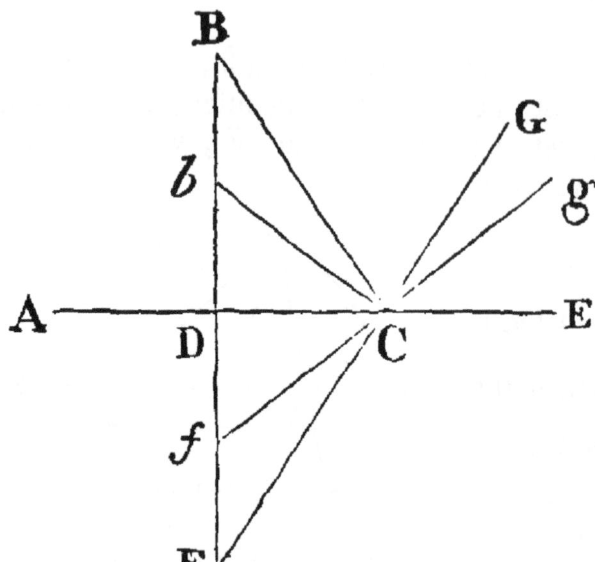

First, THAT as the *Evoluta* of the Circle is contracted into the Centre, so the Caustick, by Reflection of a right Line, is contracted into the Point F.

Secondly, THAT since if the Eye be placed any where in the reflected Ray CG, suppose at G, it receives the Rays as issuing from the Point F, it is manifest, that the Image at B will appear to the Eye as placed in the Point F.

Thirdly, AND because the Ray of Incidence is the reflected Ray to the reflected Ray, considered as a Ray of Incidence, it is evident, that the Rays of Incidence G C, *&c* converging to the Point F, will be reflected to the Point B, that is, if the Rays of Incidence converge to a Point F, beyond the Surface A E, the reflected Rays will converge to a Point on the same Side with the Rays of Incidence.

Fourthly, IF A F be a plain Speculum, in an horizontal Position, then it is evident, that the Image of B will be in F, and that of *b* in *f*, and consequently the Image will appear in an inverted Position, or upside down.

Fifthly, IF B *b* be a radiating Plane, then it is manifest, that the Image F *f*, made by a plain Speculum, is similar and equal to its Original, but in a contrary Position

Sixthly, BECAUSE CB is equal to CF, therefore GC + CF is equal to GC + CB, that is, the Distance of the Image from the Eye is equal to the Sum of the Rays of Incidence and Reflection.

EXAMPLE II.

LET ADC be an Arch of a Circle, and B a luminous Point, and let it be required to find the Point F in the reflected Ray in which it will touch the Caustick KFC

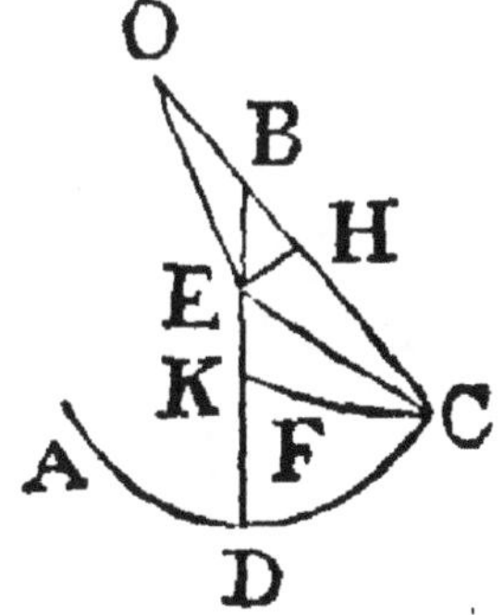

THROUGH the luminous Point B, and the Centre of the Arch F, draw the right Line BED perpendicular to the Arch in D, then it is manifest, that all the Rays of the *Evoluta* of the Circle are equal among themselves, and that the said *Evoluta* is the Centre E, whence HC $= a$, and BC $= y$, and consequently the Value of FC is equal to $\frac{ay}{2y - a}$, wherefore having produced CB to O, so that CO be equal to $2y - a$, then say, as $2y - a$ y a CF, that is, as OC BC HC CF, then the Point F will touch the Curve in the Point F Whence it follows.

First, IF the Point C be infinitely near the Point D, then BC $= y$ will be equal to BD, and HC $= a$ will be equal to ED, and the Point K, in which the reflected Ray touches the Caustick KF by Reflection, is found by saying as 2BD — ED BD ED DK, and by Division, as BE BD EK DK.

Secondly, HENCE it is evident, that if ADC be a spherical Glass, and E the Centre, and B the luminous Point, all the Rays BC falling on the concave Surface of the Glass near the Point D (the Vertex of the Glass) and being reflected, will converge to the Point K nearly.

Thirdly, AND if the Radiant Point B be at an infinite Distance from the Glass, then the Point K, to which the Rays parallel and near the Axis BD converge after their Reflection, is the middle Point between E and D, for in that Case, CK or DK equal to $\frac{ay}{2y-a}$, will become $\frac{ay}{2y} = \frac{1}{2}a, = \frac{1}{2}HC, = \frac{1}{2}ED$

Fourthly, IF EK be equal to DK, then the Rays issuing from the Point K, will be reflected by the spherical Concave Glass, parallel to the Axis DEB.

Fifthly IF the Distance of the Radiant Point B from D, the Vertex of the Glass, be less than $\frac{1}{4}$ of the Diameter of the Lens, then the reflected Rays will diverge, and the Focus K will be on the opposite Side of the Glass, in respect of the radiant Point B, for CK (supposing C at an infinite small Distance from the Vertex D) or DK is equal to $\frac{ay}{2y-a}$, and because BD or y, is supposed less than $\frac{1}{2}a$, therefore $\frac{ay}{2y-a}$ is negative, and consequently the reflected Rays CN diverge, and the Focus K may be found, by saying, as ED − 2BD is to BD, so is ED to DK, and by Composition, as EB is to BD, so is EK to DK.

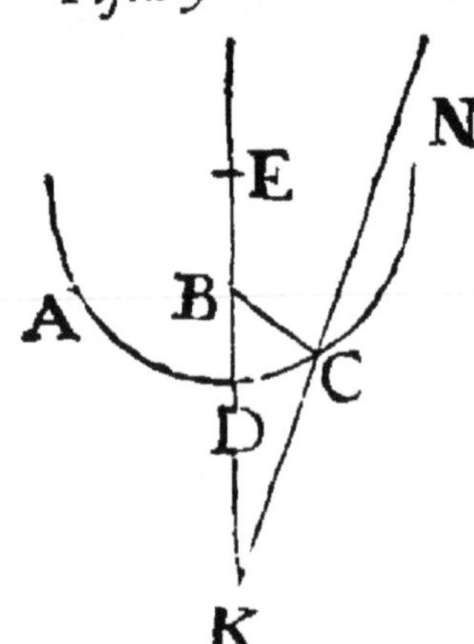

Sixthly, HENCE if Rays converging to a given Focus K be reflected by a spherical Concave Glass, the Focus F, to which the reflected Rays converge, may be found.

Seventhly, IF the Convex Surface of the Glass A D C be towards the radiant Point B, then the Focus of the reflected Rays will be on the Concave Side of the Glass, that is, the reflected Rays will diverge, for in that Case y is negative, and consequently C E or D K is equal to $\frac{-ay}{-2y-a} = \frac{ay}{2y+a}$, and because B C or B D is equal to y, when the Point C is infinitely near D, and the Ray of the *Evoluta* a constant Quantity, and C F or D E $=$ a or E C, in this Case, the Focus may be determined, by saying as 2 B D + D F : B D :: D E : D K, and by Division, as B E : B D :: E K : D K.

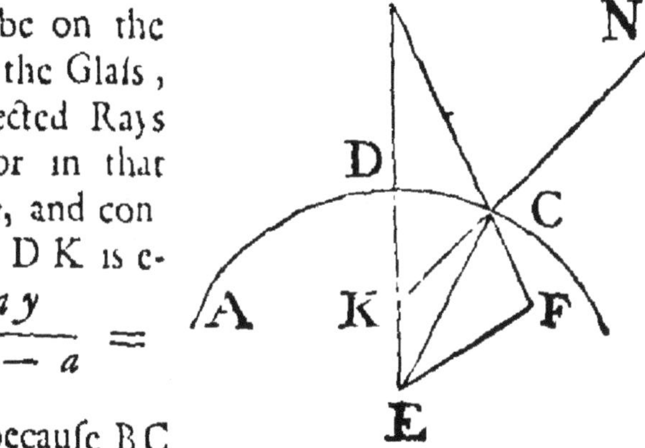

Eighthly, IF an infinite Number of Rays N C, falling on the Spherical Convex Surface of a Glass, converge to a Focus K, whose Distance D K from the Vertex is less than one Quarter of the whole Diameter of the Glass, then the Focus B, to which the reflected Rays B C converge, may be found.

EXAMPLE III.

LET the Curve A C K be a common Parabola, and suppose the Rays of Incidence B C to be perpendicular to the Axis A B, and let it be required to find the Caustick by Reflection.

LET

LET the Ray of the *Evoluta* CH be drawn, and perpendicu-

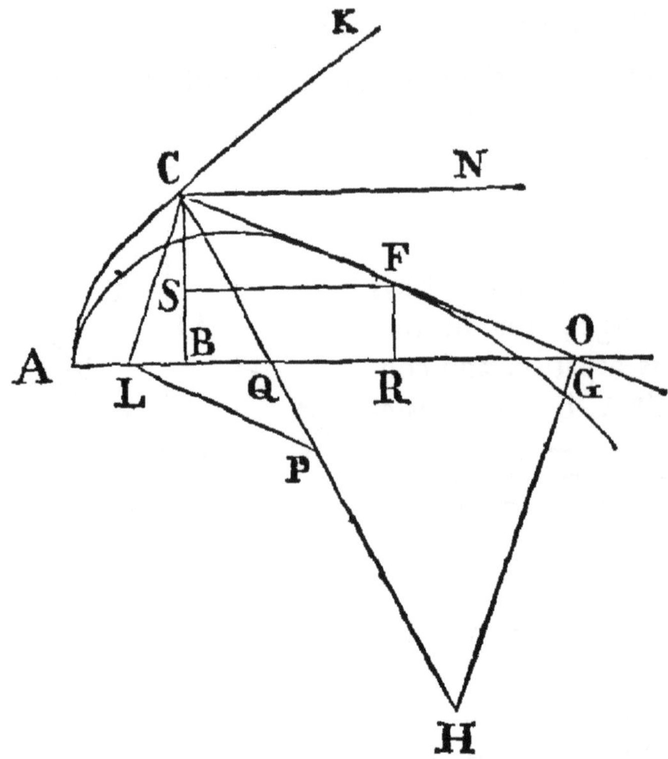

lar to the reflected Ray, the Line HG, it is manifest that C F = $\frac{1}{2}$ C G = $\frac{1}{2}$ *a*. For having drawn C N parallel to the Axis A B, and the right Line C L to the Focus L, the Angles L C B and F C N will be equal (because L C Q is equal to Q C N, and BCQ equal to Q C F by Hypothesis). Now if to each you add the Angle B C F, then the Angle L C F will be equal to B C N, equal to a right Angle; and because the Perpendicular L P bisects C H in P, and L P is equal to $\frac{1}{2}$ C G, therefore if C F be drawn equal and parallel to L P, it will be the reflected Ray to the Ray of Incidence C B, and it will touch the Caustick A F at the Point F.

AND to draw the greatest Ordinate F R that can be applied to the Caustick A F G, it is evident, that when the reflected Ray C F G runs parallel to the Axis A B, then the Ordinate F R will

will be the greatest, and in that Case the Angle CBQ will be equal to BQC, and BC equal to CQ, therefore in that Point $\dot x$ will be equal to $\dot y$

Now let the Equation expressing the Nature of the Curve ACK, be $ax = yy$, that is, $\dot y = \frac{a\dot x}{2y} = \frac{a\dot x}{2\overline{ax}^{\frac{1}{2}}}$ (by putting $\overline{ax}^{\frac{1}{2}}$ in the room of y) $= \dot x$ (because $\dot y$ is supposed equal to $\dot x$) therefore $a\dot x = 2\overline{ax}^{\frac{1}{2}} \times \dot x$, and consequently $a = 2 \times \overline{ax}^{\frac{1}{2}}$, where $x = \frac{1}{4}a$, which shews, that when the Ray of Reflection CF runs parallel to the Axis AB, and touches the Caustick in the supreme Point, then AB is equal to $\frac{1}{4}$ of the Parameter of the Curve ACK $= \frac{1}{4}a$, that is, the Point B will fall in the Focus of the Parabola, when the reflected Ray CF is parallel to the Axis, and then CB coincides with CL, LP with QL, and CF with CN, whence it is evident, that in that Case CF is equal to CL, and that if FR be drawn perpendicular to the Axis AR, AL + CF will be equal to $\frac{1}{4}a$, and in this Case the Portion of the Caustick AF is equal to BC + CF, equal to the Parameter of the Curve ACK

And because the Caustick by Reflection AFG may be infinitely produced beyond G, let it be required to investigate the Point G in the Axis AO, where the Caustick intersects the same

It is evident, that in this Case CF becomes equal to CO, therefore the Value of CO must be investigated, and made equal to CF. Let therefore the unknown Quantity CO be put equal to x; and because the Angle BCO is bisected by the Line CQ, it will be as CB : CQ :: BQ : QO, that is, as $y : z :: \frac{yy}{x} : \frac{zy}{x} = QO$, and consequently OB equal to $\frac{yy + zy}{x}$ will be equal to $\overline{zz - yy}^{\frac{1}{2}}$, and dividing both

Sides

Sides of the Equation by $z+y$, we have $\frac{\dot{y}}{\dot{x}} = \frac{\overline{zz-yy}|^{\frac{1}{2}}}{\overline{zz+2zy+yy}|^{\frac{1}{2}}}$ $= \frac{\overline{z-y}|^{\frac{1}{2}}}{\overline{z+y}|^{\frac{1}{2}}}$, whence $\frac{\dot{y}\dot{y}}{\dot{x}\dot{x}} = \frac{z-y}{z+y}$, and consequently $z\dot{x}\dot{x} - z\dot{x}\dot{x} = z\dot{y}\dot{y} + y\dot{y}\dot{y}$, whence $z\dot{x}\dot{x} - z\dot{y}\dot{y} = y\dot{x}^2 + y\dot{y}^2$, and $z = \frac{y\dot{x}\dot{x} + y\dot{y}\dot{y}}{\dot{x}\dot{x} - \dot{y}\dot{y}}$ = (by Hypothesis) to CE, $= \frac{1}{2}a = \frac{\dot{x}\dot{x} + \dot{y}\dot{y}}{-2\ddot{y}}$, therefore $-2y\ddot{y}\dot{x}^2 - 2y\ddot{y}\dot{y}^2 = \dot{x}^4 - \dot{y}^4$, and dividing by $\dot{x}\dot{x} + \dot{y}\dot{y}$, we shall have $-2y\ddot{y} = \dot{x}\dot{x} - \dot{y}\dot{y}$, that is, $\dot{y}\dot{y} - 2y\ddot{y} = \dot{x}\dot{x}$, which is a general Theorem to find the Point B; so that drawing the Ray of Incidence BC, and the reflected Ray CF, the same will touch the Caustick in the Point I, where it intersects the Axis AB.

Thus in the Parabola, because $y = x^{\frac{1}{2}}$, and $\dot{y} = \frac{1}{2}x^{-\frac{1}{2}}\dot{x}$, and (supposing $\dot{x}$ a constant Quantity) $\ddot{y} = -\frac{1}{4}x^{-\frac{3}{2}}\dot{x}\dot{x}$, and substituting these Values in the preceding Theorem $\dot{x}^2 = \dot{y}\dot{y} - 2y\ddot{y}$, there will arise $\dot{x}\dot{x} = \frac{1}{4}x^{-1}\dot{x}\dot{x} + \frac{1}{2}x^{-1}\dot{x}\dot{x}$, and by Division and Multiplication $8xx = 6x$, whence AB $= x$ is equal to $\frac{1}{4}$ of the Parameter of the Curve.

Let it now be required to investigate the Nature of the Caustick AFG, that is, to find an Equation which expresses the Relation between the Absciss AR, and the Ordinate RF, and put AR equal to s, RF equal to z, then, because CO $= \frac{y\dot{x}\dot{x} + y\dot{y}\dot{y}}{\dot{x}\dot{x} - \dot{y}\dot{y}}$, therefore BO $= \overline{CO^2 - CB^2}|^{\frac{1}{2}}$, will be equal to $\frac{2y\dot{x}\dot{y}}{\dot{x}\dot{x} - \dot{y}\dot{y}} = \frac{\dot{y}y + v\dot{y}}{\dot{x}}$ (supposing CO $= v$), and

because

because the Triangles C B O and C S F are similar, it will be as CO : CF :: CB : CS; that is, as $\frac{y\dot x\dot x+y\dot y\dot y}{\dot x\dot x-\dot y\dot y}$: $\frac{\dot x\dot x+\dot y\dot y}{-2\ddot y}$ :: $y : y-z$, but as CB : CS :: BO : SF = PR, that is, as $y : y-z$ :: $\frac{2\dot y y\dot x}{\dot x\dot x-\dot y\dot y}$: SF = PR $(s-x)=\frac{\dot x\dot y}{-\ddot y}$,

and now we have two Equations $z=y+\frac{\dot y\dot y-\dot x\dot x}{-2\ddot y}$, and $s=x+\frac{\dot x\dot y}{-\ddot y}$, which by the Help of the Equation expressing the Nature of the given Curve, will serve to find a new Equation (cleared of the flowing Quantities x and y) expressing the Relation of A R to F R, or of s to z.

For Example, if the Curve A C F be a Parabola, then $y=x^{\frac12}$, and $\dot y=\frac12 x^{-\frac12}\dot x$, and $\ddot y=-\frac14 x^{-\frac32}\dot x\dot x$ (supposing $\dot x$ a constant Quantity) therefore the Equation $z=y+\frac{\dot y\dot y-\dot x\dot x}{-2\ddot y}$, becomes $z=x^{\frac12}+\frac{\frac14 x^{-1}\dot x\dot x-\dot x\dot x}{\frac12 x^{-\frac32}\dot x\dot x}$ $=\frac{\frac12 x^{-1}\dot x\dot x+x^{-1}\dot x\dot x-2\dot x\dot x}{x^{-\frac32}\dot x\dot x}=x^{\frac12}+\frac12 x^{\frac12}-2x^{\frac32}=\frac32 x^{\frac12}-2x^{\frac32}$, and squaring both Sides of the Equation, we shall have $zz=\frac94 x-6xx+4x^3$. Again, $s=x+\frac{\dot x\dot y}{-\ddot y}=x+\frac{x^{-\frac12}\dot x\dot x}{\frac12 x^{-\frac32}\dot x\dot x}$ (by Substitution) $=x+2x=3x$ whence the Nature of the Caustick Curve A F is expressed by this Equation $zz=\frac{4}{27}s^3-\frac23 ass+\frac34 aas$. And it may be observed, that B R $(=-2x)$ is always equal to 2 A B,

 because

becauſe A R is equal to $3x$, and this Obſervation affords another Method for deſcribing the Catacauſtick A F.

EXAMPLE IV.

LET the Curve A C I D be a Semicircle, A D the Diameter, and H the Centre, and let the Ray of Incidence C B be perpendicular to the Diameter A D, and let it be required to draw the Cauſtick A F K

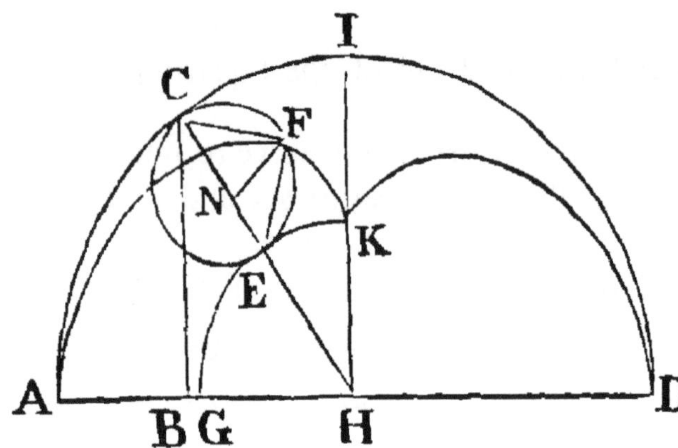

FORASMUCH as the Centre of the Circle is its *Evoluta*, and its Radius the Ray of the ſame *Evoluta*, therefore CF $= \frac{ay}{2y - a} = \frac{1}{2}a = \frac{1}{2}$ C B

Wherefore having biſected the Radius C H in E, and drawn E F perpendicular to C F, the Point F will be in the Cauſtick A F K, for the Triangles C F E and C B H are ſimilar Wherefore as C E C H C F C B Whence it follows

Firſt, THAT if the Point B falls in H, then the Point F will fall in K

Secondly, THE Portion of the Cauſtick A F is equal to 3 C F, for the Portion A F is equal to B C + C F = 3 C F (becauſe B C = 2 C F) and the Cauſtick A F K is equal to 3 I K

Thirdly, IF the Angle A H C be equal to half a right Angle, then is B C H equal to F C H, and the reflected Ray being parallel to the Diameter A D, touches the Cauſtick in the ſupreme Point F

Fourthly, THE Circle, whoſe Diameter is C E, paſſes through the Point F, for the Angle E F C is a right Angle.

Fifthly,

Fifthly, THE Caustick A F K is a Semicycloid described by the Revolution of the little Circle C F E on the Periphery or Base K E G, for the Circle C F E is described on $\frac{1}{2}$ C H, as a Diameter, and the Angle H C F is equal to H C B, equal to E H K, and consequently the Angle C N F is equal to 2 E H K, therefore the Arch E F is equal to the Arch E K, and the Curve A F K is a Semicycloid, whose beginning is in K, and whose Vertex is A.

EXAMPLE V.

LET the Curve A C D be a Semicircle, A D the Diameter, and H the Centre, and let the radiant Point A be in one of the Extremities of the Diameter, and let it be required to describe the Caustick A F K.

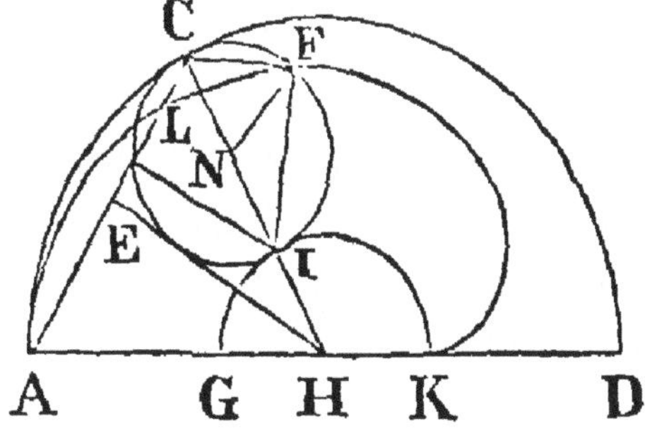

IF H E be drawn perpendicular to A C, then A E will be equal to E C, and consequently A C $=$ $y = 2a$, whence C F $= \frac{ay}{2y - a} = \frac{1}{3}y$, and consequently the reflected Ray C F will be $\frac{1}{3}$ of the incident Ray A C, and D K will be $\frac{2}{3}$ of H D, as will H K be $\frac{1}{3}$ of H D. Wherefore if A C be made equal to A H, the reflected Ray C F will be parallel to the Diameter A D, and consequently the Point F will be the supreme Point.

IF H I be made equal to $\frac{1}{2}$ H C, and I F be drawn perpendicular to C F, the Point F will be in the Caustick, for drawing I L perpendicular to A C, it is manifest, that C L is $\frac{2}{3}$ of E C $=$ $\frac{1}{3}$ of A C, because C I is $\frac{2}{3}$ of C H, therefore the Circle that has C I for its Diameter, shall pass through the Point F of the Caustick, and if from the Centre H, with the Radius H K or H I, another Circle G I K be described, it shall be equal to the Circle I F N, and the Arch I K will be equal to the Arch I F,

 for

for in the Isoscles Triangle H C A, the external Angle I H K = 2 A C H = A C F, and consequently the Arches I K, I F, being the Measures of those Angles in equal Circles, must be equal to each other, whence it follows, that the Caustick A F K is a Cycloid generated by the Rotation of the Circle C F I along the immoveable Circle G I K, whose beginning is at K, and its Vertex A.

THE Portion of the Caustick A F is equal to $\frac{4}{3}$ of A C, for the Portion A F is equal to A C + C F, = A C + $\frac{1}{3}$ A C, = $\frac{4}{3}$ A C, and the whole Caustick A F K is equal to $\frac{4}{3}$ of A D the Diameter.

IF the radiant Point A be in the Surface of a Sphere, then the reflected Rays that are nearest to the Axis A D, will converge to the Focus K, distant from H, the Centre of the Sphere, $\frac{1}{3}$ of its Semidiameter A H.

EXAMPLE VI.

LET the Curve A C D be the Logarithmetic Spiral, and suppose the Rays of Incidence to issue from the luminous Point A its Centre, and let it be required to describe the Caustick by Reflection A F K.

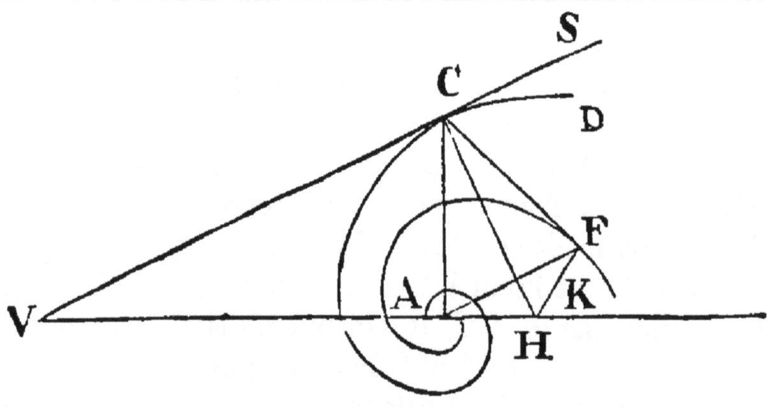

LET the Line C H be drawn perpendicular to the Curve in the Point C, and A H perpendicular to the Ray of Incidence A C, then the Point H will be in the *Evoluta* of the Curve, and

and consequently $AC = y$ is equal to a, whence $CF = \frac{ay}{2y - a}$ will be equal to y, and the Triangle ACF will be an Isosceles Triangle, and because the Angle of Incidence ACV is equal to the Angle of Reflection FCS, therefore the Angle AFC is equal to ACV, and this Angle ACV being a constant Quantity by the Nature of the Curve, therefore the Angle AFC will be a constant Quantity, and the Caustick by Reflection AFK will be a Logarithmetic Spiral, differing from the given Spiral only by Position

EXAMPLE VII

LET the Curve ACD be a Semicycloid described by the Rotation of the Semicircle NGC on the right Line PD, and supposing the Rays of Incidence CB be parallel to the Axis AP, let it be required to describe the Caustick DF by Reflection.

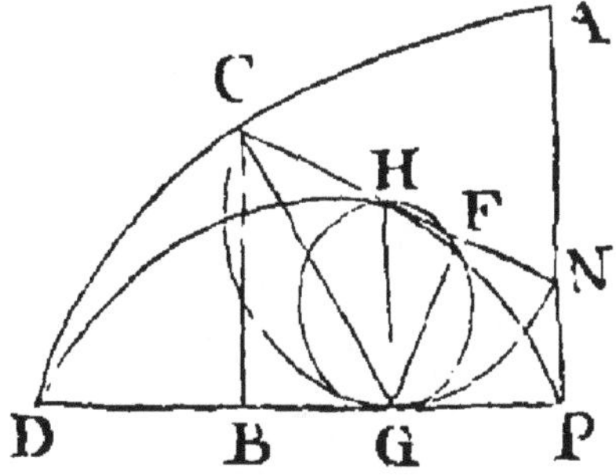

BECAUSE CG is equal to $\frac{1}{2}$ the Ray of the *Evoluta*, and GB perpendicular to CB, therefore $CF = \frac{1}{2} a = BC$, whence if GF be drawn perpendicular to the reflected Ray CF, the Point F will be a Point in the Caustick.

IF the Rays HC, HG, be drawn from H, the Centre of the generating Circle, to the generating Point C, and the Point of Contact G, it is manifest that HG will be perpendicular to the Line DP, and that the Angles GCH, CGH and GCB will be equal to each other, whence it follows, that the reflected Ray CF passes through the Centre H Now the Circle, whose Diameter is GH, passes also through the Point F, because GFH is a right Angle, therefore the Arches GN and $\frac{1}{2}$ GF, which are the Measures of the same Angle GHN, are as the Diameters CN, GH of their respective Circles, and consequently the Arch GF equal to the Arch

Arch G N, is equal to G B, whence it is manifest, that the Caustick D H P is a Cycloid described by the Rotation of the Circle G F H along the right Line D P, whence it follows, that the Space D C A P F D is equal to thrice the Area of the Circle G H F, for the Semicircle C G N is equal to twice the Area of the Circle G F H, therefore the cycloidal Space A C D P is equal to six times the Area of the Circle G F H, and the cycloidal Space P F D is equal to thrice the Area of the Circle G F H, and consequently the Space D C A P F D is equal to thrice the Area of the Circle G F H, and the Curve D F P divides the Space A C D P into two equal Parts

Let us now suppose the Ray of Incidence C B to be parallel to the Base D I.

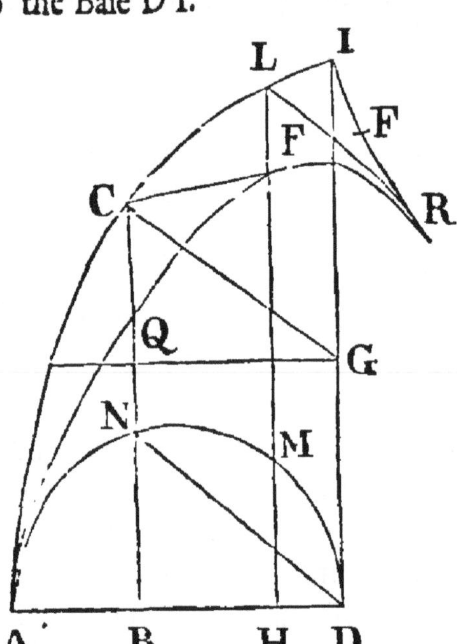

Now if Q G be drawn perpendicular to B C, then the right angled Triangles G Q C and D B N will be equal, and similar, wherefore C Q will be equal to B N, whence it follows, that C F must be assumed equal to the correspondent Ordinate B N in the generating Circle A N D

When the Point F is at an infinite Distance from the Axis A D, the Tangent C F in that Point must be parallel to the Axis, and consequently the Angle B C F will be a right Angle, and B C G or B N D half a right Angle, whence B falls in the Centre of the Circle A N D, and afterwards, as the Point B approaches nearer towards the Extremity D of the Diameter, so does the Point F approach nearer to the Axis A D, until it comes to a certain Point R, after which it recedes from thence, 'till it comes to I, so that the Caustick has a Point of Retrogression in R.

To

To determine which, we must observe, that the Part AF = BC + CF, and the Part AKR = HL + LR, and the Part KF of FKI = HL + LK − BC − CF, whence HL + LR must be a *Maximum*, and if you put AH = x, HM = y, and the Arch AM = z, then will HL + LR $= z + 2y$, whence $\dot{z} + 2\dot{y} = 0$; and $\frac{a\dot{x}}{y} + 2\dot{y} = 0$, (by substituting $\frac{a\dot{x}}{y}$ in the room of $\dot{z}$) and consequently $a\dot{x} = -2y\dot{y} = 2x\dot{x} - a\dot{x}$, by the Property of the Circle; wherefore AH = $x = \frac{3}{4}a$.

EXAMPLE VIII

Let the Curve AMD be a Semicycloid, generated by the Rotation of the Circle MGN about AGK, equal to it, the Point A the Point of Commencement, and the Point D its Vertex, and let the incident Rays issue from the Point A.

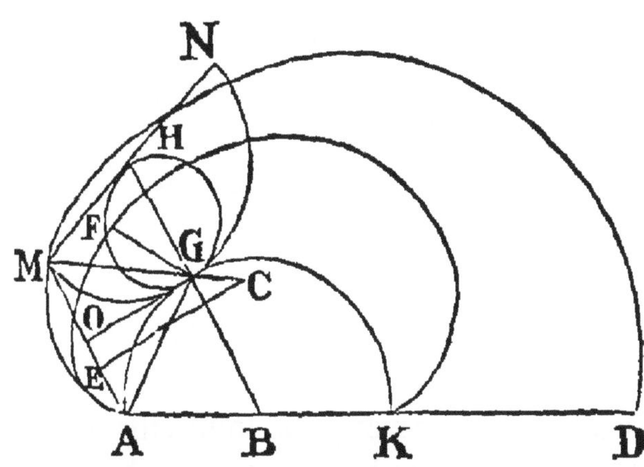

Now the Line BH that joins the Centres of the generating Circles, passes thro' the Point of Contact G, and the Arches GM, GA, as also their Chords, are always equal. Moreover, the Angles HGM and BGA are equal, as are the Angles GMA and GAM. Now the Angle HGM + BGA = GMA + GAM, because if the Angle AGM be added to each Side, there will be formed two right Angles; whence the Angle HGM will be always equal to the Angle G M A, as also to the Angle of Reflection C M F, whence it follows, that M F will always pass through H, the Centre of the immoveable Circle.

NOW if C E and G O be drawn perpendicular to the incident Ray A M, it is manifest, that M O = O A, and O E = $\frac{1}{2}$ O M, therefore M E = $\frac{3}{4}$ A M, that is, $a = \frac{3}{2} y$, and consequently M F = $\frac{a y}{2 y - a}$, in this Case, will be equal to $\frac{1}{2} y$, wherefore if G F be drawn perpendicular to M F, the Point F will be in the Caustick A F D.

THE Circle, whose Diameter is G H, passes through the Point F, and since the Arches G M and $\frac{1}{2}$ G F, the Measures of the Angles G H M, are to each other as their Diameters M N and G H, the Arch G F will be equal to G M, and consequently to the Arch G A, whence it is evident, that the Caustick A F K is a Cycloid generated by the Rotation of the moveable Circle H F G about the immoveable Arch A G K. Whence it follows

THAT if a Circle be described about the Centre B, whose Radius is equal to B H or A K, and an infinite Number of Rays, parallel to B D, fall on its Circumference, they will form the same Caustick A F K.

PROPOSITION II.

LET the Caustick H F be given, the luminous Point B, and let it be required to describe an infinite Number of Curves, such as A C, to which it is the Caustick by Reflection.

IN any Tangent, as H A, take a Point A at Pleasure for one of the Points of the Curve A C, to be found on the Centre B, with the Radius B A, describe the Arch P A, and on the same Centre B, with any other Radius, B C, describe another Arch O C q, then take A H + H E = B C

— B A

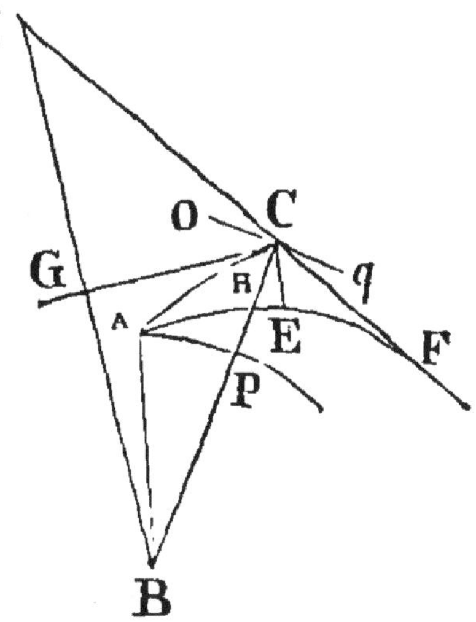

—BA=PC, and beginning at the Point E, evolve the Caustick HF, then the Point E will describe the Curve Line FC, which will intersect the little Arch *o*C*q* in the Point C, one of the Points of the Curve to be found.

For AH+HE=PC, and EF, from the Nature of Evolutions, is equal to CE, therefore PC (=BC—BA) +CF=AH+HF, and consequently the Curve HF is the Caustick by Reflection to AC. Or,

Having drawn the Tangent HA, draw another Tangent FC at Pleasure, and take FK=BA+AH+HF, and draw the Line BK, and let the same Line be bisected in G, and draw GC perpendicular to BK, and it will cut the Tangent FK in the Point C to be found, for BC+CF=BA+AH+HF, therefore the Point C is in the Curve AC to be found. Whence it follows,

If the luminous Point B be at an infinite Distance from the Curve AC, that is, if the Rays of Incidence BA, BC, be parallel to a given right Line, the first Construction will serve, if we imagine the Arches of the Circle described on the Centre B, to become straight Lines, perpendicular to the Ray of Incidence. Or,

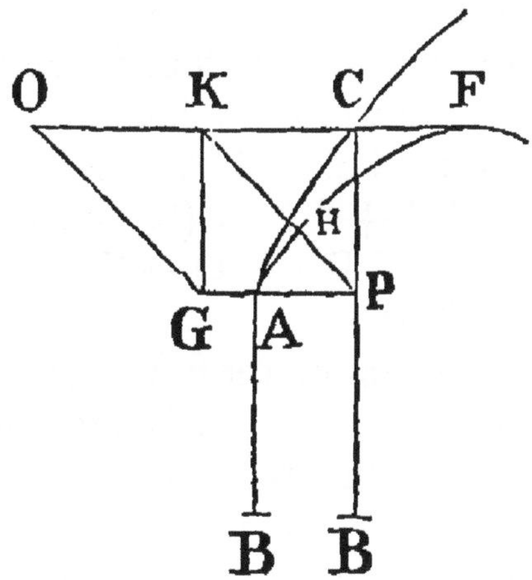

The Curve AC may be described after this manner. Take FK=AH+HF, then if the Point C be so found, that drawing CP parallel to AB, the Line CK be equal to CP,

 then

then it is manifest, that the Point C will be in the Curve A C to be found, for then P C + C F = A H + H F.

AGAIN, the Point C may be found in this manner: Draw K G perpendicular to A P, and take K O = K G, then draw O G, and parallel to it K P, also let P C be drawn parallel to G K, then C will be the Point required For because the Triangles G K O and P C K are similar, therefore P C = C K

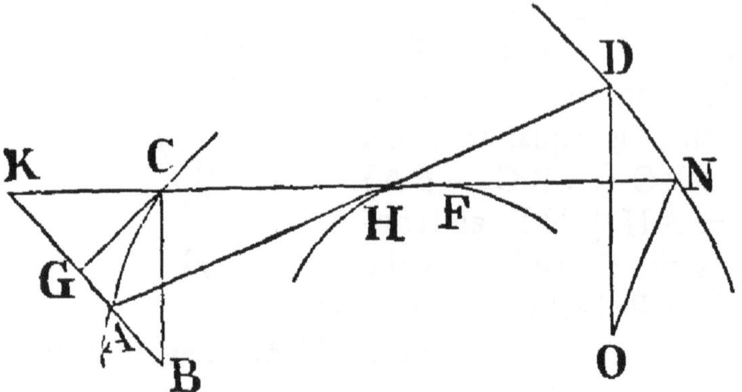

AGAIN, If the Curve Line D N, and luminous Point C, be given, to find an infinite Number of Curves, such as A C, which shall make all the double reflected Rays C B, A B, converge to a given Point B

IF we imagine the Curve H F to be the Catacaustick of the given Curve N D, C being the luminous Point, it is evident, that the same Curve H F must also be the Catacaustick to the Curve A C to be found, the luminous Point, or rather the Focus, to which the double refracted Rays converge, being in B, whence F K = B A + A H + H F, and N K = B A + A H + H F + F N = (because H D + D O = H F + F N + N O) B A + A D + D O − N O, whence there will arise this Construction

IN any of the first reflected Rays take the Point A at Pleasure for one of the Points of the Curve A C to be drawn, and in the other reflected Ray, as N C, take N K = B A + A D + D O − O N, then draw B K, and bisect the same Line in G, and draw C G perpendicular to B K, and the Point C will be in the Curve to be found

SECT

SECT. VI.

Containing the Use of FLUXIONS *in finding the* Caustick Curves *by Refraction.*

LET A C Q represent a Curve, C N a Perpendicular to the Tangent to the Curve in the Point C, B C an Incident Ray issuing from the luminous Body B, C F the same Ray re-

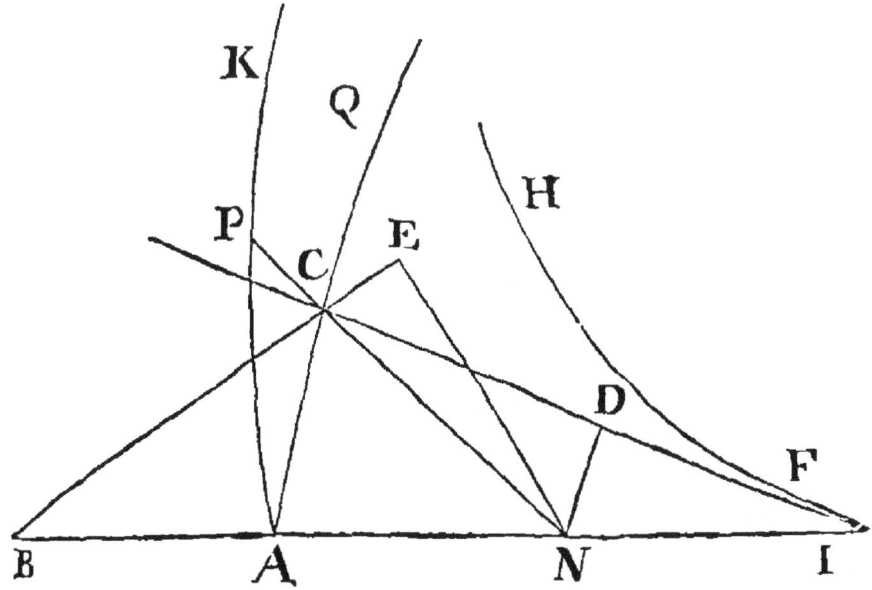

fracted to or from the Perpendicular N C, and F the focal Point Now if the extreme Point C of the Ray B C be carried along the Curve Line A C Q, and in every Point of the Curve the Sine N E of the Angle N C E, equal to the Angle of Incidence B C P, be to N D the Sine of the refracted Angle N C F in a given Ratio, suppose n to m, the Point F will describe the Curve Line F H, which is called the Diacaustick, or Caustick Curve by Refraction

WHEREFORE if the Caustick I F H be involved, beginning at the Point A, the Point A will describe the Curve A P K,

 so

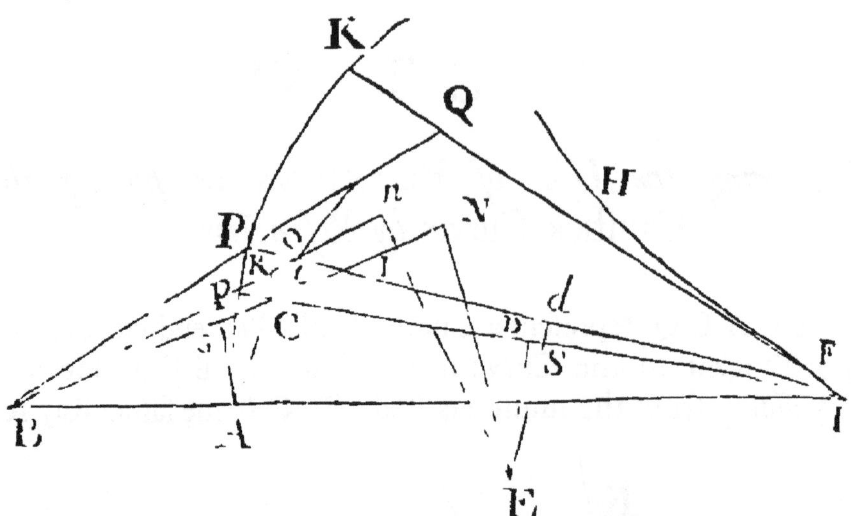

ſo that the Tangent P F, together with the Arch of the Cauſtick F I, will always be equal to the ſame right Line A I. Now if we ſuppoſe the Incident Ray B C in a flowing State to move into the Place B c, then will the Point C deſcribe the Arch C c, and the Line c F will become the new refracted Ray. Let F O be ſuppoſed equal to F C, B R = B C and B G = B A, then will the fluxionary Triangle C R c in its naſcent State be ſimilar to the Triangle C E N, for if from the equal Angles R C N and E C c, be taken the Angle N C c, a Part of each of the remaining Angles R C c and E C N will be equal. Moreover, the Triangle C O c, in its naſcent State, will be ſimilar to the Triangle C D E, for if from the equal Angles D C O, E C c, be taken the Angle N C c, a Part of each Angle, the remaining Angles O C c and D C E will be equal. Wherefore as $Rc : Oc :: NE : ED :: m : n$. Now ſince the Fluents are in the ſame Ratio with their Fluxions, it follows, that as $BC - BA : PC = AI - CF - FI :: m$ to n, and conſequently $n \times \overline{BC - BA} = m \times \overline{AI - CF - FI}$, and, by Diviſion, $\frac{n}{m} BC - \frac{n}{m} BA = AI - CF - FI$, and $FI = AI - CF + \frac{n}{m} BA - \frac{n}{m} BC$, whence it fol-

lows,

lows, that if the Arch A G be described from the Centre B, P C will be the Difference of the Incident Rays B A and B C, and if the luminous Point B become infinitely distant from the Curve A C Q, the incident Rays B A, B C, will be parallel, and the Arch A C will become a straight Line, perpendicular to the same Rays,

PROPOSITION.

THE Nature of the Curve A C Q being given, together with the luminous Point B, and the Ray of Incidence B C, let it be required to find the Point F in the refracted Ray C F, where the same Ray touches the Caustick Curve H F I by Refraction (*See the preceding Figure*)

HAVING found the Length of the Ray C E of the *Evoluta*, put B C $= y$, C N $= a$, C D $= b$, and C R $= x$, then, because of the Similitude of the Triangles C N E, C R c, C D E, C O c, B C R, B L n, it will be as C N . C D C R C O; that is, as a b x $\frac{bx}{a} =$ C O, and as B C B n equal to B N (when the Ray B c returns back into its first Place B C) C R L n, that is, as y $y + a$ x $\frac{ax + yx}{y} =$ L n, and, by the Law of Refraction, as E n E d E N E D m n, therefore as m n E n — E N ($=$ L n) E d — E D, that is, as m n . $\frac{ax + yx}{y}$ $\frac{anx - ynx}{my} =$ S d, and because the Triangles F C O and F S d are similar, it will be as C O — S d C O C S $=$ C D (in the evanascent State) C F, that is, as $\frac{bmyx - aanx - anyx}{amy}$ $\frac{bx}{a}$. b . $\frac{bbmy}{bmy - aan - any} =$ C F Wherefore,

First,

First, If the Angle N E H be made equal to D E C, and

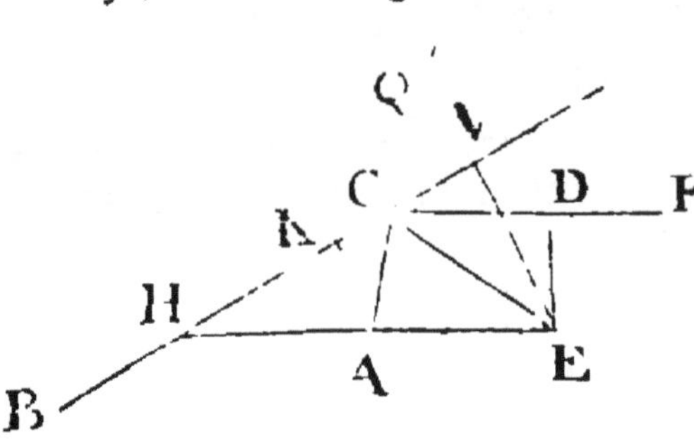

$CK = \frac{aa}{y}$, then H K is to H N as C D is to C F, wherefore the Point F will be in the Diacaustick I F H.

For the Triangles E D C and E N H are similar, whence as $ED : EN :: n : m :: (CD : NH) :: b : \frac{bm}{n}$, wherefore $HN - CN = \frac{bm}{n} - a = \frac{bm - an}{n} = HC$, and $HC - KC = HK = \frac{bmy - any - aan}{ny}$, and consequently $HK : HN :: CD : CF$, that is $\frac{bmy - any - aan}{ny} : \frac{bm}{n} :: b : \frac{bbmy}{bmy - any - aan} = CF$; whence it follows, that if the luminous Point B be on the same Side of the Curve A C Q towards N, or, which is the same thing, if the Curve be concave towards the luminous Point B, then y will become negative, and consequently C F will be $= \frac{-bbmy}{-bmy + any - aan}$ or $\frac{bbmy}{bmy - any + aan}$, and the Construction will be the same as before (*See the Figure in Page* 204)

Secondly, If we suppose the luminous Point B to be at an infinite Distance from the Curve A C Q, then the Rays of Incidence B C, B *c*, will become parallel Rays, and C F equal to $\frac{bbmy}{bmy - amy - aan}$, will become $\frac{bbmy}{bmy - any}$ (for the Term aan in this case will vanish), whence, by dividing by y, we shall have $CF = \frac{bbm}{bm - an}$, and because $\frac{aa}{y}$ becomes equal to nothing, therefore the Points C and K will coincide, and consequently it will be as HC HN CD . CF, whence the Point F is determined.

If m be infinite in respect of n, then the refracted Angle END will vanish, and consequently the refracted Ray CF, and the Ray of *Evoluta* CE, will coincide, and the Caustick by Refraction coincides with the *Evoluta* of the given Curve ACQ

Thirdly, If the Curve ACQ be convex towards the luminous Point B, and the Value of $CF = \frac{bbmy}{bmy - any - aan}$ be positive, it is manifest, that the Point F must be taken on the same Side with the Point D, in respect of C, but if the Value of CF be negative, then the refracted Ray CF must be produced on the Side towards B, and the Point F must be taken on the same Side of the Curve with the Point B whence it is manifest, that in the first case, when the Value of CF is positive, the refracted Rays converge on the Side of the Curve towards D (because it is on that Side the refracted Rays intersect each other) in order to determine the Point F, but in the last case, when the Value of CF is negative, the refracted Rays diverge, because, being produced, they intersect each other on the same Side of the Curve with B, in order to determine the Point F of the Caustick

Fourthly, If the Curve ACQ be concave towards the luminous Point B, then is the refracted Ray CF equal to $\frac{-bbmy}{-bmy + any - aan}$ or $\frac{bbmy}{bmy - any + aan}$, and consequently the refracted Rays being infinitely near, converge when the Value of CF is negative, and diverge when it is positive

Fifthly,

Fifthly, If the Curve A C Q be convex towards the luminous Point B, and if m be less than n, then $\frac{bbmy}{bmy - any - aan}$, the Value of C F will be negative, and consequently the refracted Rays diverge, and, in like manner, if the Curve A C Q be concave towards the luminous Point B, and m be greater than n, the Value of C F is positive, and consequently the refracted Rays diverge

Sixthly, If the Ray of Incidence B C touch the Curve A C Q in the Point C, then is C E $= a = 0$, and consequently C F is equal to b, whence it is manifest, that the Point F, in this case, will coincide with the Point D

Seventhly, If the Ray of Incidence B C be perpendicular to the Curve A C Q, then the refracted Ray C F will coincide with C E, the Ray of the *Evoluta*, and the right Lines C N and C D will become equal to each other, and to the Line C E, and consequently C F $= \frac{bmy}{my - ny \mp bn}$ will become $\frac{bm}{m - n}$, in which case the Rays of Incidence are parallel to each other

Eighthly, If the refracted Ray C F touch the Curve A C Q in the Point C, then is C D $= b = 0$, and consequently the Diacaustick will touch the Curve in the given Point C

Ninthly, If C E, the Ray of the *Evoluta*, be equal to nothing, the right Lines C N, C D, and consequently C F will vanish, and the Point C will be common to the Caustick, and the given Curve

Tenthly, If the Ray of the *Evoluta* C E be infinite, then the right Lines C N, C D, will also be infinite, and the Terms bmy and any will vanish, and consequently C F will be $= \frac{bbmy}{+aan}$, and because this Quantity is negative, when the Point F falls on the opposite Side of the Curve, in respect of the

the luminous Point B, and positive when B and F are on the same Side of the Curve, it is manifest, that the Point F must always be taken on the same Side of the Curve with the Point B, and consequently, that the refracted Rays will diverge. And in this Case it is plain, that the fluxionary Arch Cc is a straight Line, in which case the preceding Construction will not take Place, and therefore to determine the Point F of the Caustick H F I, when the Curve A C Q becomes a straight Line,

HAVING drawn B O perpendicular to the Ray of Incidence B C, until it intersect the right Line O C E perpendicular to A Q in O, and O L perpendicular to the refracted Ray N C L, and made the Angle BOH equal to the Angle L O C, then make B C to B H as C L to C F, I say, the Point F will be in the Diacaustick.

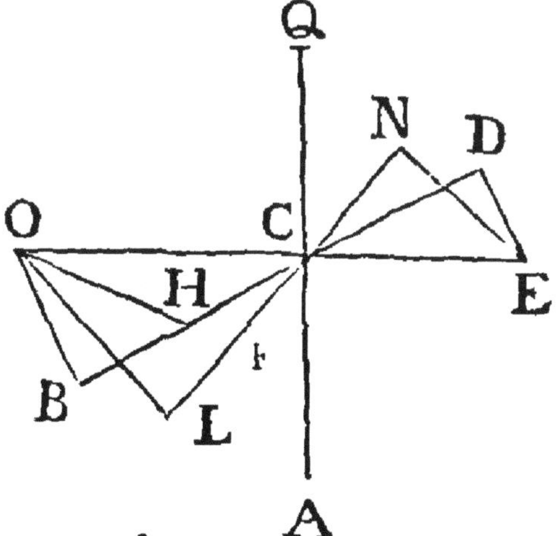

FOR the right angled Triangles C DE, C B O, C NE, and C L O are similar, and consequently, when E C is infinite, C D is to C N as B C to C L, that is, as $a : b :: y$: $\frac{by}{a} =$ C L, and because the Triangles O L C, and O B H are similar, it will be as O L to O B, so is n to m, and so is C L to B H, that is, as $n : m :: \frac{by}{a} . \frac{bmy}{an} =$ B H. It is manifest, that C B is to B H as C L is to C F, that is, as $y : \frac{bmy}{an} ::$ $\frac{by}{a} . \frac{bbmy}{aan} =$ C F.

THE same Curve A C Q can have but one Caustick by Refraction, the Ratio of m to n being given, and the Caustick is a Geometrical Curve, and may be rectified, supposing the given Curve to be a Geometrical Curve.

EXAMPLE I.

LET the Curve Line A C K be a Quadrant of a Circle, B the luminous Point, and let it be required to describe the Diacaustick H F N.

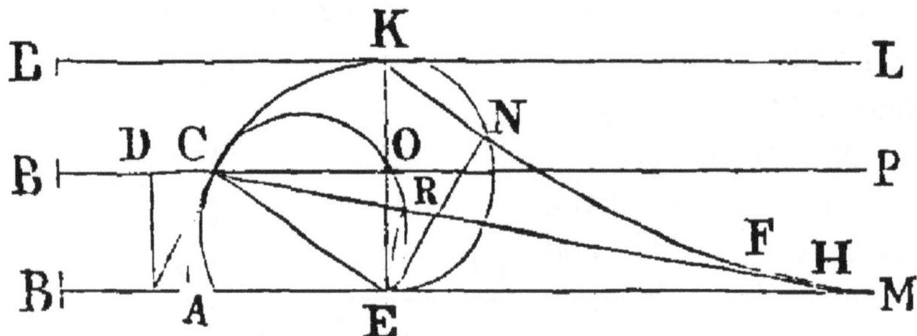

BECAUSE the Curve Line A C K is a Portion of the Circumference of a Circle, the Ray of its *Evoluta* C E is a constant Quantity. Now if the luminous Point B be placed at an infinite Distance, the Rays B A, B C, and B K will be parallel to each other, and perpendicular to K E, and supposing the Ratio of *m* to *n* to be as 3 to 2, which is the Ratio nearly of the Sine of the Angle of Incidence to the Sine of the Angle of Refraction in the Passage of a Ray of Light from Air into Glass, then because the Centre of the Circle becomes its *Evoluta*, it is manifest, that if we describe the Semicircle C O E on the Diameter C E, and make the Chord E R = $\frac{2}{3}$ E O, the Ray C R will be the refracted Ray, whose Length C F may be determined by the preceding Proposition. But,

First, To find the Point H, where the Ray B A, perpendicular to the Curve Line A C K, touches the Diacaustick H F N, we have $AH = \frac{bm}{m-n} = \frac{3b}{3-2} = 3b = 3\,AC$. And,

Secondly, IF the Semicircle E N K be described on the Diameter K E, and the Chord E N be taken equal to $\frac{2}{3}$ of E K,

E K, it is evident, that the Point N will be in the Diacaustick. And,

Thirdly, If A D be drawn parallel to E K, then the Portion of the Diacaustick F H = A H — C F — $\frac{2}{3}$ of D C, and consequently, the entire Caustick H F N is equal to $\frac{2}{3}$ of E A — K N.

Fourthly, If the parallel Rays B C, B A, fall on the concave Side of the Circumference of the Circle A C N K, and it

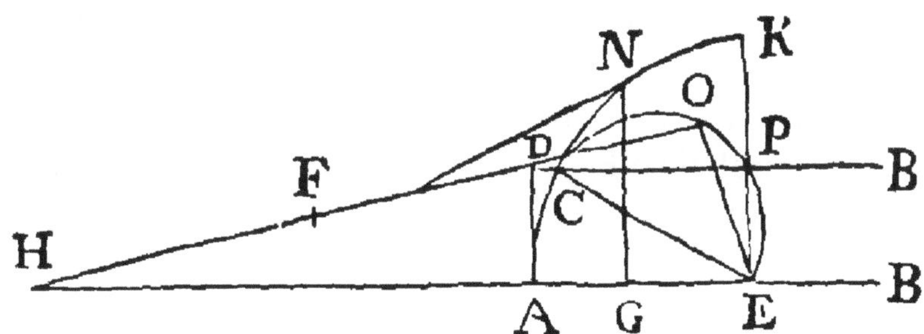

the Ratio of *m* to *n* be as 2 to 3, which is the Ratio of the Sines of the Angles of Incidence and Refraction, in passing from Glass into Air nearly, then on C E, the Ray of the *Evoluta* of the Circle, describe the Semicircle E P C, and take the Chord E O = $\frac{2}{3}$ E P, then will O C, produced towards F, be the refracted Ray, and the Point F may be determined by the preceding Proposition. But,

Fifthly, To find the Point H, where the Ray B A, perpendicular to the Curve Line A C K, passing through the Point A, touches the Diacaustick, suppose H, then A H = $\frac{bm}{m-n}$ $= \frac{2b}{2-3} = -2b$, whence it appears, that the Point H falls on the convex Side of the Curve A C N K, and the Distance of the Point H from A, the Vertex of the Curve, is equal to twice A E, or the whole Diameter of the Circle A C N K. And,

Sixthly, If we suppose C O = $\frac{1}{2}$ E P = C E, then it is manifest, that the refracted Ray C F will touch the Circle A C K in C, because, in this case, the Points O and C will coincide. Whence it is manifest, that if E P be made equal to $\frac{2}{3}$ of E K, the Point C will coincide with the Point N, where the Caustick touches the Arch of the Circle A C N K.

Seventhly, If the Line E P be more than $\frac{2}{3}$ of E K, then the Rays of Incidence B C cannot be refracted from Glass into Air, because E O, the Perpendicular to the refracted Ray O C, can never be greater than E C, and consequently all the Rays that fall between N and K will be reflected. And,

Eighthly, To find the Length of the Diacaustick H F N, draw A D parallel to E K, then the Portion of the Curve F H will be equal to A H — C F — $\frac{1}{2}$ D C, and drawing N G parallel to E K, the Caustick H F N = 2 A E + $\frac{1}{2}$ A G = $\frac{7 - \overline{5}^{\frac{1}{2}}}{2}$ E A.

Ninthly, If A C K L (*in Page* 210) be revolved about its Axis A F, the Quadrant A C K E will generate an Hemisphere, and if this Hemisphere be infinitely produced toward L and M, suppose of Glass, and the circumambient Fluid be Air, then all the Rays B O, parallel to, and infinitely near the Axis A E, will, being refracted at the spherical convex Surface of the Glass, converge to a Point H, distant from the Vertex A of the Glass three Semidiameters of the generated Sphere. And on the contrary,

Tenthly, If an infinite Number of Rays diverge from the Point H, placed at the Distance of three Semidiameters from the Vertex A of the spherical Convex Glass A C K, immerge into Air, and be refracted at the spherical convex Surface, they will, after Refraction, run parallel to the right Line H A, drawn through the radiant Point H and E, the Centre of the Sphere.

Eleventhly, If an infinite Number of Rays B C, be parallel, and infinitely near the Axis A E, and passing out of a Medium of Glass into a Medium of Air, be refracted at the spherical concave Surface of the Air, they will converge to the Point

Point H, whose Distance from the Vertex A is equal to the Diameter of the Sphere, and, on the contrary, if the Rays B C diverge from the Point H in Air, distant one Diameter of the Sphere from the Vertex of the Glass, and be refracted at the spherical convex Surface of the Glass, all the refracted Rays will run parallel to the Line H E, drawn through the luminous Point H, and E the Centre of the Sphere

In a Medium of Glass, if the Rays of Light be parallel to the Axis, and if they be refracted at the spherical convex Surface of the Air, the refracted Rays will converge to a Point in the Axis in the Medium of Glass at the Distance of one Diameter of the Sphere from the Vertex of the Glass

In a Medium of Air, if an infinite Number of Rays converge to a Point beyond the spherical convex Surface of the Air, at the Distance of one Diameter of the Sphere from the Vertex, and be refracted at the spherical concave Surface of the Glass, the refracted Rays will run parallel to the Axis of the Sphere.

In a Medium of Air, if an infinite Number of Rays, parallel to the Axis, be refracted at the spherical concave Surface of the Glass, the refracted Rays will converge to a Point in the Axis in the Air, whose Distance from the Vertex is three Semidiameters of the Sphere, and, on the contrary, in a Medium of Glass, if an infinite Number of Rays converge to a Point distant three Semidiameters beyond the spherical convex Surface of Air, be refracted at the same spherical convex Surface of Air, they will, after Refraction, run parallel to the Axis

N. B. What has been here said of parallel Rays, is to be understood of those Rays only that fall upon the Glass very near its Pole

EXAM-

EXAMPLE II.

LET the Curve A C K be a Logarithmetic Spiral, whose Centre is A, supposed to be the luminous Point from whence all the incident Rays are imagined to issue

IT is manifest, that the Point E (*See Pages* 155, 169) coin-

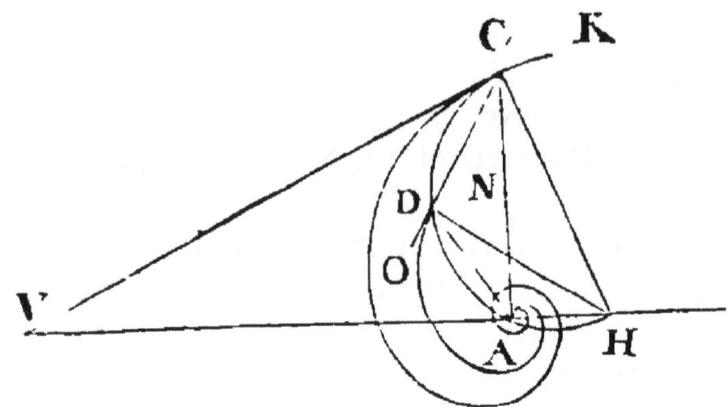

cides with the Point A, whence $a = y$, wherefore if you substitute y for a in the general Equation $\frac{bbmy}{bmy - any + aan}$, the Value of C F. (*See Page* 181) When the concave Side of the Curve is next the luminous Point, we shall have $CF = b$, wherefore the Point F will coincide with the Point D.

NOW if the Line A D be drawn, and the Tangent C V, the Angle A D O, the Complement of the Angle A D C to a Semicirle, will be equal to the Angle A C V For since the Circle, whose Diameter is H C, passes through the Points A and D, half the Arch A D C is the Measure of the Angles A D O and A C V, it is manifest, that the Caustick A D N is a Logarithmetical Spiral, differing from the given Spiral in Position only

PRO

PROPOSITION II

LET HF be a Caustick Curve by Refraction, and B the

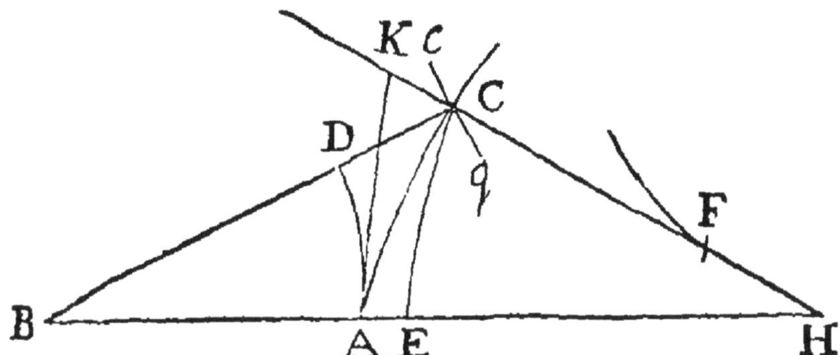

luminous Point. Now the Ratio of n to m being given, let it be required to find an infinite Number of Curves, such as AC, to which the given Curve HF shall be a Diacaustick.

DRAW any Tangent at Pleasure, HA, and take any Point A, in the same Tangent, for one of the Points of the Curve AC to be found, then on the Centre B, with the Radius BA, describe the small Arch oCq, then take $AE = \frac{n}{m} DC$, and describe the Arch AD, and on the same Centre with the Radius BC describe the Curve EC by involving the Caustick FH, until it cut the Arch oCq in the Point C, then make as DC or BC − BA : AE or CK or HA − FC − FH :: m : n, and consequently $FH = HA - FC + \frac{n}{m} BA - \frac{n}{m} BC$, and the Point C is in the Caustick to be found. Or,

IN any other Tangent FC, find the Point C, so that $HF + FC + \frac{n}{m} BC = HA + \frac{n}{m} BA$, and take $FK = \frac{n}{m} BA, + AH - FH$, and in the Line FK find the Point C; so so that C K is equal to $\frac{n}{m}$ B C; then will C be the Point to be found

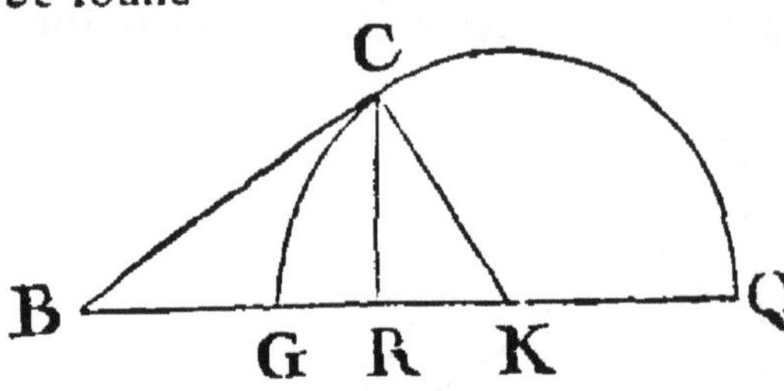

Now this may be done by describing the Curve G C, so that drawing from any Point C the Lines C B, C K, to the Points B and K, they shall always be to each other as m to n.

DRAW C R perpendicular to B K, and let the known Quantity B K $= a$, the indeterminate Quantities B R $= x$, R C $= y$, then, because the Triangles B R C and K R C are right-angled at R, B C is equal to $\overline{xx + yy}|^{\frac{1}{2}}$, and K C equal to $\overline{aa - 2ax + xx + yy}|^{\frac{1}{2}}$, but, from the Nature of the Problem, as $\overline{xx + yy}|^{\frac{1}{2}} : \overline{aa - 2ax + xx + yy}|^{\frac{1}{2}} :: m : n$, whence arises this Equation $yy = \frac{2ammx - aamm}{mm - nn} - xx$; which shews, that the Place of the Point C is in the Circumference of a Circle. Wherefore

TAKE B G $= \frac{am}{m+n}$, and B Q $= \frac{am}{m-n}$, and on the Diameter G K describe the Semi-circumference G C Q, then C will be the Place to be found, for because Q R $=$ BQ $-$ BR $= \frac{am}{m-n} - x$, and R G $=$ B R $-$ B G $= x - \frac{am}{m+n}$, by the Property of the Circle Q R $\times$ G R $=$ C R^2, and consequently $yy = \frac{2ammx - aamm}{mm - nn} - xx$.

IF the Rays of Incidence B A, B C, be parallel to a given right Line, whose Position is given, the first Solution will serve,

ſerve, but the following Conſtruction is preferable to the former.

TAKE FL = AH − HE, and draw LG parallel to AB, and perpendicular to AP, then make LO $= \frac{n}{m}$ LG, and draw LP parallel to OG, and PC

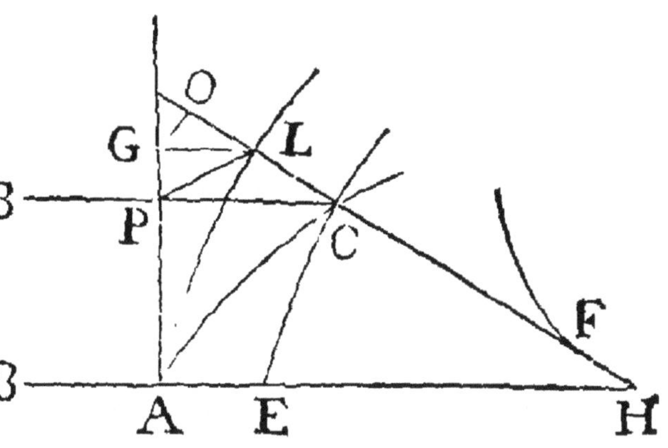

parallel to GL, then it is manifeſt, that C is a Point in the Curve to be found, for LO $= \frac{n}{m}$ LG and ML $= \frac{n}{m}$ PC. Again,

LET AK be a Curve Line, B the luminous Point, and ſuppoſing the Ratio of m to n to be given, let it be required to find a Number of Curves, ſuch as DN, which ſhall refract the Rays KN,

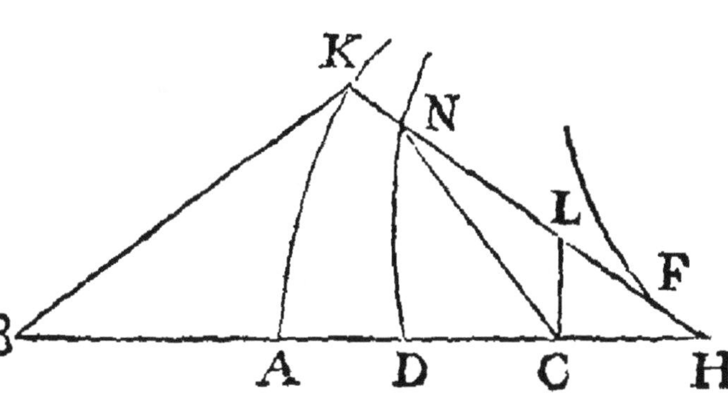

and make them converge to a given Point C.

LET the Curve FH be the Cauſtick by Refraction to the Curve AK, the luminous Point being B, it is manifeſt, that the ſame Curve FH ought to be the Cauſtick by Refraction to the Curve DN, the luminous Point being C, therefore $\frac{n}{m}BA + AH = \frac{n}{m}BK + KF + FH$, and $NF + FH - \frac{n}{m}NC = HD - \frac{n}{m}DC$, and conſequently, $\frac{n}{m}BA + AH$

Ee =

$= \frac{n}{m}BK + KN + HD - \frac{n}{m}DC + \frac{n}{m}NC$; wherefore $\frac{n}{m}BA - \frac{n}{m}BK + \frac{n}{m}DC + AD = KN + \frac{n}{m}NC$. Wherefore,

In any refracted Ray A H, if the Point D taken at Pleasure, be one of the Points of the Curve D N to be found, and in any other refracted Ray, as K F, you take $ML = \frac{n}{m}BA - \frac{n}{m}BK + \frac{n}{m}DC + AD$, and find the Point N, so that $\dot{N}L = \frac{n}{m}NC$, then the Point N will be in the Curve D N to be found

From the three last *Sections* it is evident, that the same Curve can have but one *Evoluta*, one Caustick by Reflection, and one Caustick by Refraction, when the luminous Point, the Ratio of the Angle of Incidence to the Angle of Refraction is given, and when the said given Curve is Geometrical, they are Geometrical also, and may be rectified, whereas the same Curve may be an *Evoluta*, or a Caustick by Reflection, or by Refraction to an infinite Number of Curves.

The End of the Second Part.

FLUXI-

FLUXIONS.

PART III.

CONTAINING

The Uſe of the Inverſe METHOD of FLUXIONS.

In EIGHT SECTIONS.

SECTION I.

Contains the Use of Fluxions *in the Rectification of Curves.*

SECT II.

Contains the Use of Fluxions *in the Quadrature of Curves, or in finding the Areas of Curvilinear Spaces*

SECT III.

Contains the Use of Fluxions *in finding the Values of the Surfaces of Solids generated by the Rotation of plain Surfaces about their Axis's*

SECT IV.

Contains the Use of Fluxions *in the Cubature of Solids, or in investigating Methods to find their Contents*

SECT V

Contains the Use of Fluxions *in finding the Centres of Gravity of Lines and Surfaces*

SECT VI

Contains the Use of Fluxions *in finding the Centres of Gravity of Solids*

SECT. VII

Contains the Use of Fluxions *in finding the Centres of Percussion of Lines and Surfaces*

SECT. VIII

Contains the Use of Fluxions *in finding the Centres of Percussion of Solids*

FLUXI-

FLUXIONS.

SECT. I.

Containing the Use of FLUXIONS *in the Rectification of Curves.*

PROPOSITION I

THE Fluxion of the Curve Line is to the Fluxion of the Ordinate, as the Tangent to the Ordinate

IN the following *Figure*, let A C represent a Curve, A the Vertex, A B the Absciſſe, B C the Ordinate, V C a Tangent to the Curve in the Point C, and V B the Subtangent I say,

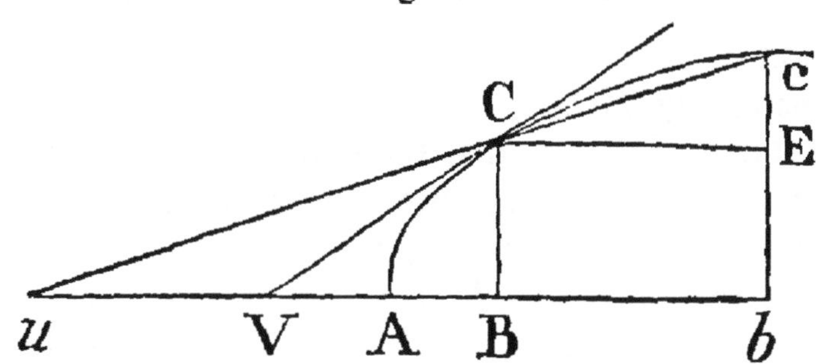

First, THAT the Fluxion of the Curve Line A C is to the Fluxion of the Ordinate B C, as the Tangent V C is to the Ordinate B C

DEMON-

DEMONSTRATION.

CONCEIVE the Ordinate B C to move along the Line A B *b*, parallel to itself 'till it arrives at the Place *b c*, and draw C E parrallel to A B *b*.

IT is manifest, that the little Arch C *c* is the nascent Augment of the Curve A C, and *c* E the nascent Augment of the Ordinate B C, generated in the same very small Particle of Time; for while the Curve Line A C flowed into, or became A C *c*, the Ordinate B C flowed into, or became *b c*

DRAW C *c* a Subtence of the little Arch C *c*, and produce it 'till it cut the Absciſſe produced in the Point *u*, then will the Triangles C *c* E, *u c b*, be similar, and it will be as C *c* : *c* E :: *u c* : *c b*, but $uc = u\text{C} + \text{C}c$, and $cb = c\text{E} + (\text{E}b =)$ C B, wherefore as C *c* : *c* E :: $uc + \text{C}c : c\text{E} + \text{CB}$

IMAGINE the Ordinate *c b* to return back into its former Place B C, at which time the Lines *c* C *u* and C V, also B *u* and B V, will coincide, the nascent Augments C *c* and *c* E will vanish, and the Triangle *c* C E, in its evanascent Form, will be similar to the Triangle C V B, and consequently the little curvilinear Arch C *c* will be to the little Line *c* E as V C to C B; but the little curvilinear Arch C *c*, and the little Line C E, in their arising State, are as the Fluxions of the Arch A C, and the Ordinate B C, whence the Fluxion of the Arch A C is to the Fluxion of the Ordinate B C, as V C the Tangent is to B C the Ordinate. *Q E D*

WHENCE it follows, that the Length of the Tangent to any Point in a Curve being known or given, the Value of the Curve Line itself may be readily found

FOR in the following *Figure*, let A B C represent the common Parabola, and suppose V C a Tangent to the Curve in the Point C, then will V B be the Subtangent.

PUT $\text{AB} = x$, $\text{BC} = y$, $\text{VB} = s$, and $\text{VC} = t$, then will $tt = ss + yy$ (*by the 47th of the 1st of* Euclid), whence

whence $t = \overline{ss + yy}^{\frac{1}{2}}$ Wherefore if z be put for the Length of the Arch itself, it will be, by the preceding Proposition, as $\dot{z} : \dot{y} :: \overline{ss+yy}^{\frac{1}{2}} : y$, whence $\dot{z} = \dot{y} \times \frac{\overline{ss+yy}^{\frac{1}{2}}}{y}$; but (*by the 3d Example of Sect.* I *Part* II.) s, the Subtangent, is equal to $2 AB = 2x$, whence $ss = 4xx$ substituting this Quantity then in the former Equation, in the room of ss, we shall have

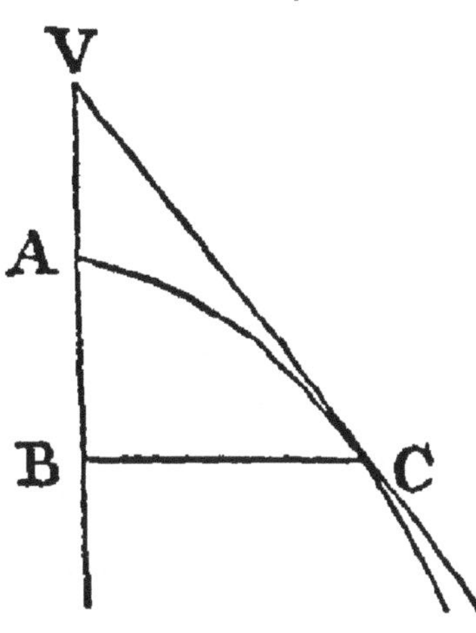

$\dot{z} = \dot{y} \times \frac{\overline{4xx + yy}^{\frac{1}{2}}}{y} = \dot{y} \times \frac{\overline{4xx + yy}^{\frac{1}{2}}}{\overline{yy}^{\frac{1}{2}}}$, but because from the Nature of the Curve, $ax = yy$ (where a stands for the Parameter), whence $aaxx = y^4$, and $xx = \frac{y^4}{aa}$, and $4xx = \frac{4y^4}{aa}$, substituting this last Equation in the room of $4xx$, and we shall have $\dot{z} = \dot{y} \times \frac{\overline{4y^4 + yyaa}^{\frac{1}{2}}}{\overline{aayy}^{\frac{1}{2}}} = \dot{y} \times \frac{\overline{4yy + aa}^{\frac{1}{2}}}{\overline{aa}^{\frac{1}{2}}} = \frac{\dot{y}}{a} \times \overline{4yy + aa}^{\frac{1}{2}}$, for the Fluxion of the Curve Line A C Now if the Square Root of $4\,\overline{yy + aa}$ be found, according to the Methods deliver'd in *Sect* II *Part* I and that Root be multiplied by $\dot{y}$, and divided by a, the Fluent of this last Quotient will give the Length of the Arch A C. *Q E I.*

PROPOSITION II.

THE Fluxion of the Curve Line is to the Fluxion of the Absciss as the Tangent is to the Subtangent.

THE same things being supposed as in the former Demonstration, it will be as $cC : CE :: cCu : ub$; but $cCu = cC + Cu$, and $ub = uB + Bb = VB + CE$, wherefore as $cC : CE :: cC + Cu : uB + CE$. Suppose now the Ordinate cb to return back again into its former Place BC, then will the nascent Augments cC, CE vanish, and the Triangle cCE, in its evanescent Form, become similar to the Triangle CVB, and the little Curve Line Cc, will be to the little Line CE, as CV to VB; but the little Curve Line Cc, and the little Line CE, in their evanescent State, are as the Fluxions of the Curve Line AC, and the Absciss AB. Wherefore the Fluxion of the Curve Line AC is to the Fluxion of the Absciss AB, as the Tangent VC is to the Subtangent VB. *Q. E. D.*

AND hence we are taught how, from the Knowledge of the Tangent and Absciss of any Curve, to find the Value of the Curve Line itself.

FOR if AB be put equal to x (*See the former Figure*) $BC = y$, $VB = s$, and $VC = t$, as before, we shall have $t = \overline{ss + yy}|^{\frac{1}{2}}$, but by *Proposition* II, as $z : x :: \overline{ss+yy}|^{\frac{1}{2}} : 2x$, whence $z = \frac{x}{2x} \times \overline{ss+yy}|^{\frac{1}{2}}$, and putting $4xx$ in the room of ss, because $s = 2x$, and ax, in the room of yy, to which it is equal from the Nature of the Curve in the former Equation, we shall have $z = \frac{x}{2x} \times \overline{4xx + ax}|^{\frac{1}{2}}$, for the Fluxion of the Curve; wherefore, if the Root of $4xx + xx$ be multiplied by x, and divided by $2x$, the Fluent arising from the Fluxion of this last Quotient, will give the Value of the Curve Line AC.

AGAIN,

AGAIN, because $x = \frac{2yy}{a}$, and $2\dot{x} = \frac{2\dot{y}y}{a}$, we shall have $\frac{\dot{x}}{2x} = \frac{2\dot{y}y}{2yy} = \frac{\dot{y}}{y}$. Substituting therefore $\frac{\dot{y}}{y}$ in the former Equation, $\dot{z} = \frac{\dot{x}}{2x} \times \overline{4xx + ax}^{\frac{1}{2}}$, in the room of $\frac{\dot{x}}{2x}$, there will arise $\dot{z} = \frac{\dot{y}}{y} \times \overline{4xx + ax}^{\frac{1}{2}}$; but because $4xx = \frac{4y^4}{aa}$, and $ax = yy$. Substituting therefore $\frac{4y^4}{aa}$ in the room of $4xx$, and yy in the room of ax, in the last Equation, and we shall have $\dot{z} = \frac{\dot{y}}{y} \times \overline{\frac{4y^4}{aa} + \frac{yy}{1}}^{\frac{1}{2}} = \frac{\dot{y}}{y} \times \frac{\overline{4y^4 + yyaa}^{\frac{1}{2}}}{\overline{aa}^{\frac{1}{2}}} = \frac{\dot{y}}{a} \times \frac{\overline{4y^4 + yyaa}^{\frac{1}{2}}}{\overline{yy}^{\frac{1}{2}}} = \frac{\dot{y}}{a} \times \overline{4yy + aa}^{\frac{1}{2}}$, for the Fluxion of the Arch A C, in the Terms of y, the same as was deduced from *Proposition* I.

PROPOSITION III.

THE Square of the Fluxion of the Curve Line is equal to the Sum of the Squares of the Fluxions of the Ordinate and Absciss.

DEMONSTRATION

PUTTING, as before, $AB = x$, $BC = y$, and the Curve Line $AC = z$, because the little Triangle CEc, in its evanescent Form, is similar to the Triangle VBC, the Angle CEc will be a right Angle; and because the Sides Cc, Ec, CE, in their arising Form, are as the Fluxions of the Curve Line,

 Ordinate,

Ordinate, and Abscisse, it follows (*from Prop* 47, *of* Euclide I) that $z\dot{z} = \dot{x}\dot{x} + \dot{y}\dot{y}$, whence $\dot{z} = \overline{\dot{x}\dot{x}+\dot{y}\dot{y}}^{\frac{1}{2}}$, and hence we are taught a direct Method to find the Value of any Curve Line from the Equation expressing the Relation of the Ordinate to the Abscisse, for if the Value of the Square of the Fluxion of the Ordinate, or Abscisse, arising from the Equation of the Curve, be substituted in the general Equation, in the room of the Square of the Fluxion of the Ordinate, or Abscisse, the new Equation thence arising will give the Fluxion of the Curve Line, whose Fluent will be the Length of the Curve Line itself

WHEREFORE if $AB = x$, $BC = y$, and the Curve Line $AC = z$, (*See the former Figure*) we shall have $\dot{z} = \overline{\dot{x}\dot{x}+\dot{y}\dot{y}}^{\frac{1}{2}}$, and supposing the Equation of the Curve to be expressed by this Equation $ax = yy$, we shall have $a\dot{x} = 2y\dot{y}$; whence $\dot{x} = \frac{2y\dot{y}}{a}$, and $\dot{x}\dot{x} = \frac{4yy\dot{y}\dot{y}}{aa}$. Substituting this last Quantity in the general Equation $\dot{z} = \overline{\dot{x}\dot{x}+\dot{y}\dot{y}}^{\frac{1}{2}}$ in the room of $\dot{x}\dot{x}$, we shall have $\dot{z} = \overline{\frac{4yy\dot{y}\dot{y}}{aa} + \dot{y}\dot{y}}^{\frac{1}{2}} =$

$$= \frac{\overline{4yy\dot{y}\dot{y} + aa\dot{y}\dot{y}}^{\frac{1}{2}}}{\overline{aa}^{\frac{1}{2}}} = \dot{y} \times \frac{\overline{4yy + aa}^{\frac{1}{2}}}{\overline{aa}^{\frac{1}{2}}} = \frac{\dot{y}}{a} \times$$

$\times \overline{4yy + aa}^{\frac{1}{2}}$, for the Fluxion of the Curve Line AC, the same as was deduced from the former Methods of Investigation And after the same manner may the Value of any Curve Line be found, as will more evidently appear from the following Examples

EXAMPLE I.

LET it be required to find the Length of the Arch AC, of the Circle AEFG.

PUT

PUT $AB = x$, $BC = y$, and $AD = 1$, then will $BF = 2 - x$, and because, from the Property of the Circle, $\overline{AB} \times \overline{BF} = BC^2$, we shall have $2x - xx = yy$, whence $2\dot{x} - 2x\dot{x} = 2y\dot{y}$, and $\dot{x} - x\dot{x} = y\dot{y}$, consequently $\dot{x} = \frac{y\dot{y}}{1 - x}$, whence $\dot{x}\dot{x} = \frac{yy\dot{y}\dot{y}}{1 - 2x + xx} = \frac{yy\dot{y}\dot{y}}{1 - yy}$ (by substituting $-yy$ in the room of $-2x + xx$, to which it is $=$)

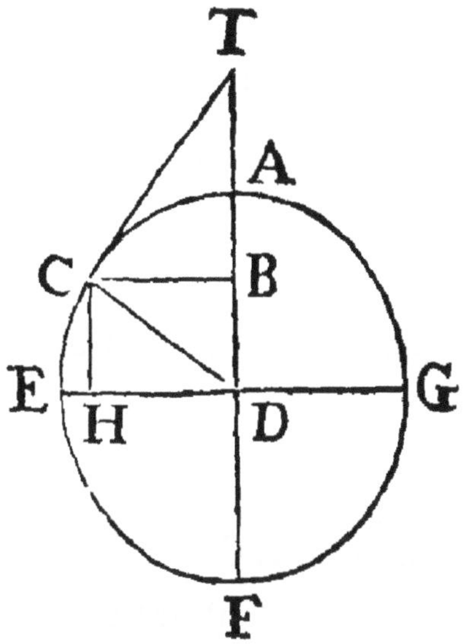

whence $\overline{\dot{x}\dot{x} + \dot{y}\dot{y}}^{\frac{1}{2}} = \overline{\frac{yy\dot{y}\dot{y}}{1 - yy} + \frac{\dot{y}\dot{y}}{1}}^{\frac{1}{2}} = \frac{\overline{yy\dot{y}\dot{y} + \dot{y}\dot{y} - yy\dot{y}\dot{y}}^{\frac{1}{2}}}{\overline{1 - yy}^{\frac{1}{2}}}$

$= \frac{\overline{\dot{y}\dot{y}}^{\frac{1}{2}}}{\overline{1 - yy}^{\frac{1}{2}}} = \frac{\dot{y}}{\overline{1 - yy}^{\frac{1}{2}}}$.

Now the Root of $\overline{1 - yy}^{-\frac{1}{2}}$ (by the Rules laid down in *Section* II *Part* I) will be found to be $1 + \frac{1}{2}y^2 + \frac{3}{8}y^4 + \frac{5}{16}y^6 + \frac{35}{128}y^8$, &c, each Term therefore of this Series being multiplied by $\dot{y}$ will produce $\dot{y} + \frac{1}{2}y^2\dot{y} + \frac{3}{8}y^4\dot{y} + \frac{5}{16}y^6\dot{y} + \frac{35}{128}y^8\dot{y}$, &c for the Fluxion of the Arch AC, whose Fluent $y + \frac{1}{6}y^3 + \frac{3}{48}y^5 + \frac{5}{112}y^7 + \frac{35}{1152}y^9$, &c.

$=y+\frac{1}{2\times3}y^3+\frac{1\times3}{2\times4\times5}y^5+\frac{1\times3\times5}{2\times4\times6\times7}y^7+\frac{1\times3\times5\times7}{2\times4\times6\times8\times9}$ y^9, *&c.* (whence the Law of Continuation is easy) will be the Length of the Arch A C.

Now if the first Term be called A, the second B, the third C, *&c.* and the first Term be multiplied by $\frac{1}{1}$, the second by $\frac{3}{3}$, the third by $\frac{5}{5}$, &c. we shall have $y+\frac{1}{2\times3}Ay^2+\frac{3}{4\times5}3By^2+\frac{5}{6\times7}5Cy^2$, &c. for the Length of the Arch A C,

Again, if from the Point C a Tangent Line, as C T, be drawn to meet the Diameter produced in T, then will B T be the Subtangent, and because the Triangles D B C and C B T are similar, it will be as B C : C D :: B T . T C; that is, B C is to C D as the Subtangent to the Tangent. But it has been proved in the second Proposition aforegoing, that the Fluxion of the Abscisse is to the Fluxion of the Curve Line, as the Subtangent is to the Tangent. Wherefore if we put the Arch $AC=z$, $BC=y$, $AB=x$, $AF=1$, then will $BF=1-x$, and $yy=x-xx$, from the Property of the Circle, wherefore it will be as $\overline{x-xx}^{\frac{1}{2}}:\frac{1}{2}(=DC)::\dot{x}:\dot{z}$, whence $\dot{z}$

$$=\frac{\dot{x}}{2\times\overline{x-xx}^{\frac{1}{2}}}=\frac{\overline{x-xx}^{-\frac{1}{2}}}{2}\dot{x}=\overline{x-xx}^{-\frac{1}{2}}\times\frac{1}{2}\dot{x}$$

will be the Fluxion of the Arch A C.

Now by extracting the Square Root of $\overline{x-xx}^{-\frac{1}{2}}$, according to the Rules laid down in *Section* II. *Part* I. we shall have $x^{-\frac{1}{2}}+\frac{1}{2}x^{\frac{1}{2}}+\frac{3}{8}x^{\frac{3}{2}}+\frac{5}{16}x^{\frac{5}{2}}+\frac{35}{128}x^{\frac{7}{2}}$, &c.

and

and multiplying this Root by $\frac{1}{2}\dot{x}$, we shall have $\frac{1}{2}x^{-\frac{1}{2}}\dot{x} + \frac{1}{4}x^{\frac{1}{2}}\dot{x} + \frac{3}{16}x^{\frac{3}{2}}\dot{x} + \frac{5}{32}x^{\frac{5}{2}}\dot{x} + \frac{35}{256}x^{\frac{7}{2}}\dot{x}$, &c. whose Fluent $x^{\frac{1}{2}} + \frac{1}{6}x^{\frac{3}{2}} + \frac{3}{40}x^{\frac{5}{2}} + \frac{5}{112}x^{\frac{7}{2}} + \frac{35}{1152}x^{\frac{9}{2}}$, &c. or $x^{\frac{1}{2}} \times \overline{1 + \frac{1}{6}x + \frac{3}{40}x^{2} + \frac{5}{112}x^{3} + \frac{35}{1152}x^{4}}$, &c or $x^{\frac{1}{2}} \times \overline{1 + \frac{1}{2\times3}x + \frac{1\times3}{2\times4\times5}x^{2} + \frac{1\times3\times5}{2\times4\times6\times7}x^{3} + \frac{1\times3\times5\times7}{2\times4\times6\times8\times9}x^{4}}$, &c will give the Length of the Arch A C.

AGAIN, if B D be put equal to x, and A D $= 1$, then C B $= \overline{1 - xx}^{\frac{1}{2}}$ (*by the 47th of* Euclid I) wherefore, by the first *Proposition* of this *Section*, it will be as $\overline{1-xx}^{\frac{1}{2}} : 1 :: \dot{x} : \dot{z}$; wherefore $\dot{z} = \frac{1}{\overline{1-xx}^{\frac{1}{2}}}\dot{x}$. Or, because A B $\times$ B F $=$ B C^{2}, therefore $\overline{1-x}$ ($=$ A B) $\times$ $\overline{1+x}$ ($=$ B F) $= 1 - xx = yy$, whence $-2x\dot{x} = 2y\dot{y}$, and $-x\dot{x} = y\dot{y}$; whence $-\dot{y} = \frac{x\dot{x}}{y}$, and $\dot{y}\dot{y} = \frac{xx\dot{x}\dot{x}}{yy} = \frac{xx\dot{x}\dot{x}}{1-xx}$. Wherefore if this Quantity $\frac{xx\dot{x}\dot{x}}{1-xx}$ be substituted in the general Equation $\dot{z} = \overline{\dot{x}\dot{x} + \dot{y}\dot{y}}^{\frac{1}{2}}$, in the room of $\dot{y}\dot{y}$, we then shall have $\dot{z} = \overline{\frac{\dot{x}\dot{x}}{1} + \frac{xx\dot{x}\dot{x}}{1-xx}}^{\frac{1}{2}} = \frac{\overline{\dot{x}\dot{x}}^{\frac{1}{2}}}{\overline{1-xx}^{\frac{1}{2}}} = \frac{1}{\overline{1-xx}^{\frac{1}{2}}}\dot{x}$, whose Fluent $x + \frac{1}{6}x^{3} + \frac{3}{40}x^{5} + \frac{5}{112}x^{7}$, &c will be the Length of the Arch C E, the Complement of the Arch A C

If

If $AB = 1$, and $x = \frac{1}{2}$, then will the Arch CE be equal to $\frac{1}{2} + \frac{1}{6}$ of $\frac{1}{8} + \frac{3}{40}$ of $\frac{1}{32} + \frac{5}{112}$ of $\frac{1}{128} + \frac{35}{1152}$ of $\frac{1}{512}$, *&c.* = .523598, but when x is equal to $\frac{1}{2}$ AD, then the the Arch CE will be $\frac{1}{6}$ of the Semi circumference, and $6 \times .523988$, *&c* equal to 3.141588, or rather 3.14159, will be the Semi-circumference, when the Radius is assumed equal to Unity, or the whole Circumference when the Diameter it self is put equal to Unity.

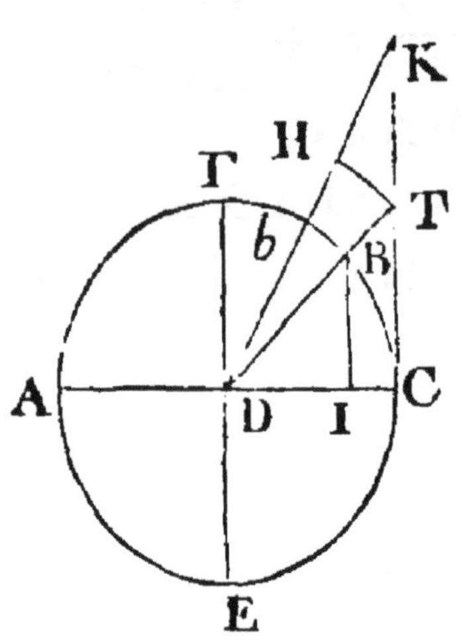

Again, if in the adjacent *Figure* we put the Arch $BC = z$, the Tangent $CT = t$, and the Radius $DB = DC = 1$, we shall have the Secant $DT = \overline{1+tt}^{\frac{1}{2}}$ (*by the 47th of* Euclid I.) Now if we imagine the Secant DT to move about the Centre D, till it comes into the Place DK, and in the same Time as the Point T does describe the little Arch TH (which we will assume equal to v) the Tangent CT will become CK, and the Arch BC will become Cb, and consequently the nascent Augments TK and Bb, will be as the Fluxions of CT and CB, that is, as $\dot{t}$ to $\dot{z}$, and because the Triangle THK, in its nascent Form, is similar to the Triangle TCD, it will be as $\dot{t} : v :: \overline{1+tt}^{\frac{1}{2}} : 1$. And again, because the nascent Triangles DHT and DbB are similar, it will be as $v : \dot{z} :: \overline{1+tt}^{\frac{1}{2}} : 1$, multiplying therefore these two Sets of Proportionals together, we shall have as $v \times \dot{t} : v \times \dot{z} :: 1+tt : 1$, and dividing the two first Terms by v, it will be as $\dot{t} : \dot{z} :: 1 + tt : 1$, whence $\dot{z} \times \overline{1+tt} = \dot{t}$, and $\dot{z} = \frac{\dot{t}}{1+tt}$, but

but by the Rules deliver'd in *Section* II. *Part* I) $\frac{\dot{t}}{1+tt} = \dot{t} - t^2\dot{t} + t^4\dot{t} - t^6\dot{t} + t^8\dot{t}$, &c. Whence by *Section* VIII. *Part* I, we shall have the Fluent $z = t - \frac{1}{3}t^3 + \frac{1}{5}t^5 - \frac{1}{7}t^7 + \frac{1}{9}t^9$, &c for the Length of the Arch of the Circle CB

Now if we consider the Arch BC as an Arch of 30 Degrees, or $\frac{1}{12}$ of the whole Circumference, the right Sine BI, in the present Case, is equal to $\frac{1}{2}$, consequently DI $= \overline{DB^2 - BI^2}^{\frac{1}{2}}$ will be equal to $\sqrt{1-\frac{1}{4}} = \sqrt{\frac{3}{4}}$, and because the Triangles DIB and DCT are similar, it will be as DI : IB :: DC : CT, that is, as $\sqrt{\frac{3}{4}} : \sqrt{\frac{1}{4}} :: \sqrt{1} : \sqrt{\frac{1}{3}}$, equal, in this Case, to t, whence the Length of the correspondent Arch BC $= z$ is equal (because $\frac{1}{3}$ is the Square of $\sqrt{\frac{1}{3}}$) to $\sqrt{\frac{1}{3}} - \frac{\frac{1}{3}\sqrt{\frac{1}{3}}}{3} + \frac{\frac{1}{9}\sqrt{\frac{1}{3}}}{5} - \frac{\frac{1}{27}\sqrt{\frac{1}{3}}}{7} + \frac{\frac{1}{81}\sqrt{\frac{1}{3}}}{9}$, &c. $= \sqrt{\frac{1}{3}} - \frac{1}{9}\sqrt{\frac{1}{3}} + \frac{1}{45}\sqrt{\frac{1}{3}} - \frac{1}{189}\sqrt{\frac{1}{3}} + \frac{1}{729}\sqrt{\frac{1}{3}}$, &c. and because the Arch of 30 Degrees is $\frac{1}{6}$ of the Semi-circumference, therefore $6 \times \sqrt{\frac{1}{3}} = \sqrt{\frac{36}{3}} = \sqrt{12}$, will give the Semi-circumference itself. Wherefore if the Square Root of 12 be divided continually by 3, and the several Quotients again by the odd Numbers successively, *viz* the first by 3, the second by 5, the third by 7, &c. the Sum of all the last Quotients (regard being had to the negative and positive Terms) will give the Length of the Semi-circumference in such Parts as the Radius is Unity, or the whole Circumference, the Diameter being supposed equal to Unity, equal to 3.14159265389. +

It has been shewn, that if t be put for the Length of the Tangent of any Arch, and z for the Length of the correspondent

dent Arch, that $z = t - \frac{1}{3}t^3 + \frac{1}{5}t^5 - \frac{1}{7}x^7 + \frac{1}{9} - t^9$, &c whence the Length of the Tangent being given, the Length of the Arch may be found Hence, and by the Help of the Rules laid down in Page 40, for the Reversion of Series, may the Series be found for finding the Length of the Tangent from the Length of the Arch supposed to be known or given; for because $z = t - \frac{1}{3}t^3 + \frac{1}{5}t^5 - \frac{1}{7}t^7$, *&c.* therefore $z^3 = t^3 - t^5 + \frac{42}{45}t^7$, *&c.* whence $z + \frac{1}{3}z^3$, *&c* $= t - \frac{2}{15}t^5 + \frac{53}{315}t^7$, &c. Again, because $z^5 = t^5 - \frac{5}{3}t^7$, *&c.* therefore $z + \frac{1}{3}z^3 + \frac{2}{15}z^5$, &c. $= t - \frac{2}{9}t^7$, &c. and because $z^7 = t^7$, &c. therefore $z + \frac{1}{3}z^3 + \frac{2}{15}z^5 + \frac{17}{315}z^7$, &c. $= t$ whence t, the Tangent, is equal to $z + \frac{1}{3}z^3 + \frac{2}{15}z^5 + \frac{17}{315}z^7$, &c. or by putting $z = At + Bt + Ct$, &c. after the manner taught in Page 41, the same Series would arise.

AGAIN, because $DT = \overline{TC^2 + DC^2}^{\frac{1}{2}}$ (*See the Figure in Page* 230.) if to the Square of $z + \frac{1}{3}z^3 + \frac{2}{15}z^5 + \frac{17}{315}z^7$, &c. which is $z^2 + \frac{2}{3}z^4 + \frac{17}{45}z^6 + \frac{62}{315}z^8$, *&c.* be added 1, the Square Root of the Sum $1 + z^2 + \frac{2}{3}z^4 + \frac{17}{45}z^6$ +

$+\frac{62}{315}z^8$, *&c.* viz. $1+\frac{1}{2}z^2+\frac{5}{24}z^4+\frac{61}{720}z^6+\frac{277}{8064}z^8$, &c. will be the Length of the Secant of the same Arch, and because as DT : TC :: DB : BI, whence $BI=\frac{TC\times DB}{DT}$ If $z+\frac{1}{3}z^3+\frac{2}{15}z^5+\frac{17}{315}z^7$, &c. be divided by $1+\frac{1}{2}z^2+\frac{5}{24}z^4+\frac{61}{720}z^6$, *&c.* the Quotient $z-\frac{1}{6}z^3+\frac{1}{120}z^5-\frac{1}{5040}z^7$, &c. will give the Length of the Sine of the same Arch, and by reversing these last Series for finding the Secant and Sine of any Arch, you will have new Series arise, for finding the Length of the corresponding Arch from the Sine or Secant supposed to be known or given. For Example, if y be put for the Sine of any Arch, because $y=z-\frac{1}{6}z^3+\frac{1}{120}z^5-\frac{1}{5040}z^7$, *&c.* we shall find, by the Method of infinite Series, that $y^3=z^3-\frac{1}{2}z^5+\frac{13}{120}z^7$, *&c.* Whence $y+\frac{1}{6}y^3=z-\frac{3}{40}z^5+\frac{3}{168}z^7$, &c. and because $y^5=z^5-\frac{5}{6}z^7$, &c. $y+\frac{1}{6}y^3+\frac{3}{40}y^5=z+\frac{5}{112}z^7$, &c. And inasmuch as $y^7=z^7$, *&c.* we shall have $y+\frac{1}{6}y^3+\frac{3}{40}y^5+\frac{5}{112}y^7$, &c. $=z$, which is a Series for finding the Length of the Arch corresponding to the Ordinate or right Sine y, the same as was directly investigated in Page 227. And after

 the

the ſame manner may the Arch correſponding to $1 + \frac{1}{2} z^2 + \frac{5}{24} z^4$, &c its Secant, be found, whence Variety of Series may be inveſtigated for finding the Length of the ſame circular Arch.

EXAMPLE II

LET it be required to find the Length of any Arch of the Ellipſis

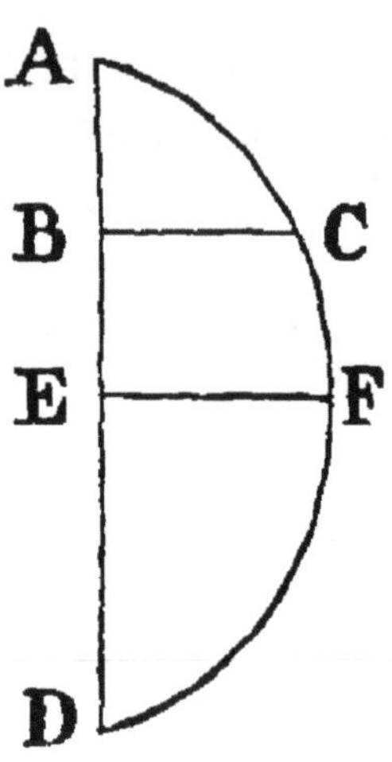

IN the adjacent *Figure*, which repreſents a Semi-Ellipſis, put $FE = c$, $AE = a$, $AB = x$, then will $BD = 2a - x$, let $BC = y$, and the Arch, whoſe Length is required, be $= z$

NOW becauſe from the Nature of the Ellipſis, as $AB \times BD$ ($AE \times ED =$) AE^2 : BC^2 :: FE^2, therefore as $x \times \overline{2a - x} = 2ax - xx : aa :: yy : cc$, whence $cc \times \overline{2ax - xx} = aayy$, conſequently $2ax - xx = \frac{aa}{cc} \times yy$, conſequently $2a\dot{x} - 2x\dot{x} = \frac{aa}{cc} \times 2y\dot{y}$, and $a\dot{x} - x\dot{x} = \frac{aa}{cc} \times y\dot{y}$, and $\overline{a - x}\,\dot{x} = \frac{aa \times y\dot{y}}{cc}$, whence $\dot{x} = \frac{aay\dot{y}}{cca - ccx}$, and

$$\dot{x}\dot{x} = \frac{a^4 yy\dot{y}\dot{y}}{c^4 aa - 2c^4 ax + c^4 xx} = \frac{a^4 yy\dot{y}\dot{y}}{c^4 aa - c^4 \times \overline{2ax - xx}},$$

and becauſe from the Nature of the Curve $cc \times \overline{2ax - xx} = aayy$, and $c^4 \times \overline{2ax - xx} = aaccyy$, if we ſubſtitute $aaccyy$ in the former Equation, in the room of $c^4 \times \overline{2ax - xx}$, to which

which it is equal, we shall have $xx = \frac{a^4 yyyy}{c^4 aa - aaccyy}$, and (by dividing by aa) $xx = \frac{aayyyy}{c^4 - ccyy}$, consequently $zz = xx + yy = \frac{a^2 yyyy}{c^4 - ccyy} + yy$, by adding yy to each Side of the Equation, whence $zz = \frac{aayyyy + c^4 yy - ccyyyy}{c^4 - ccyy}$

$$= \frac{\overline{c^4 + aa - cc} \times yy}{c^4 - ccyy} \times yy = \frac{\overline{c^4 + aa - cc} \times yy}{cc - yy} \times \frac{yy}{cc}$$

whence $z = \frac{y}{c} \times \frac{\overline{c^4 + aa - cc \times yy}^{\frac{1}{2}}}{\overline{cc - yy}^{\frac{1}{2}}}$. Now if we assume $c = 1$, then $z = y \times \frac{\overline{1 + aa - 1 \times yy}^{\frac{1}{2}}}{\overline{1 - yy}^{\frac{1}{2}}}$, and if $aa - 1$ be put equal to d, we shall have $z = y \times \frac{\overline{1 + dyy}^{\frac{1}{2}}}{\overline{1 - yy}^{\frac{1}{2}}} = y$

$$\times \frac{1 + \frac{1}{2} dyy - \frac{1}{8} ddy^4 + \frac{1}{16} d^3 y^6 - \frac{5}{128} d^4 y^8 + \frac{7}{256} d^5 y^{10}}{1 - \frac{1}{2} yy - \frac{1}{8} y^4 - \frac{1}{16} y^6 - \frac{5}{128} y^8 - \frac{7}{256} y^{10}},$$

&c for the Fluxion of the Arch A C, whose Fluent $y + \frac{dy^3}{2\times3} + \frac{dy^5}{2\times5} - \frac{d^2 y^5}{2\times2\times2\times5} + \frac{dy^7}{2\times7} - \frac{d^2 y^7}{2\times2\times7} + \frac{d^3 y^7}{2\times2\times2\times2\times7}$, &c. will give the Length of the Arch itself.

Now if the Length of the Arch F C be required, put A F $= a$, E F $= c$, BC $= y$, and BE $= x$, then will A B $= a - x$, and BD $= a + x$, and consequently, from the Property of the

Curve, it will be as $\overline{a+x}\times\overline{a-x} : a\times a :: yy : cc$, that is, as $aa-xx : aa :: yy : cc$, whence $\overline{aa-xx}\times cc = aayy$, and $aacc - ccxx = aayy$, and $ccxx = aacc - aayy$, and $2ccx\dot{x} = -2aay\dot{y}$, and $ccx\dot{x} = -aay\dot{y}$, and $\dot{x} = \frac{aay\dot{y}}{-ccx}$, and $\dot{x}\dot{x} = \frac{a^4yy\dot{y}\dot{y}}{c^4xx}$, and because $ccaa - ccxx = aayy$, whence $xx = \frac{aacc-aayy}{cc}$, therefore $c^4xx = aac^4 - aaccyy$, substituting therefore this Quantity in the former Equation in the room of c^4xx, and we shall have $\dot{x}\dot{x} = \frac{a^4yy\dot{y}\dot{y}}{aac^4-aaccyy} = \frac{aayy\dot{y}\dot{y}}{c^4-ccyy}$ (by dividing by aa), whence $\dot{z}\dot{z} = \dot{x}\dot{x}+\dot{y}\dot{y} = \frac{aayy\dot{y}\dot{y}}{c^4-ccyy}+\dot{y}\dot{y}$ (by adding $\dot{y}\dot{y}$ to each Side of the Equation) and $\dot{z}\dot{z}$

$$= \frac{aayy\dot{y}\dot{y}+c^4\dot{y}\dot{y}-ccyy\dot{y}\dot{y}}{c^4-ccyy} = \frac{aayy+c^4-ccyy}{c^4-ccyy}\times\dot{y}\dot{y}$$

$$= \frac{c^4+\overline{aa-cc}\times yy}{c^4-ccyy}\times\dot{y}\dot{y} = \frac{c^4+\overline{aa-cc}\times yy}{cc-yy}\times\frac{\dot{y}\dot{y}}{cc},$$

whence $\dot{z} = \overline{\frac{c^4+\overline{aa-cc}\times yy}{cc-yy}}^{\frac{1}{2}}\times\frac{\dot{y}}{c}$, will be the Fluxion of the Arch C F, the same with the Fluxion of the Arch A C, when A B was supposed equal to x, and consequently the Fluent of this Fluxion must be the same with the Fluent of A C.

But if instead of putting A E $= a$, we put the whole transverse Diameter A D $= a$, and B C $= x$, as before, the Length of the Arch C F will be

$+$ x

$$+x$$
$$+\frac{cc}{2aa}\times\frac{x^3}{3a}$$
$$+\frac{cc}{2aa}-\frac{c^4}{8a^4}\times\frac{x^5}{5a^4}$$
$$+\frac{cc}{2aa}-\frac{c^4}{4a^4}+\frac{c^6}{16a^6}\times\frac{x^7}{7a^6}$$
$$+\frac{cc}{2aa}-\frac{c^4}{8a^4}+\frac{3c^6}{16a^6}+\frac{5c^8}{128a^8}\times\frac{x^9}{9a^8},\ \&c$$

AND because $yy=\overline{aa-xx}\times\frac{cc}{aa}$, therefore $y=\overline{aa-xx}^{\frac{1}{2}}\times\frac{c}{a}$, whence $\dot{y}=\frac{-x\dot{x}}{\overline{\overline{aa-xx}}^{\frac{1}{2}}}\times\frac{c}{a}=\frac{-x}{\overline{\overline{aa-xx}}^{\frac{1}{2}}}\times\frac{c}{a}\times\dot{x}$, whence $\dot{y}\dot{y}=\frac{xx}{aa-xx}\times\frac{cc}{aa}\times\dot{x}\dot{x}$, and $\dot{z}\dot{z}=\dot{x}\dot{x}+\dot{y}\dot{y}$ $=1+\frac{cc}{aa}\times\frac{xx}{aa-xx}\times\dot{x}\dot{x}$, whence $\overline{1+\frac{cc}{aa}\times\frac{xx}{aa-xx}}\Big|^{\frac{1}{2}}$ $\dot{x}=\dot{z}$ the Fluxion of the Arch C F, equal to $\dot{x}\times 1+\frac{1}{2}\frac{cc}{aa}$ $\times\frac{xx}{aa-xx}-\frac{1}{8}\times\frac{c^4}{a^4}\times\frac{\overline{xx}^2}{\overline{\overline{aa-xx}}^2}+\frac{1}{16}\times\frac{c^6}{a^6}\times\frac{\overline{xx}^3}{\overline{\overline{aa-xx}}^3}$ $-\frac{5}{128}\times\frac{c^8}{a^8}\times\frac{\overline{xx}^4}{\overline{\overline{aa-xx}}^4}=\dot{x}+\frac{1}{2}\dot{x}\times\frac{cc}{aa}\times\frac{x^2}{a^2}+\frac{x^4}{a^4}+\frac{x^6}{a^6}$ $+\frac{x^8}{a^8},\ \&c$

$$-\frac{1}{8}\dot{x}\times\frac{c^4}{a^4}\times\frac{x^4}{a^4}+\frac{2x^6}{a^6}+\frac{x^8}{a^8},\ \&c$$
$$+\frac{1}{16}\dot{x}\times\frac{c^6}{a^6}\times\frac{x^6}{a^6}+\frac{3x^8}{a^8},\ \&c$$

$-\frac{5}{128}\dot{x}\times\frac{c^8}{a^8}\times\frac{x^8}{a^8}$, &c whose Fluent will be x

$+\frac{1}{2}\times\frac{cc}{aa}\times\frac{x^3}{3aa}+\frac{x^5}{5a^4}+\frac{x^7}{7a^6}+\frac{x^9}{9a^8}$, &c.

$-\frac{1}{8}\times\frac{c^4}{a^4}\times \qquad \frac{x^5}{5a^4}+\frac{2x^7}{7a^6}+\frac{x^9}{9a^8}$, &c.

$+\frac{1}{16}\times\frac{c^6}{a^6}\times \qquad +\frac{x^7}{7a^6}+\frac{3x^9}{9a^8}$, &c.

$-\frac{5}{128}\times\frac{c^8}{a^8}\times \qquad \frac{x^9}{9a^8}$, &c. being equal to the Series first proposed.

EXAMPLE III.

LET it be required to find the Length of any Arch AC of the Parabola ACE.

PUT AB $= x$, BC $= y$, and the Parameter $= a$. Now because, from the Nature of the Curve, $ax = yy$, therefore $a\dot{x} = 2\dot{y}y$, and $\dot{x} = \frac{2y\dot{y}}{a}$; whence $\dot{x}\dot{x} = \frac{4y^2\dot{y}^2}{aa}$ and substituting this Value of $\dot{x}\dot{x}$ in the general Equation $\dot{z} = \sqrt{\dot{x}\dot{x}+\dot{y}\dot{y}}$ in the room of $\dot{x}\dot{x}$, we shall have

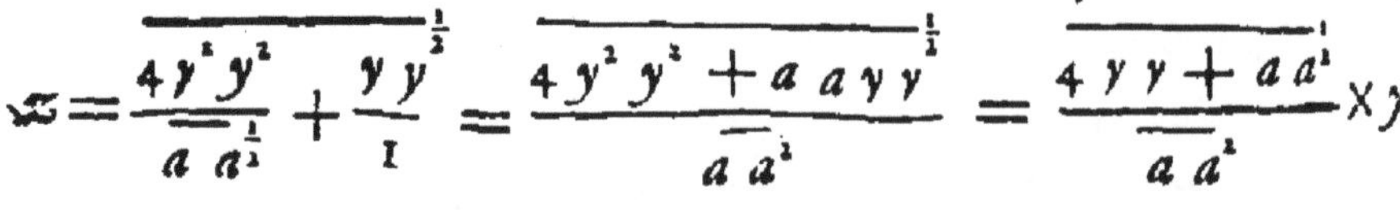

$$\dot{z} = \overline{\frac{4y^2\dot{y}^2}{aa}+\frac{\dot{y}\dot{y}}{1}}^{\frac{1}{2}} = \overline{\frac{4y^2\dot{y}^2+aa\dot{y}\dot{y}}{aa}}^{\frac{1}{2}} = \overline{\frac{4yy+aa}{aa}}^{\frac{1}{2}}\times\dot{y}$$

$= \overline{4yy+aa}^{\frac{1}{2}}\times\frac{\dot{y}}{a}$, for the Fluxion of the Arch AC, but the Square Root of $\overline{aa+4yy}$ (by *Section* II. *Part* I) is is $a + \frac{2y^2}{a} - \frac{2y^4}{a^3} + \frac{4y^6}{a^5} -$, &c. This therefore being multiplied by $\frac{\dot{y}}{a}$ will give $\dot{y} + \frac{2y^2\dot{y}}{aa} - \frac{2y^4\dot{y}}{a^4} + \frac{4y^6\dot{y}}{a^6} -$, &c whose Fluent $y + \frac{2y^3}{3aa} - \frac{2y^5}{5a^4} + \frac{4y^7}{7a^6}$, &c. will be the Length of the Curve Line A C. Now if we put $DE = c$, and the Parameter equal to 1, when A B flows into, or becomes A D, that is, when the Points B and D coincide, then y becomes equal to c, and consequently we shall have $c + \frac{2}{3}c^3 - \frac{2}{5}c^5 + \frac{4}{7}c^7$, &c for the Length of the whole Curve Line A C E.

Let us suppose $1x^2 = y^3$, which is the Property of the Cubic Parabola, the Parameter being supposed Unity, then will $2x\dot{x} = 3yy\dot{y}$, and $\dot{x} = \frac{3yy\dot{y}}{2x}$; whence $\dot{x}\dot{x} = \frac{9y^4\dot{y}\dot{y}}{4xx}$, and by substituting this in the general Equation $\dot{z} = \overline{\dot{x}\dot{x} + \dot{y}\dot{y}}^{\frac{1}{2}}$, in the room of $\dot{x}\dot{x}$, we shall have $\dot{z}\dot{z} = \frac{9y^4\dot{y}\dot{y}}{4xx} + \dot{y}\dot{y}$; and because $1x^2 = y^3$, whence $4x^2 = 4y^3$. If we substitute this last Quantity $4y^3$ in the room of $4xx$ in the last Equation, we shall have $\dot{z}\dot{z} = \frac{9y^4\dot{y}\dot{y}}{4y^3} + \dot{y}\dot{y}$ $= \frac{9y\dot{y}\dot{y}}{4} + \dot{y}\dot{y} = \frac{9y\dot{y}\dot{y} + 4\dot{y}\dot{y}}{4} = \frac{9y+4}{4} \times \dot{y}\dot{y}$, whence $\dot{z} = \frac{\overline{9y+4}^{\frac{1}{2}}}{2} + \dot{y} = \overline{9y+4}^{\frac{1}{2}} \times \frac{\dot{y}}{2}$ for the Fluxion on of the Curve, whose Fluent will be $\frac{1}{27}\times\overline{9y+4}\times\overline{9y+4}|^{\frac{1}{2}}$ and to find whether any thing is to be added or taken from this, put $y=0$, and there will remain $\frac{4}{27}\times\overline{4}|^{\frac{1}{2}}=\frac{8}{27}$, wherefore the Length of the Curve Line will be $\frac{1}{27}\times\overline{9y+4}\times\overline{9y+4}|^{\frac{1}{2}}-\frac{8}{27}$.

Now if we suppose $y^m = x$, which is the general Equation for all kinds of Parabola's, we shall have $\dot{x}=my^{m-1}\dot{y}$, whence $\dot{x}\dot{x}=m^2y^{2m-2}\dot{y}^2$, and putting $2m-2=n$, we shall have $\dot{x}^2=m^2y^n\dot{y}^2$, and substituting this Quantity $m^2y^n\dot{y}^2$ in the general Equation $\dot{z}=\overline{\dot{x}^2+\dot{y}^2}|^{\frac{1}{2}}$ in the room of $\dot{x}\dot{x}$, we shall have $\dot{z}=\overline{m^2y^n\dot{y}^2+\dot{y}^2}|^{\frac{1}{2}}=\dot{y}\times\overline{m^2y^n+1}|^{\frac{1}{2}}$ for the Fluxion of the Arch, whose Fluent $y+\frac{m^2y^{n+1}}{2\,\overline{n+1}}-\frac{m^4y^{2n+1}}{2\times4\times\overline{2n+1}}+\frac{1\times3m^6y^{3n+1}}{2\times4\times6\times\overline{3n+1}}-\frac{1\times3\times5m^8y^{4n+1}}{2\times4\times6\times8\times\overline{4n+1}}$, *&c* will be the Length of the Curve of any kind of Parabola whatsoever; and if in the room of n we substitute its Value $2m-2$, we shall have $y+\frac{m^2y^{2m-1}}{2\times\overline{2m-1}}-\frac{m^4y^{4m-3}}{2\times4\times\overline{4m-3}}+\frac{1\times3m^6y^{6m-5}}{2\times4\times6\times\overline{6m-5}}-\frac{1\times3\times5m^8y^{8m-7}}{2\times4\times6\times8\times\overline{8m-7}}$, *&c* for the Value of the Curve Line.

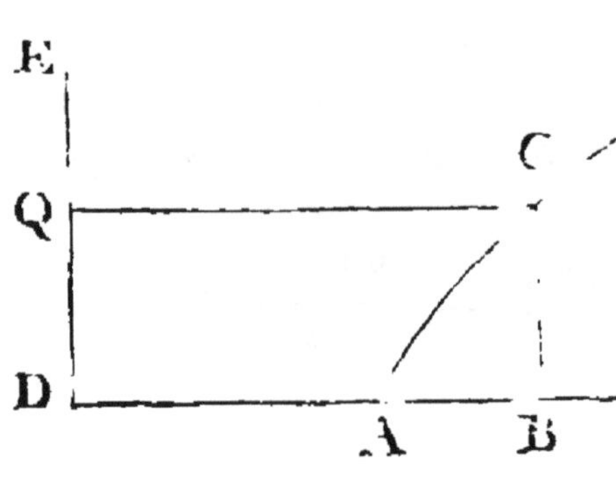

If DA = DE, the Semi-Conjugate Axis of an Equilateral Hyperbola be put equal to a, the Parameter of the Parabola, and the Ordinate BC = $2y$, and the Abscisse QC = DB = x, then will AB = $x-a$, consequently $xx-aa=4yy$, and $xx=4yy+aa$, whence $x=$

whence $x = \overline{4yy+aa}^{\frac{1}{2}}$, whence the Fluxion of the Hyperbolic Space D E C A will be $\dot{y}\times\overline{4yy+aa}$, the same with the Fluxion of the Curve of the Parabola, whence the Rectification of the Parabolic Curve depends upon the Quadrature of the Hyperbolic Space, whence the Rectification of a Curve may be compar'd with the Quadrature of a Curve, by supposing the Fluxion of the Curve to be rectified as an Ordinate, and the variable Quantity in that Fluxion as an Absciss to that Ordinate.

EXAMPLE IV.

LET it be required to find the Length of the Curve A C of the Hyperbola A C H.

LET I be the Centre, and put the Transverse Axis A E $= 2a$, the Semi Conjugate Axis I D $= c$, B C $= y$, and A B $= x$, then will E B $= 2a + x$, and because, from the Nature of the Curve, as E I $\times$ I A : E B $\times$ A B :: $\overline{ID}^2 : \overline{BC}^2$, therefore as $aa : 2ax + xx :: cc : yy$, whence $\overline{2ax+xx}\times cc = aayy$, and $2ax + xx = \frac{aayy}{cc} = \frac{aa}{cc}\times yy$, consequently $2a\dot{x} + 2x\dot{x} = \frac{aa}{cc}\times 2y\dot{y}$; whence $a\dot{x} + x\dot{x} = \frac{aa}{cc}\times y\dot{y}$, and $\dot{x} = \frac{aay\dot{y}}{cc\times\overline{a+x}} = \frac{aay\dot{y}}{cca+ccx}$, whence $\dot{x}\dot{x}$ is equal to $\frac{a^4yy\dot{y}\dot{y}}{aac^4+2ac^4x+c^4xx}$, and because, from the Pro-

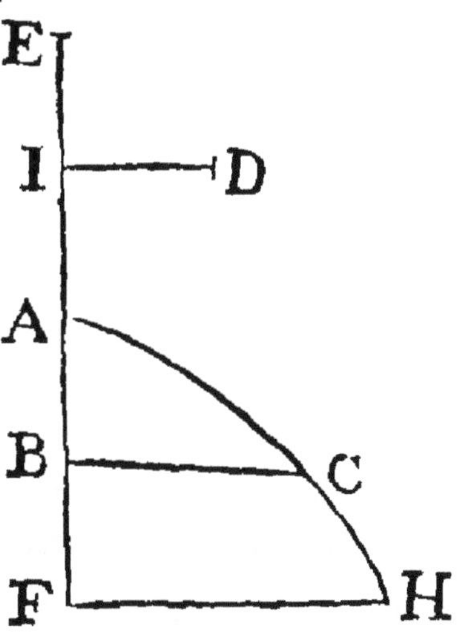

perty of the Curve $cc \times \overline{2ax+xx} = aayy$; whence $c^4 \times \overline{2ax+xx} = 2ac^4x + c^4xx = aaccyy$. If we substitute $aaccyy$, in the former Equation, in the room of $2ac^4x + c^4xx$, to which it is equal, we shall have $\dot{x}\dot{x}$

$$= \frac{a^4yy\dot{y}\dot{y}}{aac^4+aaccyy} = \frac{aayy\dot{y}\dot{y}}{c^4+ccyy}$$ (by dividing by aa),

this Quantity therefore being substituted in the room of $\dot{x}\dot{x}$ in the general Equation $\dot{z}\dot{z} = \dot{x}\dot{x} + \dot{y}\dot{y}$, we shall have $\dot{z}\dot{z}$

$$= \frac{aayy\dot{y}\dot{y}}{c^4+ccyy} + \dot{y}\dot{y}, \text{ whence } \dot{z}\dot{z} =$$

$$= \frac{aayy\dot{y}\dot{y} + c^4\dot{y}\dot{y} + ccyy\dot{y}\dot{y}}{c^4+ccyy} = \frac{c^4\dot{y}\dot{y} + \overline{aa+cc}\times yy\dot{y}\dot{y}}{c^4+ccyy}$$

$$= \frac{c^4+\overline{aa+cc}\times yy}{c^4+ccyy} \times \dot{y}\dot{y} = \frac{c^4+\overline{aa+cc}\times yy}{cc+yy} \times \frac{\dot{y}\dot{y}}{cc},$$

whence $\dot{z} = \dfrac{\overline{c^4+\overline{aa+cc}\times yy}^{\frac{1}{2}}}{\overline{cc+yy}^{\frac{1}{2}}} \times \dfrac{\dot{y}}{c}$, the Fluxion of the Arch A C, being the same Expression as that in the Ellipsis in *Example* II, except that in the Ellipsis, the Quantity c^2yy is negative, consequently the Fluent of this Fluxion will be the same with that of the Ellipsis, except in the Change of the Sign, when the Quantity c^2yy is concerned.

If the Hyperbola be an Equilateral Hyperbola, then $2ax + xx = yy$, whence $2a\dot{x} + 2x\dot{x} = 2y\dot{y}$, and $a\dot{x} + x\dot{x} = y\dot{y}$, and $\dot{x} = \dfrac{y\dot{y}}{a+x}$, whence $\dot{x}\dot{x} = \dfrac{yy\dot{y}\dot{y}}{aa+2ax+xx}$, and by substituting yy in the room of $2ax+xx$, in the last Equation, to which it is equal, we shall have $\dot{x}\dot{x} = \dfrac{yy\dot{y}\dot{y}}{aa+yy}$, substituting this Quantity therefore in the general Equa-

tion

tion $z\dot{z} = x\dot{x} + y\dot{y}$ in the room of $\dot{x}x$, we shall have $z\dot{z} = \frac{yyy\dot{y}}{aa+yy} + y\dot{y} = \frac{yyy\dot{y}+aay\dot{y}+yyy\dot{y}}{aa+yy} = \frac{aa+2yy}{aa+yy} \times y\dot{y}$, whence $\dot{z} = \frac{\overline{aa+2yy}^{\frac{1}{2}}}{\overline{aa+yy}^{\frac{1}{2}}} \times \dot{y}$, for the Fluxion of the Curve Line A C, and if we make the Parameter, which is supposed equal to a, to be equal to Unity, we shall have $\dot{z} = \dot{y} \times \frac{\overline{1+2yy}^{\frac{1}{2}}}{\overline{1+yy}^{\frac{1}{2}}}$; but the Root of $1+2yy$ is $1+yy$, &c and the Root of $1+yy$ is $1+\frac{1}{2}yy$, & these therefore being divided by each other, will produce $1+\frac{1}{2}yy$, &c and this being multiplied by $\dot{y}$, will produce $\dot{y}+\frac{1}{2}yy\dot{y}$, whose Fluent $y+\frac{1}{2\times3}y^3$, &c. will be the Length of the Curve Line A C of the Hyperbola.

EXAMPLE V.

LET it be required to find the Length of any Arch of the Equiangular, or Logarithmical Spiral.

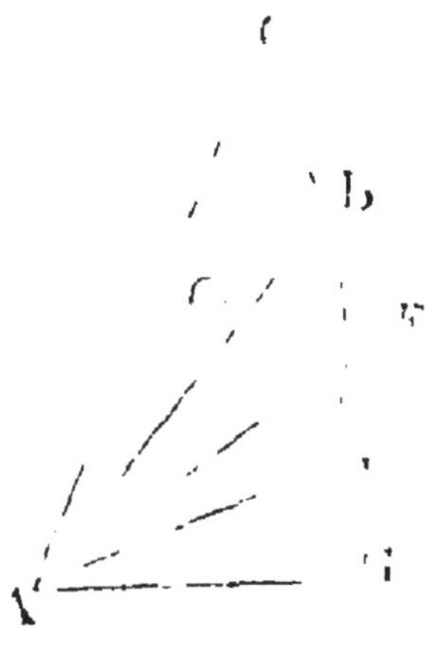

LET the Lines B I and F G touch the Spiral in the Points B and F, and draw the Lines A F and A G, so as to form right Angles with the Tangents B I and F G, and on A, as a Centre, describe the Arch Q F.

PUT $AF = a$, $AC = b$, and $BQ = AB - AF = y$, and $FG = c$. Now since, from the Nature of the Curve, any Radius, A F, forms the same Angle A F G with the Tangent F G, there-

fore

fore any Triangle, as A B E, will be similar to the given Triangle A F G, whence, by the first *Proposition* aforegoing, F G will be to A F as the Fluxion of A B to the Fluxion of the Arch, wherefore as $c . a :: \dot{y} : \frac{a\dot{y}}{c}$, the Fluxion of the Part F B of the Curve Line, whose Fluent $\frac{ay}{c}$ will be the Length of the Part F B, and putting $b - a = y$, to which it is equal, we shall have $\frac{ba - aa}{c}$ for the Length of F C, wherefore, by converting the Equation into an Analogy, it will be as $c : a :: b - a :$ F C, that is, as F G . A F :: A C — A F : F C, the Length of the Curve.

EXAMPLE VI.

LET it be required to find the Length of any Portion, D B, of the *Archimedian* Spiral Line A B D.

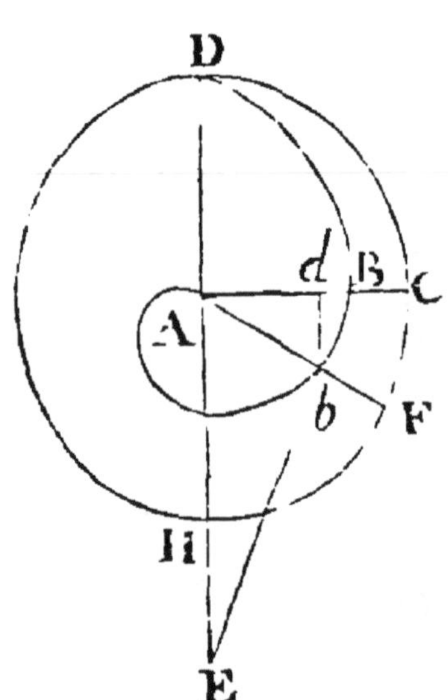

LET A D C H be the generating Circle, and put A D = A C = a, the Circumference D C H D = c, the Arch D C = x, the Ordinate A B = y, and let the Tangent to the Spiral in the Point B be drawn, and produc'd 'till it cut the Diameter D A H produced in the Point E.

IMAGINE the Ray A C to revolve about the Point A, and to move 'till it comes into the Place A F. Now because the nascent Triangles A C F, and A B b are similar, it will be as $a : \dot{x} :: y : \frac{y\dot{x}}{a} = $ B b, and again, because the nascent Triangle d b B, in its arising

State

State is similar to the Triangle AEB, it will be as $y : \frac{yx}{a} \quad y$ $\frac{yyx}{ay} = AE$; but because, from the Nature of the Curve, $ax = cy$, therefore $ax = cy$, whence $x = \frac{cy}{a}$, which being substituted in the room of x, in the former Equation, we shall have the Subtangent $AE = \frac{cyy}{aa}$ Again, because the Triangle EAB is right angled at the Point A, therefore $\frac{ccy^4}{a^4} + yy = \frac{ccy^4 + a^4yy}{a^4} = ccyy + a^4 \times \frac{yy}{a^4}$ (*by the 47th of* Euclid) is equal to EB^2, whence the Tangent $EB = \overline{ccyy + a^4}^{\frac{1}{2}} \times \frac{y}{aa}$ Again, because the nascent Triangle Bbd, in its arising State, is similar to the Triangle BEA, and the Sides dB and Bb of the nascent Triangle Bdb, are as the Fluxions of the Ordinate AB, and the Part AB of the Spiral Curve ABD, it will be as $y \quad \overline{a^4 + ccyy}^{\frac{1}{2}} \times \frac{y}{aa} \quad y \quad \overline{a^4 + ccyy}^{\frac{1}{2}} \times \frac{y}{aa}$, the Fluxion of the Part AB of the Spiral Line ABD

Now if we suppose the Radius AC of the generating Circle to be Unity, and put z for the Length of the Arch, then z will be equal $\overline{1 + ccyy}^{\frac{1}{2}} \times y$, but the Root of $1 + ccyy$ is $1 + \frac{1}{2}c^2y^2 - \frac{1}{8}c^4y^4 + \frac{1}{16}c^6y^6 - \frac{5}{128}c^8y^8 + \frac{7}{256}c^{10}y^{10}$, &c. This Root therefore being multiplied be y, will produce $y + \frac{1}{2}c^2y^2y - \frac{1}{8}c^4y^4y + \frac{1}{16}c^6y^6y - \frac{5}{128}c^8y^8y$ +

$+\frac{7}{256}c^{10}y^{10}\dot{y}$, &c. whose Fluent $y+\frac{1}{6}c^2y^3-\frac{1}{40}c^4y^5+\frac{1}{112}c^6y^7-\frac{5}{1152}c^8y^9+\frac{7}{2816}c^{10}y^{11}$, &c or $y+\frac{1}{2\times3}c^2y^3-\frac{1\times1}{2\times4\times5}c^4y^5+\frac{1\times1\times3}{2\times4\times6\times7}c^6y^7-\frac{1\times1\times3\times5}{2\times4\times6\times8\times9}c^8y^9+\frac{1\times1\times3\times5\times7}{2\times4\times6\times8\times10\times11}c^{10}y^{11}$, &c. will be the Length of the Spiral Arch A B

EXAMPLE VII

LET it be required to find the Length of any Part of the reciprocal Spiral A B E.

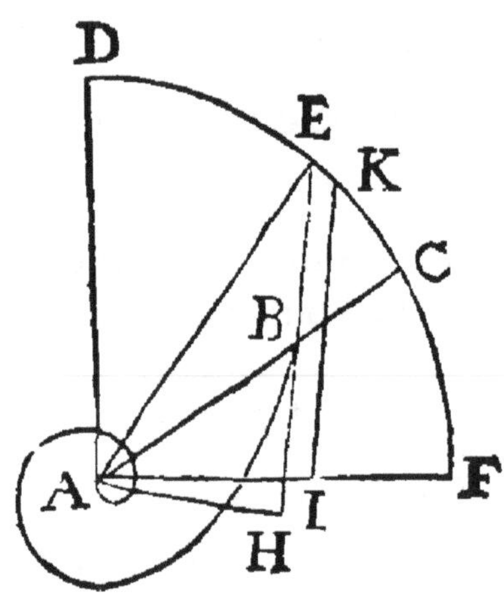

ABOUT the Centre A, with the Distance A E, describe the Quadrantal Arch D E C F, and produce A B to C, and because, from the Nature of the Curve, any Radius A E is reciprocally as the Angle D A E, it forms with the first Radius AD, or as the Arch D E, it will be as A B : A E :: D E : D C, whence AB × DC = A E × D E

Now if A D = A E = a, the Arch D E = c, the Arch D C = y, and A B = x then will $ac = xy$. Draw B H to touch the Curve in B, and at right Angles to B H draw A H, wherefore by *Proposition* II aforegoing, it will be $a : y :: x : \frac{yx}{a}$, and as $y : \frac{yx}{a} :: \dot{y} : \frac{y\dot{y}x}{ay}$, but because, from the Nature of the Curve $ac = xy$, therefore $x = \frac{acy}{yy}$, which

being

being put in the room of x in the former Expression $\frac{yy\dot{x}}{a\dot{y}}$, we shall have A H$=c$; that is, the Line drawn from the Centre A, perpendicular to any Radius A B of the Spiral, to intersect the Tangent to that Spiral at the Extremity of that Radius, will be a standing Quantity equal to the Arch D E, which Arch will become a strait Line perpendicular to the first Radius A D, when the Point E is at an infinite Distance, and the Angle D A E infinitely small, that is, it will be equal to A I, the Distance of the Asymptote I K from the Centre, whence $\dot{x}\,\overline{cc+yy}^{\frac{1}{2}} = \frac{\dot{y}}{y}\times\overline{cc+yy}^{\frac{1}{2}}$, the Fluxion of the Portion A B.

Now by extracting the Root of $cc+yy$, we shall have $c+\frac{yy}{2c}-\frac{y^4}{8c^3}+\frac{y^6}{16c^5}-\frac{5y^8}{128c^7}+\frac{7y^{10}}{256c^9}$, &c. and multiplying this Series by $\frac{\dot{y}}{y}$, we shall have $\frac{c\dot{y}}{y}+\frac{y\dot{y}}{2c}-\frac{y^3\dot{y}}{8c^3}+\frac{y^5\dot{y}}{16c^5}-\frac{5y^7\dot{y}}{128c^7}+\frac{7y^9\dot{y}}{256c^9}$, &c whose Fluent $c+\frac{yy}{4c}-\frac{y^4}{32c^3}+\frac{y^6}{96c^5}-\frac{5y^8}{1024c^7}+\frac{7y^{10}}{2560c^9}$, &c. Or,

$$c+\frac{\overline{1\times y^2}}{2\times 2c}-\frac{\overline{1\times 1y^4}}{2\times4\times4c^3}+\frac{\overline{1\times1\times3y^6}}{2\times4\times6\times6c^5}-\frac{\overline{1\times1\times3\times5y^8}}{2\times4\times6\times8\times8c^7}+\frac{\overline{1\times1\times3\times5\times7y^{10}}}{2\times4\times6\times8\times10\times10c^9},$$

&c. will be the Length of the Portion of the Curve A B.

EXAM-

EXAMPLE VIII.

LET it be required to find the Length of any Portion of the Logarithmetic Curve.

LET D P, B Q be Ordinates perpendicular to the Asymptote E P.

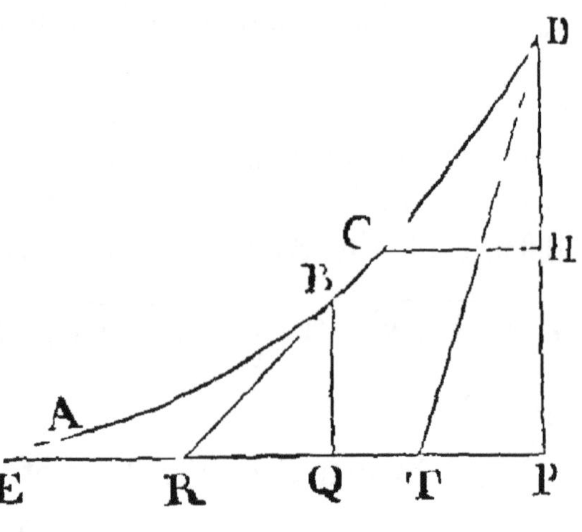

PUT D P $= z$, B Q $= y$, and P T $=$ Q R $= c$, whence B R$^2 =$ R Q^2 + Q B^2 $= cc + yy$, and B R $= \overline{cc+yy}|^{\frac{1}{2}}$, but by *Proposition* I aforegoing, it will be as

B Q : B R :: $y : \overline{cc+yy}|^{\frac{1}{2}} :: \dot{y} : \dot{z}$, whence $\dot{z} = \frac{\dot{y}}{y} \times \overline{cc+yy}|^{\frac{1}{2}}$ for the Fluxion of the Curve, but by extracting the Square Root of $\overline{cc+yy}$, we shall have $c + \frac{yy}{2c} - \frac{y^4}{8c^3} + \frac{y^6}{16c^5} - \frac{5y^8}{128c^7} + \frac{7y^{10}}{256c^9}$, &c. and multiplying this Series by $\frac{\dot{y}}{y}$, we shall have $\frac{c\dot{y}}{y} + \frac{y\dot{y}}{2c} - \frac{y^3\dot{y}}{8c^3} + \frac{y^5\dot{y}}{16c^5} - \frac{5y^7\dot{y}}{128c^7} + \frac{7y^9\dot{y}}{256c^9}$, &c. whose Fluent $c + \frac{y^2}{4c} - \frac{y^4}{32c^3} + \frac{y^6}{96c^5} - \frac{5y^8}{1024c^7} + \frac{7y^{10}}{2560c^9}$, &c. or $c + \frac{1 \times y^2}{2 \times 2 \times c} - \frac{1 \times 1\,y^4}{2 \times 4 \times 4 \times c^3} + \frac{1 \times 1 \times 3\,y^6}{2 \times 4 \times 6 \times 6 \times c^5} - \frac{1 \times 1 \times 3 \times 5\,y^8}{2 \times 4 \times 6 \times 8 \times 8c^7} + \frac{1 \times 1 \times 3 \times 5 \times 7\,y^{10}}{2 \times 4 \times 6 \times 8 \times 10 \times 10c^9}$, &c. will give the Length of the Arch.

EXAM-

EXAMPLE IX

LET it be required to find the Length of any Portion of the Cycloid.

PUT AH, the Diameter of the generating Circle, $= 1$, and $AB = x$, then will $BH = 1 - x$, and $BC^2 = 1 - x \times x$, $= x - xx$, by the Property of the Circle, whence $BC = \overline{x - xx}^{\frac{1}{2}}$. Again, because as $AC : AB :: AH : AC$, that is, as $AC : x :: 1 : AC$, whence $AC^2 = x$, and $AC = x^{\frac{1}{2}}$, it will be (by *Proposition* II of this *Section*) as $AB : AC$, that is, as $x : x^{\frac{1}{2}} :: x : \frac{x^{\frac{1}{2}} x}{x} = z$;

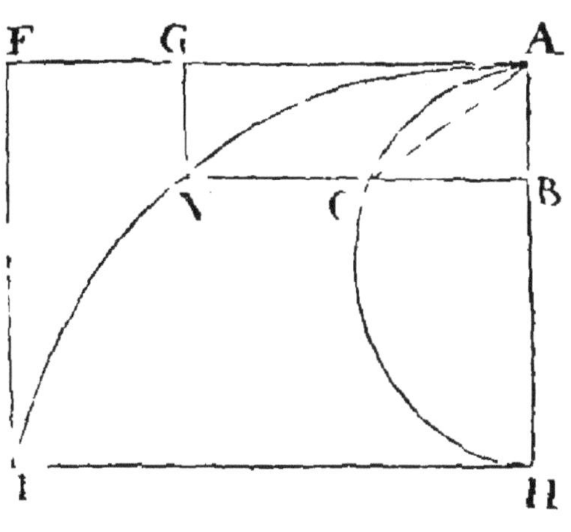

whence $z = \frac{x}{x^{\frac{1}{2}}}$, by dividing by $x^{\frac{1}{2}}$, consequently $z = x^{-\frac{1}{2}} x$ will be the Fluxion of the Portion AN of the Cycloid, whose Fluent $2 x^{\frac{1}{2}} = 2 AC$, will be equal to the Arch AN, whence it follows, that the Length of the Semi-cycloid is equal to 2 AH, the Diameter of the generating Circle. For when BN, by flowing, arrives at HF, AC will become equal to AH.

EXAMPLE X

LET it be required to find the Length of any Portion of the Cissoid of *Diocles*.

LET AD, the Diameter of the generating Circle (*See Figure* [illegible]) be put $= d$, AE $= x$, the Arch AC $= z$, BC $= y$, and [illegible], then will DE = BC $= d -$ [illegible] and because from the

A Nature of the Curve, $y = \overline{d-x} \times \frac{\overline{d-x}^{\frac{1}{2}}}{x^{\frac{1}{2}}} = \frac{\overline{d-x}^{\frac{3}{2}}}{x^{\frac{1}{2}}}$, equal to $x^{-\frac{1}{2}} \times \overline{d-x}^{\frac{3}{2}}$, and because the Fluxion of $x^{-\frac{1}{2}} = -\frac{1}{2}x^{-\frac{1}{2}-1}\dot{x} = -\frac{1}{2}x^{-\frac{3}{2}}\dot{x}$, and the Fluxion of $\overline{d-x}^{\frac{3}{2}} = \frac{3}{2}\overline{d-x}^{\frac{3}{2}-1} \times -\dot{x} = -\frac{3}{2}\overline{d-x}^{\frac{1}{2}}\dot{x}$; therefore $\dot{y} = -\frac{1}{2}x^{-\frac{3}{2}}\dot{x} \times \overline{d-x}^{\frac{3}{2}} - \frac{3}{2}\overline{d-x}^{\frac{1}{2}}\dot{x} \times x^{-\frac{1}{2}} = -\frac{1}{2}x^{-\frac{3}{2}} \times \overline{d-x}^{\frac{3}{2}} - \frac{3}{2}x^{-\frac{1}{2}} \times \overline{d-x}^{\frac{1}{2}} \times \dot{x} = -\frac{1}{2} \times \frac{\overline{d-x}^{\frac{3}{2}}}{x^{\frac{3}{2}}} - \frac{3}{2} \times \frac{\overline{d-x}^{\frac{1}{2}}}{x^{\frac{1}{2}}} \times \dot{x} = -\frac{1}{2} \times \frac{\overline{d-x}}{x} \times \frac{\overline{d-x}^{\frac{1}{2}}}{x^{\frac{1}{2}}} - \frac{3}{2} \times \frac{\overline{d-x}^{\frac{1}{2}}}{x^{\frac{1}{2}}} \times \dot{x} = -\frac{1}{2} \times \frac{\overline{d-x}}{x} - \frac{3}{2} \times \frac{\overline{d-x}^{\frac{1}{2}}}{x^{\frac{1}{2}}} \times \dot{x} = \frac{\overline{-d+x}}{2x} - \frac{3}{2} \times \frac{\overline{d-x}^{\frac{1}{2}}}{x^{\frac{1}{2}}} \times \dot{x} = \frac{\overline{-2d+2x-6x}}{4x} \times \frac{\overline{d-x}^{\frac{1}{2}}}{x^{\frac{1}{2}}} \times \dot{x} = \frac{-2d-4x}{4x} \times \frac{\overline{d-x}^{\frac{1}{2}}}{x^{\frac{1}{2}}} \times \dot{x} = \frac{-d-2x}{2x} \times \frac{\overline{d-x}^{\frac{1}{2}}}{x^{\frac{1}{2}}} \times \dot{x}$, whence $\dot{y}\dot{y} = \frac{dd+4dx+4xx}{4xx} \times \frac{d-x}{x} \times \dot{x}\dot{x} = \frac{d^3+4d^2x+4dx^2-d^2x-4dx^2-4x^3}{4x^3} \times \dot{x}\dot{x} = \frac{d^3+3ddx-4x^3}{4x^3} \times \dot{x}\dot{x}$, whence $\dot{z}\dot{z} = \dot{y}\dot{y} + \dot{x}\dot{x} = \frac{d^3+3ddx-4x^3}{4x^3} \times \dot{x}\dot{x} + \dot{x}\dot{x} =$

=

$$=\frac{d^3\dot{x}\dot{x}+3dd\dot{x}\dot{x}\,x-4x^3\dot{x}\dot{x}+4x^3\dot{x}\dot{x}}{4x^3}=\frac{ddd+3ddx}{4x^3}$$

$\times\,\dot{x}\dot{x}=\frac{dd}{4xx}\times\frac{d+3x}{x}\times\dot{x}\dot{x}$, whence $\dot{z}=\frac{d}{2x}\times\frac{\overline{d+3x}^{\frac{1}{2}}}{x^{\frac{1}{2}}}$ $\times\,\dot{x}=\frac{d\dot{x}}{2x}\times\frac{\overline{d+3x}^{\frac{1}{2}}}{x^{\frac{1}{2}}}=\frac{d\dot{x}}{2x^{\frac{3}{2}}}\times\overline{d+3x}^{\frac{1}{2}}$ Now the Square Root of $d+3x$ is $d^{\frac{1}{2}}+\frac{3x}{2d^{\frac{1}{2}}}-\frac{9xx}{8d^{\frac{3}{2}}}+\frac{27x^3}{16d^{\frac{5}{2}}}$ $-\frac{405x^4}{128d^{\frac{7}{2}}}$, &c which being multiplied by $\frac{d\dot{x}}{2x^{\frac{3}{2}}}$, will produce $\frac{d^{\frac{3}{2}}\dot{x}}{2x^{\frac{3}{2}}}+\frac{3d^{\frac{1}{2}}x\dot{x}}{4x^{\frac{3}{2}}}-\frac{9x^2\dot{x}}{16d^{\frac{1}{2}}x^{\frac{3}{2}}}+\frac{27x^3\dot{x}}{32d^{\frac{3}{2}}x^{\frac{3}{2}}}-\frac{405x^4\dot{x}}{256d^{\frac{5}{2}}x^{\frac{3}{2}}}$, &c whose Fluent $\frac{d^{\frac{3}{2}}x}{2x^{\frac{3}{2}}}+\frac{3d^{\frac{1}{2}}xx}{8x^{\frac{3}{2}}}-\frac{3x^3}{16d^{\frac{1}{2}}x^{\frac{3}{2}}}+\frac{27x^4}{128d^{\frac{3}{2}}x^{\frac{3}{2}}}$ $-\frac{81x^5}{256d^{\frac{5}{2}}x^{\frac{3}{2}}}$, &c. Or $\frac{1}{2}d^{\frac{3}{2}}x^{-\frac{1}{2}}+\frac{3}{8}d^{\frac{1}{2}}x^{\frac{1}{2}}-\frac{3}{16}d^{-\frac{1}{2}}x^{\frac{3}{2}}$ $+\frac{27}{128}d^{-\frac{3}{2}}x^{\frac{5}{2}}-\frac{81}{256}d^{-\frac{5}{2}}x^{\frac{7}{2}}$, &c. Or $\frac{1}{1\times2}d^{\frac{3}{2}}x^{-\frac{1}{2}}$ $+\frac{1\times3}{2\times2\times2}d^{\frac{1}{2}}x^{\frac{1}{2}}-\frac{1\times1\times3\times3}{2\times4\times2\times3}d^{-\frac{1}{2}}x^{\frac{3}{2}}+\frac{1\times1\times3\times3\times3\times3}{2\times4\times6\times2\times4}$ $d^{-\frac{3}{2}}x^{\frac{5}{2}}$, &c. will give the Length of the Arch.

SECT. II.

Containing the Use of FLUXIONS *in the Quadrature of Curves, or in finding the Areas of Curvilinear Spaces.*

PROPOSITION IV

THE Fluxions of the Areas A B C, and A B D G, described by the uniform Motion of the Ordinates B C and B D, along the Base A B, are to each other as the generating or describing Ordinates B C, B D

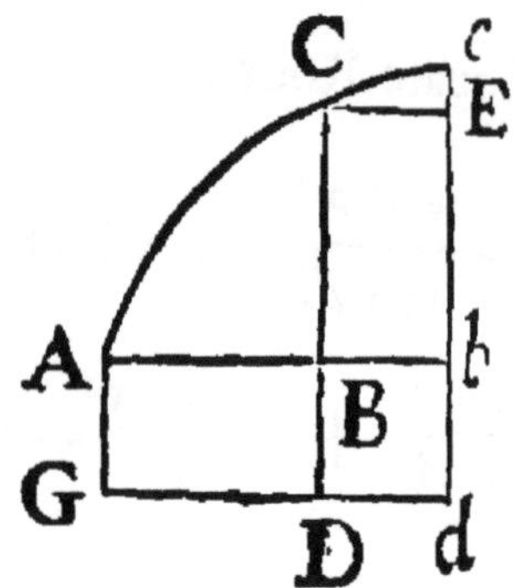

DEMONSTRATION.

CONCEIVE the Line C B D to move with an uniform Motion along the Line A B *b*, constantly parallel to itself, 'till it comes into the Place *c b d*, then will the Ordinates B C and B D describe the little Spaces B C *c b* and B *b d* D, which are the nascent Augments of the Spaces A B C and A B D G, generated in the same very small Particle of Time, for while the Space A B C flowed into or become A *c b*, the Space A B D G flowed into or became A *b d* G

FROM the Point C draw the Line C E parallel to the Base Line A B *b*, then will the nascent Augment of the Curvilinear Area A B C be equal to the Rectangle C E *b* B + the trilinear Space C *c* E, and inasmuch as Fluxions are in the last Ratio of their evanescent Decrements, if we imagine the right Line

Line *c b d*, or, which is the same thing, the Ordinates *b c* and *b d*, to return back towards their first Situation B C and B D, it is manifest, that the nearer *b c* approaches to B C, the nearer they will approach to an Equality, and the lesser will be the trilinear Space *c* C E, 'till at last, when *b c* arrives at, or becomes coincident with B C, the trilinear Space C *c* E will vanish, and the Fluxion of the Curvilinear Space A B C will be to the Fluxion of the rectangular Space A B D G, in the evanescent State, as the describing Ordinate B C to the describing Ordinate B D

AND inasmuch as the Ordinate B D is supposed to move with an uniform Motion constantly of the same Length, and parallel to itself, the Fluxion of the generated Rectangle A B D G will be a constant Quantity, and consequently the Fluxion of the Curvilinear Area A B C will be every where as the describing Ordinate B C Wherefore,

IF the Fluxion of the Abscisse A B be multiplied by the Ordinate B C, the Product will be the Fluxion of the Area. And again, if in this Product the Value of the Ordinate arising from the Equation expressing the Nature of the Curve, be substituted instead of the Ordinate itself, the Fluent of this last Fluxion will give the Area of the Curvilinear Space A B C

NOW if we imagine the Line A D to be carried along the Line A B, constantly parallel to itself, and the Point A moving along the Line A B, to move with an uniform Motion, moving over equal Portions A *b*, &c in equal Times, while the Ordinates *b c*, &c increase in a Subduplicate Ratio of the same Spaces A *b*, &c I say, the Fluxion of the Area of the Curvilinear Space A B C (supposing A B $= x$) described by the generating or

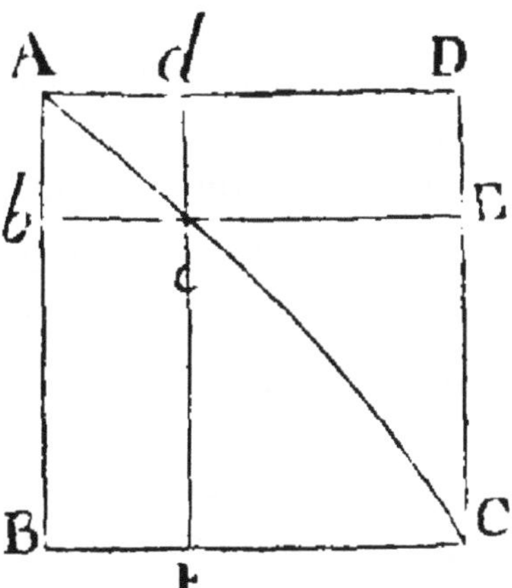

descri-

describing Ordinate B C will be $x^{\frac{1}{2}} x$, and the Fluent $\frac{2}{3} x^{\frac{1}{2}} x$ will be the Area itself

But if we suppose the Line A B (*See the former Figure*) to be carried according to the Direction B C or A D, and the Point A to move with an uniform Motion, moving over equal Portions A *d*, *&c* in equal Times, while the Ordinates *d c*, *&c* increase in a duplicate Ratio, or as the Squares of the Portions A *d*, *&c* I say, the Fluxion of the Area of the Curvilinear Space A D C *c* (supposing A D = *x*) will be $x^2 x$, and consequently its Fluent $\frac{x^2 x}{3} = \frac{1}{3} x^2 x$, will be the Area, and this is called the Supplemental Part

Now if, for Distinctions sake, we express the Ordinate B C in the first Case, to which the Line A D, generated by the Motion of the Point A is equal, by a different Symbol, suppose *y*; then the Fluxion of the Area A C B A, in the first Case, will be $y x$, and the Area itself $\frac{2}{3} x y$, and in the second Case the Fluxion of the Area A C D A, the Supplemental Space $x y$, and the Area itself, will be $\frac{1}{3} x y$, which being added together, will produce $x y$ equal to the Area of the circumscribing Parallelogram A B C D. Wherefore

If the Value of *y* in the Equation expressing the Nature of the Curve, be multiplied by $\dot{x}$, the Fluent arising from this Fluxionary Product will give the Area of the Curvilinear Space Or

If the Value of *x* in the Equation expressing the Nature of the Curve, be multiplied by *y*, the Fluent arising from this Fluxionary Fact, will give the Area of the Supplemental Space Wherefore,

If A B, the Abscisse of any Curve, be put equal to *x*, B C, the corresponding Ordinate, equal to *y*, the Area A B C of the same Curvilinear Space equal to *z*, and the Equation, expressing the Nature of the Curve, be $a x^{\frac{m}{n}} = y$, where the Quantity

tity a is supposed to be a standing Quantity. I say, that $a x^{\frac{m}{n}} \dot{x} = \dot{z}$, is the Fluxion of the Area, and $\frac{n}{m+n} a x^{\frac{m+n}{n}} = \frac{n}{m+n} x y$, the Fluent thence arising, will be equal to z the Area, for if m be put equal to 1, and n equal to 2, then $a x^{\frac{1}{2}}$ will be equal to y, consequently $\frac{n}{m+n} x y = \frac{2}{1+2} x y = \frac{2}{3} x y$, will be the Area of the Curve agreeing with the former Investigation.

AND that this may still the more evidently appear, let us find the Value of the Ordinate y, in the Terms of x, in the Equation expressing the Nature of the Curve, the relation between the Ordinate x, and the Area of the Curve z, being given or assumed at Pleasure.

LET therefore ACB represent a Curvilinear Space. Put the Absciss $AB = x$, the Ordinate $BC = y$, and the Area, as before, equal to z, also $Bb = o$, $BD = v$, then will the Rectangle $BDdb$, which we suppose equal to the Space $BCcd$, be equal to ov, and the whole Area $ACcb$ will be equal to $z + ov$. Let the Area ABC be represented by this Expression $\frac{2}{3} x^{\frac{3}{2}}$, then will $\frac{2}{3} x^{\frac{3}{2}} = z$ and $\frac{4}{9} x^3 = z^2$, and because while AB flows into or becomes Ab, x flows into or becomes $x + o$, and the Curvilinear Space ABC flows into or becomes $Abc = z + ov$. Substitute these Values in the room of x, and z in the former Equation, and we shall have $\frac{4}{9} \overline{x^3 + 3x^2 o + 3 x o^2 + o^3} = z^2 + 2 z o v + o^2 v^2$, from whence taking away $\frac{4}{9} x = z z$, and dividing the remaining Terms by o, we shall have $3x^2 + 3 x o + o o = 2 z v + o v$. Let us now suppose bc to return again into

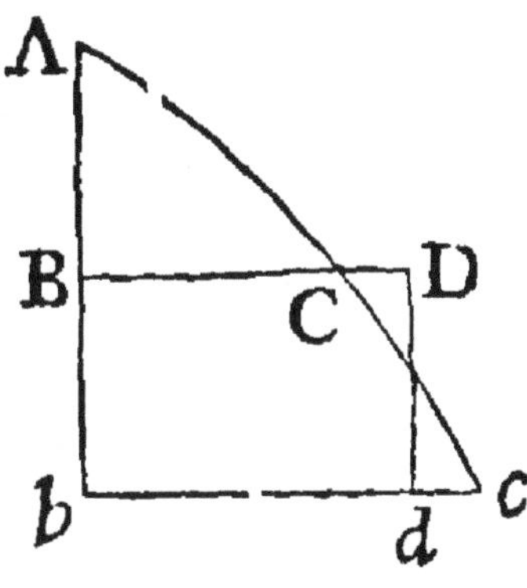

into its former Place BC, then will the Quantity o become equal to nothing, and consequently all the Terms into which it is multiplied will vanish, whence $\frac{4}{9}3xx = 2zv$, that is, $\frac{12}{9}xx = 2zv$; that is $\frac{6}{9}$ or $\frac{2}{3}xx = zv = zy$. For when bc returns again into the Place of BC, bd or BD becomes each equal to BC, whence $\frac{2}{3}xx = \frac{2}{3}x^{\frac{1}{2}}y$ (by substituting $\frac{2}{3}x^{\frac{3}{2}}$ in the room of z, to which it is equal) and $xx = x^{\frac{1}{2}}y$, and $x^{\frac{1}{2}} = y$, for $x^{\frac{1}{2}} \times x^{\frac{1}{2}} = x^{\frac{2}{2}} = x^{1}$, and on the contrary, if $x^{\frac{1}{2}} = y$, then $\frac{2}{3}x^{\frac{3}{2}} = z$ the Area.

AND universally if $\frac{n}{m+n} \times ax^{\frac{m+n}{n}} = z$, putting $\frac{na}{m+n} = c$, and $m+n = d$, we shall have $cx^{\frac{d}{n}} = z$, and $c^{n}x^{d} = z^{n}$.

LET us now imagine the Ordinate BC to flow into, and become bc, and putting $Bb = o$, and $BD = v$, as before, we shall have $Ab = x + o$, and the Space $AbcA = z + ov$, and substituting these in the former Equation $c^{n}x^{d} = z^{n}$, in the room of x and z, there will arise $c^{n} \times x^{d} + dx^{d-1}o + d \times \frac{d-1}{2} x^{d-2}o^{2}$, &c $= z^{n} + nz^{n-1}ov + n \times \frac{n-1}{2} z^{n-2}o^{2}v^{2}$, &c. from whence substracting $c^{n} \times x^{d} = z^{n}$, and dividing the remaining Quantities by o, we shall have $c^{n} \times dx^{d-1} + d \times \frac{d-1}{2} \times x^{n-2}o = nz^{d-1} + n \times \frac{n-1}{2} z^{n-2}ov$

LET the Ordinate bc return again into the Place BC, then will the Quantity o vanish, and all the Terms into which it is multiplied become equal to nothing, and consequently $c^{n}dx^{d-1} = nyz^{d-1}$ (for when the Point c comes into the Place C, v becomes equal y) $= \frac{nyz^{n}}{z}$ (by multiplying nyz^{n-1} by $\frac{z}{z}$)

(=

$= \frac{n y c^n x^d}{c x^{\frac{d}{n}}}$ (by substituting $c^n x^d$ in the room of z^n, and $c x^{\frac{d}{n}}$ in the room of z) whence $c^n d x^{d-1} = \frac{n y c^n x^d}{c x^{\frac{d}{n}}}$, and by dividing each Side of this Equation by $c^n x^d$, we shall have $d x^{-1} = \frac{n y}{c x^{\frac{d}{n}}}$ Now by multiplying each Side by $c x^{\frac{d}{n}}$, we shall have $d c x^{\frac{d-n}{n}} = n y$, and by putting $\frac{n a}{m+n}$ in the room of c, $m+n$ in the room of d, and m in the room of $d-n$, we shall have $m+n \times \frac{n a}{m+n} x^{\frac{m}{n}} = n y$, whence $n a x^{\frac{m}{n}} = n y$, and $a x^{\frac{m}{n}} = y$, the Relation between the Absciffe and the Ordinate, or the Equation expressing the Nature of the Curve. Whence, on the contrary, if $a x^{\frac{m}{n}} = y$, then $\frac{n}{m+n} a x^{\frac{m+n}{n}}$ = to z the Area.

AND hence we are taught how to find the Area of any Surface, the Equation of the Curve being known or given, as shall be shewn at large in the following Examples.

EXAMPLE I

LET it be required to find the Area of the Rectangular Quadrilateral Space B C D A.

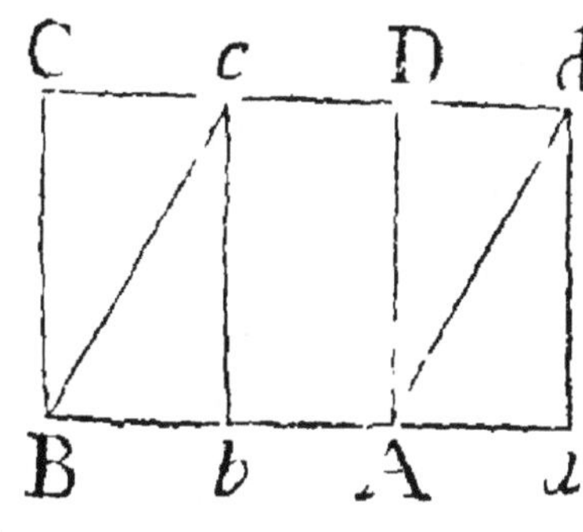

IMAGINE the Line B C to be carried with an uniform Motion, according to the Direction of the Line B A, and to move always parallel to itself,

K k and

and at right Angles to the Line B A, the Space B C D A, generated by the describing Line B C is called a rectangular Parallelogramic Space, and if we put A B = *b*, and B C = *a*, then the Area of the Space A B C D will be expounded by *a b*, or *a* × *b*.

BUT if the generating or describing Line doth not move in a Situation perpendicular to the Base A B, but inclined to it at a given Angle, as *c* B A, and of such a Length, that the Height or Distance of its Extremity *c*, above the Base B A, be equal to the upright describing Line B C, and the Line thus inclined be imagined to be carried along the Line A B, according to the Direction A B, and to move in a Position always parallel to itself, and to its first Position or Inclination B *c* I say, this Line thus moved will describe or generate a Parallelogramic Space B *c d* A, equal in Area to the Parallelogramic Space B C D A, inasmuch as the generating Lines B C, B *c*, are supposed to move with an equal Velocity, and the Spaces B C D A and B *c d* A are described in the Time expounded by the Line B A, that is, in the same Time that the generating Line B C arrives at, or coincides with A D, the generating or describing Line B *c* arrives at, or coincides with A *d*, and the Line *c b* arrives at, or coincides with *d a* And

HENCE it is that Parallelograms standing upon the same or equal Bases, and having the same or equal Altitudes, contain equal Quantities of Space, or are equal in Area.

As the principal End of the Science of Geometry is to find out the Relations that Magnitudes of the same Kind have to each other, according to Quantity; that is, as how oft the one contains, or is contained in the other, so the rectangular Parallelogram has been pitch'd upon as the Standard to which Surfaces of all Kinds are referred. And to find the Quadrature of any Curvilinear Space, is to find what Proportion it has to its circumscribing Parallelogram, and by knowing what Proportion they have to their circumscribing Parallelograms, we know what Proportion they have to each other. For Example, as it will be shewn in the Sequel of this Section, the

Tr.

Triangle will be found to be one half of its circumscribing Parallelogram, and the Parabolic Space will be shewn to be $\frac{2}{3}$ of its circumscribing Parallelogram Whence (supposing the Parallelogramic Space equal to 1) the Triangular Space is to the Parabolic Space, each standing upon the same Base, and having the same Altitude, as $\frac{1}{2}$ to $\frac{2}{3}$, or as $\frac{3}{6}$ to $\frac{4}{6}$, or as 3 to 4, and by the same Method we may compare all kinds of Surfaces amongst themselves And 'tis for this reason that I have begun with the Generation of Parallelogramic Spaces, and shewed how they may be estimated and valued, it being the Basis upon which the following Part of this *Section* is founded.

EXAMPLE II.

LET it be required to find the Area of the Triangle A D E.

DRAW A F a Perpendicular to D E, and through B, a Point taken at Pleasure, draw C B C parallel to the Base D E.

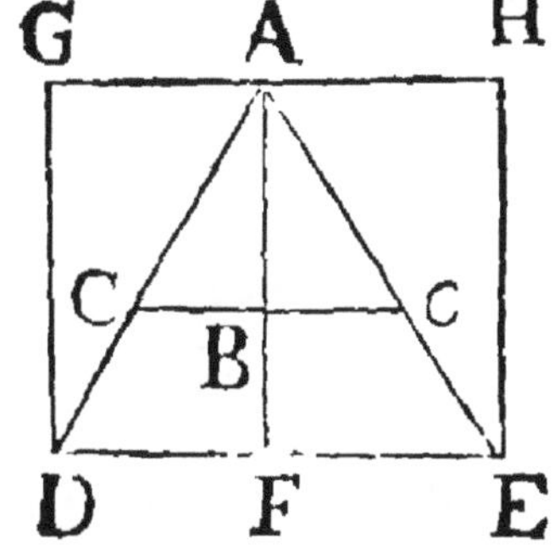

PUT A F $= a$, D E $= b$, A B $= x$, and C B C $= y$, and because, from the Nature of the Triangle, $bx = ay$, and $y = \frac{bx}{a}$, therefore $\frac{bx\dot{x}}{a}$ is the Fluxion of the Area, and consequently $\frac{bxx}{2a} = \frac{yx}{2}$ (by substituting y in the room of $\frac{bx}{a}$, to which it is equal) will be the Area of the Space A C B C.

BUT when the Point B by flowing arrives at F, A B will become equal to A F, and the Line C B C will coincide with the Line D F E, consequently x will become $= a$, and y become equal to b, and the Area of the Triangle A D E will be equal to $\frac{ab}{2}$, or $\frac{1}{2}\, a \times b$

But by the preceding Example, the Area of the circumscribing Parallelogram D E H G has been shewn to be equal to ab, wherefore the Triangle D A E is $\frac{1}{2}$ of its circumscribing Parallelogram, and consequently the Spaces are to each other as 1 to 2.

EXAMPLE III.

Let it be required to find the Area of the Circle A E F G.

From any Point, as C, in the Circumference draw C B parallel to E D, or perpendicular to A F, and put B C $= y$, A B $= x$, A F $= a$, then will B F $= a - x$, and because, from the Property of the Circle, A B $\times$ B F $=$ C B^2, therefore $x \times \overline{a - x} = ax - xx = yy$, and $y = \overline{ax - xx}^{\frac{1}{2}} = x^{\frac{1}{2}} \times \overline{a - x}^{\frac{1}{2}}$, and consequently $y\dot{x} = \dot{x} \times x^{\frac{1}{2}} \times \overline{a - x}^{\frac{1}{2}}$, will be Fluxion of the Area.

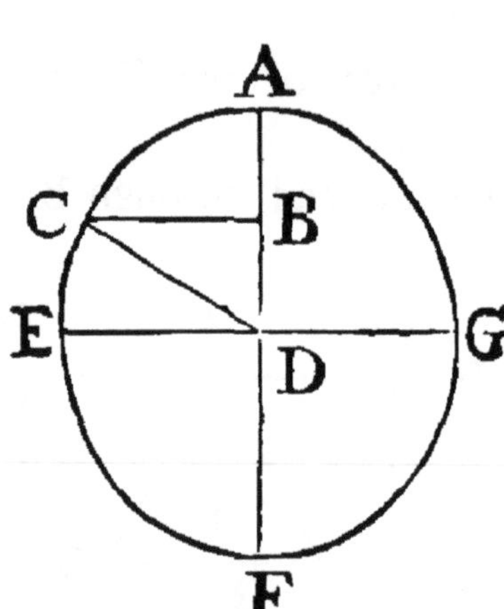

But the Square Root of $\overline{a - x}$ is $a^{\frac{1}{2}} - \frac{1}{2}\, a^{-\frac{1}{2}}\, x - \frac{1}{8}\, a^{-\frac{3}{2}}\, x^{\frac{3}{2}} - \frac{1}{16}\, a^{-\frac{5}{2}}\, x^{\frac{5}{2}} - \frac{5}{128}\, a^{-\frac{7}{2}}\, x^{\frac{7}{2}}$, &c. This Series therefore being multiplied by $x^{\frac{1}{2}}\, \dot{x}$, will give $a^{\frac{1}{2}}\, x^{\frac{1}{2}}\, \dot{x} - \frac{1}{2}\, a^{-\frac{1}{2}}\, x^{\frac{3}{2}}\, \dot{x} - \frac{1}{8}\, a^{-\frac{3}{2}}\, x^{\frac{5}{2}}\, \dot{x} - \frac{1}{16}\, a^{-\frac{5}{2}}\, x^{\frac{7}{2}}\, \dot{x} - \frac{5}{128}\, a^{-\frac{7}{2}}\, x^{\frac{9}{2}}\, \dot{x}$ for the

the Fluxion of the Area A B C, whose Fluent $\frac{2}{3}a^{\frac{1}{2}}x^{\frac{3}{2}} - \frac{1}{5}a^{-\frac{1}{2}}x^{\frac{5}{2}} - \frac{1}{28}a^{-\frac{3}{2}}x^{\frac{7}{2}} - \frac{1}{72}a^{-\frac{5}{2}}x^{\frac{9}{2}} - \frac{5}{704}a^{-\frac{7}{2}}x^{\frac{11}{2}}$, &c will be the Area itself.

LET us now put $a = 1$, and imagine the Point B to move 'till it comes into the Place D, at which Time the Ordinate, or right Line BC, will coincide, or become equal to the Radius D E, and x will become equal to $\frac{1}{2}a$, which we will suppose equal to r, and consequently $\frac{2}{3}r^{\frac{3}{2}} - \frac{1}{5}r^{\frac{5}{2}} - \frac{1}{28}r^{\frac{7}{2}} - \frac{1}{72}r^{\frac{9}{2}} - \frac{4}{704}r^{\frac{11}{2}}$, &c. will be the Area of the Quadrant A D L. This Series therefore being multiplied by 4, will give $4\times\frac{2}{3}r^{\frac{3}{2}} - \frac{1}{5}r^{\frac{5}{2}} - \frac{1}{28}r^{\frac{7}{2}} - \frac{1}{72}r^{\frac{9}{2}} - \frac{5}{704}r^{\frac{11}{2}}$, &c. $= 4r^{\frac{1}{2}}\times\frac{2}{3}r - \frac{1}{5}r^{2} - \frac{1}{28}r^{3} - \frac{1}{72}r^{4} - \frac{5}{704}r^{5} = 4r^{\frac{1}{2}}\times\frac{1\times2}{1\times3}r - \frac{1\times2}{2\times5}r^{2} - \frac{1\times1\times2}{2\times4\times7}r^{3} - \frac{1\times1\times3\times2}{2\times4\times6\times9}r^{4} - \frac{1\times1\times3\times5\times2}{2\times4\times6\times8\times11}r^{5}$, &c for the Area of the whole Circle A E F G.

AGAIN, if we put B C $= y$, as before, D B $= x$, and D C $= r$, because $rr - xx = yy$ (by *the* 47*th of* Euclid I.) Therefore $y = \overline{rr - xx}^{\frac{1}{2}}$, consequently $\dot{x}y = \dot{x}\times\overline{rr - xx}^{\frac{1}{2}}$ will be the Fluxion of the Area of the Space E D B C.

BUT the Square Root of $rr - xx$ is $r - \frac{xx}{2r} - \frac{x^{4}}{8r^{3}} - \frac{x^{6}}{16r^{5}} - \frac{5x^{8}}{128r^{7}}$, this therefore multiplied by $\dot{x}$, will

give

give $r\dot{x} - \frac{xx\dot{x}}{2r} - \frac{x^4\dot{x}}{8r^3} - \frac{x^6\dot{x}}{16r^5} - \frac{x^8\dot{x}}{128r^7}$, &c. whose Fluent $rx - \frac{x^3}{6r} - \frac{x^5}{40r^3} - \frac{x^7}{112r^5} - \frac{x^9}{1152r^7}$, &c will give the Area of the same Zone E D B C

Now if we imagine the Ordinate B C in a flowing State, and to move 'till the Point B coincides with the Point A, then will D B become equal to D A, consequently x will become equal to r, and we shall have $r^2 - \frac{1}{6}r^2 - \frac{1}{40}r^2 - \frac{1}{112}r^2 - \frac{5}{1152}r^2$, &c. $= r^2 \times 1 - \frac{1}{6} - \frac{1}{40} - \frac{1}{112} - \frac{5}{1152}$, &c $= r^2 \times 1 - \frac{1}{2\times3} - \frac{1\times1}{2\times4\times5} - \frac{1\times1\times3}{2\times4\times6\times7} - \frac{1\times1\times3\times5}{2\times4\times6\times8\times9}$, &c for the Area of the Quadrantal Space A D E, and consequently $4r^2 \times 1 - \frac{1}{2\times3} - \frac{1\times1}{2\times4\times5} - \frac{1\times1\times3}{2\times4\times6\times7}$, &c (or $1 - \frac{1}{2\times3} - \frac{1\times1}{2\times4\times5} - \frac{1\times1\times3}{2\times4\times6\times7}$, &c when the Diameter A F is supposed equal to 1) will give the Area of the whole Circular Space

Again, as the extreme Point B of the right Line A B will, when it revolves about the fix'd Point A, describe the Circumference of the Circle B c, while the whole Line A B, being carried about the same immoveable Point B, will describe the circular Space A B c B, so any Point, as D, will in the same Time describe the Circumference D d D, while the Line A D will describe the Circular Space A D d D.

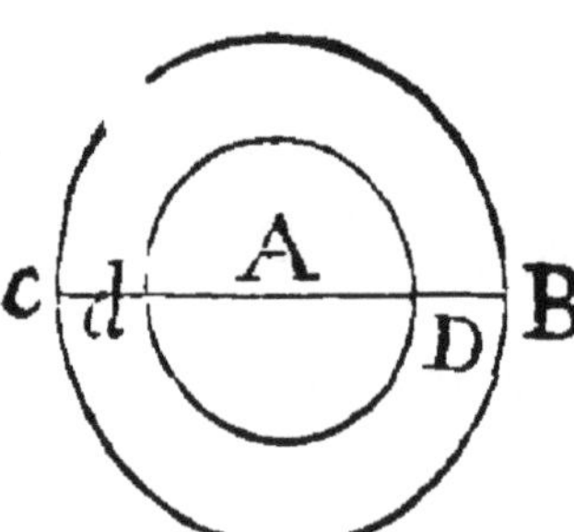

Put

Put therefore the Circumference $B c B = c$, the Radius $AB = r$, the Circumference $D d D = y$, and the Radius $AD = x$.

Now because, from the Nature of the Circle, $c x = r y$, and $y = \frac{c x}{r}$, therefore $\frac{c x \dot{x}}{r}$ is the Fluxion of the Area, and $\frac{c x x}{2 r}$, the Fluent thence arising, will be the Area itself, and by substituting y in this last Equation in the room of $\frac{c x}{r}$, we shall have $\frac{y x}{2}$ for the Area of the Circular Space $A D d D$.

Imagine the Point D to move into the Place of B, then will the Radius A D become equal to A B, the Circumference $d D d$ will coincide with the Circumference $c B c$, x will become equal to r, and y will become equal to c, and the Area of the Circular Space A B C B will be equal to $\frac{r c}{2}$. Or,

Put the Radius $A C = r$, the Circumference $B C D = c$, and the Arch $B C = x$, then will $\frac{r \dot{x}}{2}$ be the Fluxion of the Area of the Sector A B C, and consequently $\frac{r x}{2}$ will be equal to the Area of the Sector itself

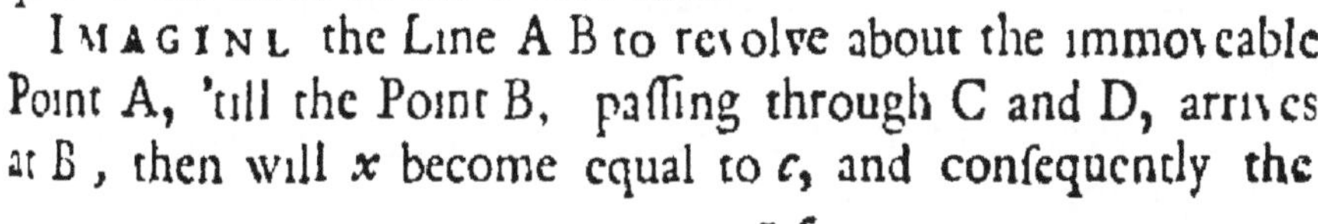

Imagine the Line A B to revolve about the immoveable Point A, 'till the Point B, passing through C and D, arrives at B, then will x become equal to c, and consequently the Area of the Circular Space will be $\frac{r c}{2}$, or $\frac{1}{2} r c$, the same as by the former Investigation Whence it follows,

First, That every Circle is equal to a Triangle, whose Base is equal to the Circumference, and Perpendicular equal to the Radius

Secondly,

Secondly, THAT the Square of the Diameter of any Circle is to the Area of the same Circle, as the Diameter is to $\frac{1}{4}$ of the Circumference.

FOR let d represent the Diameter of any Circle, of which A is the Area, and let the Proportion of the Diameter to the Circumference be as n to m. Now because as $n : m :: d : \frac{md}{n}$ therefore $\frac{d}{2} \times \frac{md}{2n} = \frac{mdd}{4n} = A$, whence as $n : \frac{1}{4}m :: dd : A$.

Thirdly, Circles are to each other as the Squares of their Diameters, since the Squares of the Diameters are to the Areas of their respective Circles in a constant Ratio, *viz.* of n to $\frac{1}{4}m$.

IT has been shewn in the preceding *Section*, Page 230, that if the Diameter of a Circle be put equal to 1, the Circumference of the same Circle will be 3.14159, &c. consequently its $\frac{1}{4}$ will be .785397, &c. Wherefore as 1 is to .785397, so is the Square of the Diameter of any Circle to its Area, consequently if the Square of the Diameter of any Circle be multiplied by .785397, &c. the Product will give the Area of the same Circle.

AGAIN, because $dd = 4rr$, therefore as $n : m :: rr : A$. Whence it follows,

Fourthly, THAT the Area of every Circle is to the Square of its Radius as the Diameter is to the Circumference. And consequently,

Fifthly, CIRCLES are to each other as the Square of their respective Radii.

AGAIN, because as $m : n :: c : \frac{nc}{m} = d$, therefore $\frac{c}{2} \times \frac{nc}{2m} = \frac{ncc}{4m} = A$, and consequently as $m : \frac{1}{4}n :: cc : A$. Whence it follows,

Sixthly,

Sixthly, THAT the Area of any Circle is to the Square of its Circumference as $\frac{1}{4}$ of the Diameter to the Circumference. And consequently,

Seventhly, CIRCLES are to each other as the Squares of their Circumferences.

EXAMPLE IV.

LET it be required to find the Area of the Ellipsis ACEF.

PUT DE $= c$, BC $= y$, BD $= x$, and AD $= r$, then will AB $= r - x$, and FB $= r + x$, and because, from the Nature of the Curve, as $\overline{AD}^2 : \overline{AB} \times \overline{BF} :: \overline{DE}^2 : \overline{BC}^2$, therefore it will be as $rr : \overline{r - x} \times \overline{r + x} :: cc : yy$, whence $rryy = cc \times \overline{rr - xx}$, and $yy = \frac{cc}{rr} \times \overline{rr - xx}$, and $y = \frac{c}{r} \times \overline{rr - xx}^{\frac{1}{2}}$, consequently $y\dot{x} = \frac{c}{r} \times \overline{rr - xx}^{\frac{1}{2}} \times \dot{x}$ will be the Fluxion of the Space CBDE, but the Square Root of $\overline{rr - xx}$ is $r - \frac{xx}{2r} - \frac{x^4}{8r^3} - \frac{x^6}{16r^5} - \frac{5x^8}{128r^7} - \frac{7x^{10}}{256r^9}$, &c. This Series therefore being multiplied by $\dot{x}$, will produce $r\dot{x} - \frac{x^2\dot{x}}{2r} - \frac{x^4\dot{x}}{8r^3} - \frac{x^6\dot{x}}{16r^5} - \frac{5x^8\dot{x}}{128r^7} - \frac{7x^{10}\dot{x}}{256r^9}$, &c. whose Fluent $rx - \frac{x^3}{6r} - \frac{x^5}{40r^3} - \frac{x^7}{112r^5}$ —

$-\frac{5x^7}{1152r^7}-\frac{7x^{11}}{2816r^9}$, &c being multiplied by $\frac{c}{r}$ will produce $cx-\frac{cx^3}{2r^2}-\frac{cx^5}{40r^4}-\frac{cx^7}{112r^6}-\frac{5cx^9}{1152r^8}-\frac{7cx^{11}}{2816r^{10}}$, &c for the Area of the Elliptical Zone CBDE.

Now if we imagine the Ordinate BC in a flowing State, and to move in the Direction BA, 'till the Point B arrives at, or is coincident with the Point A, then DB will become equal to DA, x will become equal to r, and consequently the Series $cx-\frac{cx^3}{6r^2}$, &c will become $rc-\frac{cr^3}{6r^2}-\frac{cr^5}{40r^4}-\frac{cr^7}{112r^6}-\frac{5cr^9}{1152r^8}-\frac{7cr^{11}}{2816r^{10}}$, &c $=cr-\frac{cr}{6}-\frac{cr}{40}-\frac{cr}{112}-\frac{5cr}{1152}-\frac{7cr}{2816}$, &c $=cr\times\overline{1-\frac{1}{6}-\frac{1}{40}-\frac{1}{112}-\frac{5}{1152}-\frac{7}{2816}}$, &c equal to the Area of the Quadrant ADL. This therefore being multiplied by 4, will give $4cr\times\overline{1-\frac{1}{6}-\frac{1}{40}-\frac{1}{112}-\frac{5}{1152}-\frac{7}{2816}}$, &c Or $4cr\times\overline{1-\frac{1}{2\times3}-\frac{1\times1}{2\times4\times5}-\frac{1\times1\times3}{2\times4\times6\times7}-\frac{1\times1\times3\times5}{2\times4\times6\times8\times9}}$, &c. for the whole Elliptical Space.

Now if instead of putting DB $=x$, we put AB $=x$, then will BF $=2r-x$, consequently because from the Property of the Curve, as $\overline{AD}^2 : \overline{AB\times BF} :: \overline{DE}^2 : \overline{BC}^2$, it will be as $rr : x\times\overline{2r-x} :: cc : yy$, whence $yyrr=cc\times\overline{2rx-xx}$, and $yy=\frac{cc}{rr}\times\overline{2rx-xx}$, and $y=\frac{c}{r}$

$\times\overline{2rx - xx}^{\frac{1}{2}}$, and $y = \frac{2c}{2r}\times\overline{2rx - xx}^{\frac{1}{2}}$. Now if we put $2c$, or the conjugate Diameter $2ED = a$, and $2r$, the transverse Diameter $AF = d$, we shall have $y = \frac{a}{d}\times\overline{dx - xx}$;

whence $yx = \frac{a}{d}\times\overline{dx - xx}\times x$, for the Fluxion of the Elliptical Space ABC, but the Square Root of $\overline{dx - xx}$ is $d^{\frac{1}{2}}x^{\frac{1}{2}} - \frac{x^{\frac{3}{2}}}{2d^{\frac{1}{2}}} - \frac{x^{\frac{5}{2}}}{8d^{\frac{3}{2}}} - \frac{x^{\frac{7}{2}}}{16d^{\frac{5}{2}}} - \frac{5x^{\frac{9}{2}}}{128d^{\frac{7}{2}}}$, &c. This therefore being multiplied by x, will produce $d^{\frac{1}{2}}x^{\frac{1}{2}}x - \frac{x^{\frac{3}{2}}x}{2d^{\frac{1}{2}}} - \frac{x^{\frac{5}{2}}x}{8d^{\frac{3}{2}}} - \frac{x^{\frac{7}{2}}x}{16d^{\frac{5}{2}}} - \frac{5x^{\frac{9}{2}}x}{128d^{\frac{7}{2}}}$, &c. whose Fluent $\frac{2}{3}d^{\frac{1}{2}}x^{\frac{3}{2}} - \frac{x^{\frac{5}{2}}}{5d^{\frac{1}{2}}} - \frac{x^{\frac{7}{2}}}{28d^{\frac{3}{2}}} - \frac{x^{\frac{9}{2}}}{72d^{\frac{5}{2}}} - \frac{5x^{\frac{11}{2}}}{704d^{\frac{7}{2}}}$, &c being multiplied $\frac{a}{d}$ will give $\frac{a}{d}\times\frac{2}{3}d^{\frac{1}{2}}x^{\frac{3}{2}} - \frac{x^{\frac{5}{2}}}{5d^{\frac{1}{2}}} - \frac{x^{\frac{7}{2}}}{28d^{\frac{3}{2}}} - \frac{x^{\frac{9}{2}}}{72d^{\frac{5}{2}}} - \frac{5x^{\frac{11}{2}}}{704d^{\frac{7}{2}}}$, &c. for the Area of the Elliptical Segment ABC.

Now if we put d, the transverse Diameter, $= 1$, and imagine the Ordinate BC in a flowing State, and to move according to the Direction BF, 'till the Point B arrives at, or is coincident with the Point D, then will AB become equal to AD, x will become equal to r, and the Series $a\times\frac{2}{3}d^{\frac{1}{2}}x^{\frac{3}{2}} - \frac{x^{\frac{5}{2}}}{5d^{\frac{1}{2}}}$, &c will become $a\times\frac{2}{3}r^{\frac{3}{2}} - \frac{1}{5}r^{\frac{5}{2}} - \frac{1}{28}r^{\frac{7}{2}} - \frac{1}{72}r^{\frac{9}{2}} - \frac{5}{704}r^{\frac{11}{2}}$, &c $= a\times r^{\frac{1}{2}}\times\frac{2}{3}r - \frac{1}{5}r^{2} - \frac{1}{28}r^{3} - \frac{1}{72}r^{4} - \frac{5}{704}r^{5}$, &c equal to the Area of the Elliptical Quadrant

ADE, and being multiplied by 4, will give $a \times 4 r^{\frac{1}{2}} \times \frac{2}{3} r - \frac{1}{5} r^2 - \frac{1}{28} r^3 - \frac{1}{72} r^4 - \frac{5}{704} r^5$, &c $= a \times 4 r^{\frac{1}{2}} \times \frac{1 \times 2}{1 \times 3} r - \frac{1 \times 2}{2 \times 5} r^2 - \frac{1 \times 1 \times 2}{2 \times 4 \times 7} r^3 - \frac{1 \times 1 \times 3 \times 2}{2 \times 4 \times 6 \times 9} r^4 - \frac{1 \times 1 \times 3 \times 5 \times 2}{2 \times 4 \times 6 \times 8 \times 11} r^5$, &c for the Area of the whole Ellipsis.

And universally if we put m for the Exponent of the Power of AB, and n for the Exponent of the Power of BF; d for the Diameter AF, and b for the Parameter, we shall have $\frac{dy^{m+n}}{b} = x^m \times \overline{d - x}^n$, which is a general Equation for all Sorts of Ellipses whatsoever, and putting the transverse Diameter $d = 1$ we shall have $\frac{y^{m+n}}{b} = x^m \times \overline{1 - x}^n$, and $y^{m+n} = b x^m \times \overline{1 - x}^n$, and $y^{m+n} = b \times \overline{x^m - x^{m+1}}^n$, and $y = b^{\frac{1}{m+n}} \times \overline{x^m - x^{m+1}}^{\frac{n}{m+n}}$, consequently $y\dot{x} = b^{\frac{1}{m+n}} \times \overline{x^m - x^{m+1}}^{\frac{n}{m+n}} \times \dot{x}$, will be Fluxion of the Segment ABC.

Put $m + n = s$, then will $b^{\frac{1}{s}} \times \overline{x^m - x^{m+1}}^{\frac{n}{s}} \times \dot{x}$, be the Fluxion of the same Space, but the $\frac{n}{s}$ Root of $x^m - x^{m+1}$ is $x^{\frac{mn}{s}} - \frac{n}{s} x^{\frac{mn}{s}+1} - \frac{n}{s} \times \frac{n-s}{2s} \times x^{\frac{mn}{s}+2} - \frac{n}{s} \times \frac{n-s}{2s} \times \frac{n-2s}{3s} x^{\frac{mn}{s}+3} - \frac{n}{s} \times \frac{n-s}{2s} \times \frac{n-2s}{3s} \times \frac{n-3s}{4s} x^{\frac{mn}{s}+4}$, &c

This Series therefore being multiplied by $b^{\frac{1}{s}} \times \dot{x}$, will produce

duce $b^{\frac{1}{s}} \times x^{\frac{mn}{s}} \dot{x} - \frac{n}{s} x^{\frac{mn}{s}+1} \dot{x} - \frac{n}{s} \times \frac{n-s}{2s} \times x^{\frac{mn}{s}+2} \dot{x} - \frac{n}{s}$ $\times \frac{n-s}{2s} \times \frac{n-2s}{3s} \times x^{\frac{mn}{s}+3} \dot{x} - \frac{n}{s} \times \frac{n-s}{2s} \times \frac{n-2s}{3s} \times \frac{n-3s}{4s}$ $x^{\frac{mn}{s}+4} \dot{x}$, &c. whose Fluent $b^{\frac{1}{s}} \times \frac{s}{mn+s} x^{\frac{mn}{s}+1} - \frac{n}{s}$ $\times \frac{s}{mn+2s} x^{\frac{mn}{s}+2} - \frac{n}{s} \times \frac{n-s}{2s} \times \frac{s}{mn+3s} x^{\frac{mn}{s}+3} - \frac{n}{s}$ $\times \frac{n-s}{2s} \times \frac{n-2s}{3s} \times \frac{s}{mn+4s} \times x^{\frac{mn}{s}+4} - \frac{n}{s} \times \frac{n-s}{2s}$ $\times \frac{n-2s}{3s} \times \frac{n-3s}{4s} \times \frac{s}{mn+5s} \times x^{\frac{mn}{s}+5}$, &c. $= b^{\frac{1}{s}}$ $\times \frac{s}{mn+s} x^{\frac{mn}{s}+1} - \frac{n}{mn+2s} x^{\frac{mn}{s}+2} - \frac{n}{2s} \times \frac{n-s}{mn+3s}$ $x^{\frac{mn}{s}+3} - \frac{n}{2s} \times \frac{n-s}{3s} \times \frac{n-2s}{mn+4s} \times x^{\frac{mn}{s}+4} - \frac{n}{2s} \times \frac{n-s}{3s}$ $\times \frac{n-2s}{4s} \times \frac{n-3s}{mn+5s} x^{\frac{mn}{s}+5}$, &c. $= b^{\frac{1}{s}} \times x^{\frac{mn}{s}} \times \frac{s}{mn+s}$ $x - \frac{n}{mn+2s} x^2 - \frac{n}{2s} \times \frac{n-s}{mn+3s} x^3 - \frac{n}{2s} \times \frac{n-s}{3s}$ $\times \frac{n-2s}{mn+4s} \times x^4 - \frac{n}{2s} \times \frac{n-s}{3s} \times \frac{n-2s}{4s} \times \frac{n-3s}{mn+5s} x$, &c. will be the Area of the same Space A B C

Now if m and n be put each equal to 1 (as in the common Ellipsis) and x be supposed equal to r, as it will be when the Ordinate B C moves into the Place D E, we shall have $b \times r^{\frac{1}{2}} \times \frac{2}{3} r - \frac{1}{5} r^2 - \frac{1}{28} r^3 - \frac{1}{72} r^4 - \frac{5}{704} r^5$, for the Area of the Elliptical Quadrant A D E, the same as was before investi-

investigated, and consequently $4b \times r^{\frac{1}{2}} \times \frac{2}{3}r - \frac{1}{5}r^2 - \frac{1}{28}r^3$, &c will give the whole Elliptical Area

BUT it has been shewn in the last Example, that $4r^{\frac{1}{2}} \times \frac{2}{3}r - \frac{1}{5}r^2 - \frac{1}{28}r^3$, &c was equal to the Area of a Circle, whose Diameter was Unity and Radius r, as it is in the present Case of the circumscribing Circle A F H.

PUT therefore A equal to the Area of the circumscribing Circle, and a equal to the Area of the inscribed Ellipsis, then $a = \frac{c}{d}$ A, and $ad = c$A, whence as d : c :: A : a, and consequently the Area of the circumscribing Circle is to the Area of the inscribed Ellipsis as 2 A D to 2 E D, that is, as the longest Diameter of the Ellipsis is to the shortest. Or,

BECAUSE as $\overline{AD}^2 : \overline{AB \times BD + DF} :: \overline{DH}^2 : \overline{BK}^2$, in the Circle, and as $\overline{AD}^2 : \overline{AB \times BD + DF} :: \overline{DE}^2 : \overline{BC}^2$, in the Ellipsis, therefore as $\overline{DH}^2 : \overline{DE}^2 :: \overline{BK}^2 : \overline{BC}^2$, and consequently as DH : DE :: BK : BC, whence any Ordinate in the Circle is to its correspondent Ordinate in the Ellipsis in a constant Ratio of D H to D E, or of 2 D H to 2 D E, that is, of the longest Diameter of the Ellipsis to the shortest

BUT in the same time that the generating Ordinate B K, by its Motion along the Line A F, describes the Semi-circle, in the same time the generating correspondent Ordinate B C will describe the Semi Ellipsis Whence it follows, that as the longest Diameter of any Ellipsis is to the shortest, so is the Area of the circumscribed Circle to the Area of the inscribed Ellipsis, and so is the Area of any Segment of the Circle to the Area of the corresponding Elliptical Segment, since the Doubles are in the same Proportion with their Halves Whence it follows

First,

First, THAT the Quadrature of the Ellipsis depends upon the Quadrature of the Circle.

Secondly, THAT the Ellipsis is to its circumscribing Parallelogram as the Circle is to its circumscribing Square.

AND inasmuch as by the same Method of Reasoning it may be proved, that the Ellipsis is to its inscribed Circle, as the longest Diameter is to the shortest, it follows,

Thirdly, THAT the Ellipsis is a mean Proportional between the circumscribed and inscribed Circle.

EXAMPLE V.

To find the Area of the Parabola.

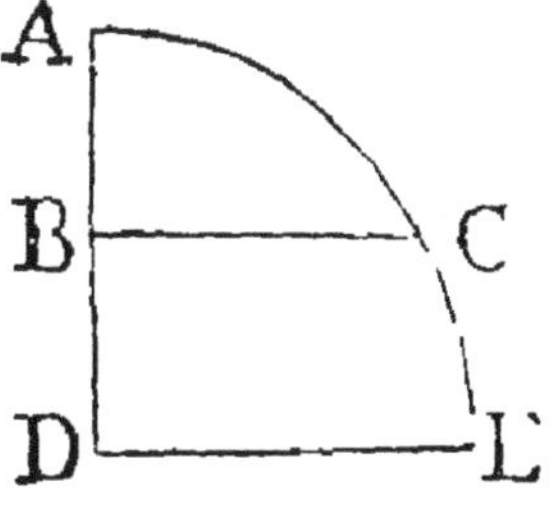

LET ADE represent a Semi-Parabola, AD its Axis, BC, DE Ordinates rightly applied. Put AB = x, BC = y, AD = a, DE = b, and the Parameter = 1. Now because, from the Nature of the Curve, $1x = yy$, therefore $x^{\frac{1}{2}} = y$, and consequently $x^{\frac{1}{2}}\dot{x}$ will be the Fluxion of the Space ABC, whose Fluent $\frac{2}{3}x^{\frac{3}{2}}$ equal to $\frac{2}{3}$ of xy, by substituting y in the room of $x^{\frac{1}{2}}$, to which it is equal, will be the Area of the same Space ABC. Now if we imagine the Ordinate BC to be in a flowing State, and to move into the Place of DE, at the same time AB will flow into, or become equal to AD, x will become equal to a, and y will become equal to b, and consequently we shall have $\frac{2}{3}ab$ for the Area of the whole Space ADE.

AGAIN, put $1x = y^m$, which expresses the Nature of all kinds of Parabolic Spaces, then will $y = x^{\frac{1}{m}}$, and $x^{\frac{1}{m}}\dot{x}$ be the Fluxion of the Area, whence $\frac{m}{1+m}x^{\frac{1}{m}}x = \frac{m}{1+m}yx$ (by substituting y in the room of $x^{\frac{1}{m}}$, to which it is equal) will be the Area itself.

If $m = 2$, then A, the Area, is equal to $\frac{2}{3} y x$, the Circumscribing Parallelogram, and the Curve A B C is the common *Apolonian* Parabola, and consequently the Supplemental Part must be $\frac{1}{3}$, which may be investigated directly after the manner following

For because $y^m = x$, therefore $y^m \dot{y}$ will be the Fluxion of the Supplemental Part, and consequently $\frac{1}{m+1} y^m y$ $= \frac{1}{m+1} x y$ (putting x in the room of y^m, to which it is equal) will be equal to the Area of the Supplemental Part, equal to $\frac{1}{3}$ of $x y$, or the Circumscribing Parallelogram, when $m = 2$, as in the Case of the common Parabola. Whence it follows

First, That the Triangle E A E is to the Circumscribing Parabola as 3 to 4, and to the Supplemental Space as 3 to 2

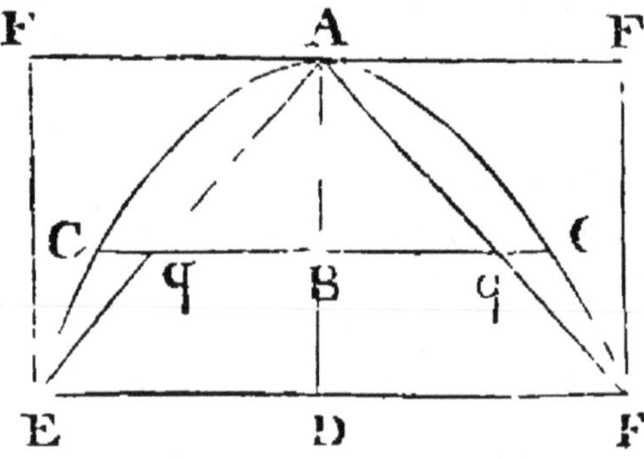

Secondly, That the Space comprehended between the Chords A F, A E, and the Curves A C E, A C E, is $\frac{1}{6}$ of the whole Parallelogramic Space F F F E.

Thirdly, That the Spaces A C E q, A q E D, A C E D, and A F F D, are as the Numbers 1, 2, 3, 4.

EXAMPLE VI

To find the Area of an Hyperbola

Let A D F (*See the following Figure*) represent a Semi Hyperbol, A E the transverse Diameter, A D the Axis, A B the

the Absciffe, B C an Ordinate. Put A B $= x$, B C $= y$, A D $= b$, A E $= a$, D F $= d$, and the Parameter $= c$

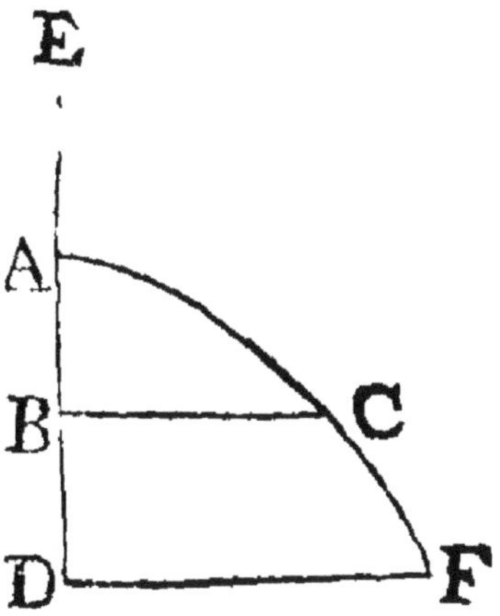

Now becaufe, from the Nature of the Curve, as $x \times \overline{a + x} : yy :: a : c$, therefore $\overline{ax + xx} \times c = ayy$, and $yy = \frac{c}{a} \times \overline{ax + xx}$, and putting $a = 1$, we fhall have $y = c^{\frac{1}{2}} \times \overline{x + xx}|^{\frac{1}{2}}$, whence $c^{\frac{1}{2}} \times \overline{x + xx}|^{\frac{1}{2}} \dot{x}$, will be the Fluxion of the Area

But the Square Root of $\overline{x + xx}$, is $x^{\frac{1}{2}} + \frac{1}{2} x^{\frac{3}{2}} - \frac{1}{8} x^{\frac{5}{2}} + \frac{1}{16} x^{\frac{7}{2}} - \frac{5}{128} x^{\frac{9}{2}}$, &c. This Series therefore being multiplied by $\dot{x}$, will produce $x^{\frac{1}{2}} \dot{x} + \frac{1}{2} x^{\frac{3}{2}} \dot{x} - \frac{1}{8} x^{\frac{5}{2}} \dot{x} + \frac{1}{16} x^{\frac{7}{2}} \dot{x} - \frac{5}{128} x^{\frac{9}{2}} \dot{x}$, &c. whofe Fluent $\frac{2}{3} x^{\frac{3}{2}} + \frac{1}{5} x^{\frac{5}{2}} - \frac{1}{28} x^{\frac{7}{2}} + \frac{1}{72} x^{\frac{9}{2}} - \frac{5}{704} x^{\frac{11}{2}}$, &c being multiplied by $c^{\frac{1}{2}}$, will give $c^{\frac{1}{2}} \times \frac{2}{3} x^{\frac{3}{2}} + \frac{1}{5} x^{\frac{5}{2}} - \frac{1}{28} x^{\frac{7}{2}} + \frac{1}{72} x^{\frac{9}{2}} - \frac{5}{704} x^{\frac{11}{2}}$, &c $= c^{\frac{1}{2}} \times x^{\frac{1}{2}} \times \frac{2}{3} x + \frac{1}{5} x^{2} - \frac{1}{28} x^{3} + \frac{1}{72} x^{4} - \frac{5}{704} x^{5}$, &c. for the Area of the Space A B C.

Now if we imagine the Ordinate B C in a flowing State, and to move 'till it arrives at, or coincides with the Ordinate D F, then A B will become equal to A D, and x will become equal to b, and we shall have $c^{\frac{1}{2}} \times b^{\frac{1}{2}} \times \frac{2}{3} b + \frac{1}{5} b^2 - \frac{1}{28} b^3 + \frac{1}{72} b^4 - \frac{5}{704} b^5$, &c. for the Area of the Semi Hyperbolic Space A D F.

AND universally if we put m for the Exponent of the Power of A B, and n for the Exponent of the Power of B C, we shall have $\frac{a y^{m+n}}{c} = x^m \times \overline{a+x}^n$, whence putting $a = 1$, we shall have $y^{m+n} = c x^m \times \overline{1+x}^n$, and $y^{m+n} = c \times \overline{x^m + x^{m+1}}^n$, and $y = c^{\frac{1}{m+n}} \times \overline{x^m + x^{m+1}}^{\frac{n}{m+n}}$, and $y = c^{\frac{1}{s}} \times \overline{x^m + x^{m+1}}^{\frac{n}{s}}$ (by substituting s in the room of $m + n$), whence $y x = c^{\frac{1}{s}} \times \overline{x^m + x^{m+1}}^{\frac{n}{s}} \times x$, will be the Fluxion of the Space A B C.

BUT the $\frac{n}{s}$ Root of $\overline{x^m + x^{m+1}}$ is $x^{\frac{mn}{s}} + \frac{n}{s} x^{\frac{mn}{s}+1} - \frac{n}{s} \times \frac{n-s}{2s} x^{\frac{mn}{s}+2} + \frac{n}{s} \times \frac{n-s}{2s} \times \frac{n-2s}{3s} x^{\frac{mn}{s}+3} - \frac{n}{s} \times \frac{n-s}{2s} \times \frac{n-2s}{3s} \times \frac{n-3s}{4s} x^{\frac{mn}{s}+4}$ &c. Multiplying therefore this Series by $c^{\frac{1}{s}} x$, we shall have $c^{\frac{1}{s}} \times x^{\frac{mn}{s}} x + \frac{n}{s} x^{\frac{mn}{s}+1} x - \frac{n}{s} \times \frac{n-s}{2s} \times x^{\frac{mn}{s}+2} x + \frac{n}{s} \times \frac{n-s}{2s} \times \frac{n-2s}{3s} x^{\frac{mn}{s}+3} x - \frac{n}{s} \times \frac{n-s}{2s} \times \frac{n-2s}{3s} \times \frac{n-3s}{4s} x^{\frac{mn}{s}+4} x$, for the Fluxion of the same Space A B C, and consequently its Fluent $c^{\frac{1}{s}}$

×

$\times \frac{s}{mn+s} x^{\frac{mn}{s}+1} + \frac{n}{s} \times \frac{s}{mn+2s} \times x^{\frac{mn}{s}+2} - \frac{n}{s} \times \frac{n-s}{2s} \times \frac{s}{mn+3s} x^{\frac{mn}{s}+3} + \frac{n}{s} \times \frac{n-s}{2s} \times \frac{n-2s}{3s} \times \frac{s}{mn+4s} \times x^{\frac{mn}{s}+4} - \frac{n}{s} \times \frac{n-s}{2s} \times \frac{n-2s}{3s} \times \frac{n-3s}{4s} \times \frac{s}{mn+5s} \times x^{\frac{mn}{s}+5} +$, &c $= c^{\frac{1}{s}} \times x^{\frac{mn}{s}} \times \frac{s}{mn+s} x + \frac{n}{s} \times \frac{s}{mn+2s} x^2 - \frac{n}{s} \times \frac{n-s}{2s} \times \frac{s}{mn+3s} x^3 + \frac{n}{s} \times \frac{n-s}{2s} \times \frac{n-2s}{3s} \times \frac{s}{mn+4s} \times x^4 - \frac{n}{s} \times \frac{n-s}{2s} \times \frac{n-2s}{3s} \times \frac{n-3s}{4s} \times \frac{s}{mn+5s} \times x^5$, &c $= c^{\frac{1}{s}} \times x^{\frac{mn}{s}} \times \frac{s}{mn+s} x + \frac{n}{mn+2s} x^2 - \frac{n}{2s} \times \frac{n-s}{mn+3s} x^3 + \frac{n}{2s} \times \frac{n-s}{3s} \times \frac{n-2s}{mn+4s} x^4 - \frac{n}{2s} \times \frac{n-s}{3s} \times \frac{n-2s}{4s} \times \frac{n-3s}{mn+5s} x^5$, &c will give the Hyperbolic Space A B C.

Now if we imagine the Ordinate B C in a flowing State, and to move 'till it arrives at, or coincides with the Ordinate D F, then A B will become equal to A D, and x will become equal to b, and we shall $c^{\frac{1}{s}} \times b^{\frac{mn}{s}} \times \frac{s}{mn+s} b + \frac{n}{mn+2s} b^2 - \frac{n}{2s} \times \frac{n-s}{mn+3s} b^3 + \frac{n}{2s} \times \frac{n-s}{3s} \times \frac{n-2s}{mn+4s} b^4 - \frac{n}{2s} \times \frac{n-s}{3s} \times \frac{n-2s}{4s} \times \frac{n-3s}{mn+5s} b^5$, &c for the Semi-Hyperbolic Space A D E

EXAMPLE VI

To find the Area, or Space inclosed between the Hyperbola and its Asymptotes, or the Relation of the Supplemental Space to the Square or Rhombus.

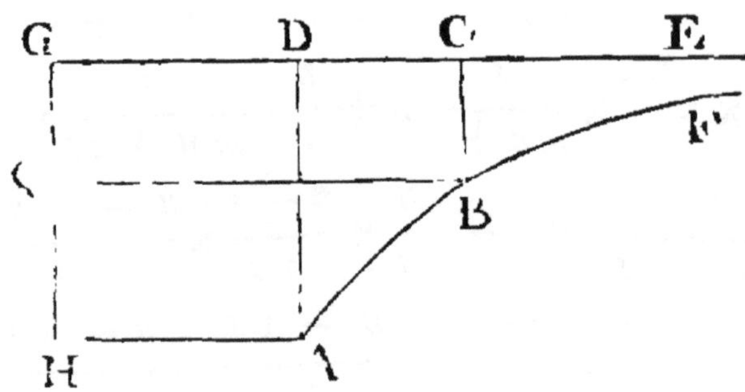

LET A B F represent a Semi Hyperbola G E, G H its Asymptotes, and having drawn any Ordinate, as B C, put G C $= x$, B C $= y$, G H $=$ D A $= a$, and because, from the Nature of the Curve, $y = x^{-1}$, therefore $x^{-1}\dot{x}$ will be the Fluxion of the Area. Whence $x^{-1+1} = y\,x$ (by putting y in the room of x^{-1}, to which it is equal) $= a\,a$, will be the Area, for when G C becomes equal to G D, C B becomes equal to D A, and x and y become each equal to a, and this is called the Equilateral Hyperbola.

AND universally, if G D be put equal to b, D A $= a$, and m for the Exponent of the Power of y, we shall have $y^m = x$, and $y = x^{\frac{1}{m}}$, and $x^{\frac{1}{m}}\,\dot{x}$ for the Fluxion of the Area, whence $\frac{m}{m+1}\,x^{\frac{1}{m}}\,x = \frac{m}{m+1}\,y\,x$ (by putting y in the room of $x^{\frac{1}{m}}$) $= \frac{m}{m+1}\,a\,b$, will be the Area, for when G C becomes equal to G D, then C B flows into or becomes equal to A D, consequently x will become equal to b, and y become equal to a.

THIS general Theorem $\frac{m}{m+1}\,a\,b$, expresses as well the Proportion of the Parabola to its circumscribed Parallelogram, as the Hyperbola to the Asymptotical Parallelogram; for if

$m = 2$,

$m = 2$, then $y\,y = x$, which is the Property of the common *Apollonian* Parabola, and the Area will be $\frac{2}{3}$, if $m = 3$, then $y = x$, which is the Property of the Cubic Parabola, and the Area will be $\frac{3}{4}$, *&c.* of the circumscribing Parallelogram.

If the Exponent m be negative, the Expression $\frac{m}{m+1}\,a\,b$ will serve for finding the Areas of all sorts of Hyperbolic Spaces, and the Theorem will be $\frac{-m}{-m+1}\,a\,b$, or $\frac{m}{m-1}\,a\,b$, whence it appears, that if m be greater than 1, the Space is finite if $m = 1$, the Space is infinite, and if m be less than 1, it is more than infinite.

If $-m = -1$, that is, if it be $y^{-1} = x$, or $1 = x\,y$, the Curve will be the common *Apollonian* Hyperbola, and the Area, or Space E G H A B F $= \frac{m}{m-1}\,a\,b = \frac{1}{0}\,a\,b$, is infinite in respect of the Parallelogram G H A D.

If $m = 2$, that is, if $y^{-2} = x$, or $1 = x\,y^2$, then the Area of the Hyperbolic Space E G H A B F $= \frac{m}{m-1} - a\,b$ is equal to $2\,a\,b$, equal to twice the Parallelogram G H A D. But

If $m = -\frac{1}{2}$, then $y^m = x$, is $y^{-\frac{1}{2}} = x$, or $1 = x\,y^{\frac{1}{2}}$, and $\frac{m}{m-1}\,a\,b$ is $\frac{\frac{1}{2}}{\frac{1}{2}-1}\,a\,b = -\frac{1}{2}\,a\,b$, which shews, that the Area of the Hyperbolic Space E G H A B F is more than infinite in respect of the Space G H A D.

If about the same transverse Axis A B (*See the following Figure*) be described two Hyperbolas, the one an Equilateral one, as N A N, the other upon any given Base C B C, the Area of the Equilateral Hyperbola, will be the Area of the Hyperbola C A C, as the Ordinate B N to the Ordinate B C

FOR

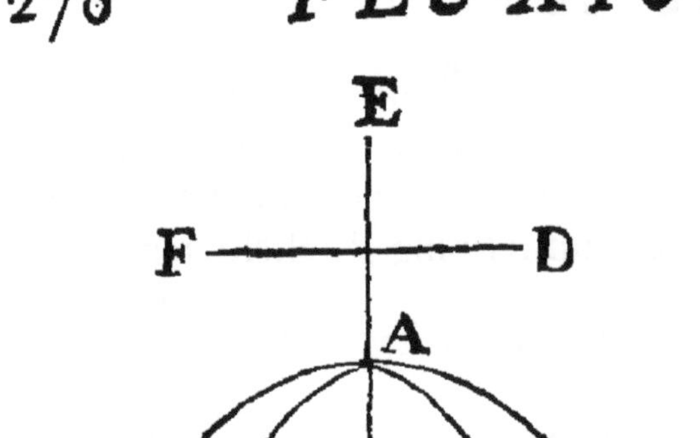

For putting $AE = a$, $FD = b$, $AB = x$, $BC = y$, and $BN = z$.

Because, from the Nature of the Hyperbola, as $ax + xx \; yy \; aa \; bb$ in the given Hyperbola, and $ax + xx \; zz \; aa \; aa$ in the Equilateral Hyperbola, therefore as $yy \; zz \; bb . aa$; that is, as $y \; z \; b \; a$, and because in the Time that the Equilateral Hyperbola N A N is generated by the Motion of the Ordinate B N, in the same time the Hyperbola C A C is generated by the Motion of C B, whence the Equilateral Hyperbola N A N, is to the Hyperbola C A C, as E A to F D, or as B N to B C

Hence it follows, that Hyperbolas described about the same common Axis, having the same transverse Diameter, are as their conjugate Diameters, or as their correspondent Ordinates directly

EXAMPLE VII.

To find the Area of the Logarithmetic Space A C D F E.

The Logarithmic Curve may be generated after thi manner.

Conceive the right Line D F (*See the following Figure*) to move uniformly along the Line F E, so that while the Point F moves over equal Spaces in equal Times, the Line D F decrease, or, which is the same thing, the extream Point is carried towards F, with a Velocity, in a Geometric Ratio of the same Time, the Point D, by these two Motions, will describe the

the Curve A C D, which is call'd the Logarithmic Curve, as will the Ordinate D F describe the Logarithmic Space A C D F E in the same Time.

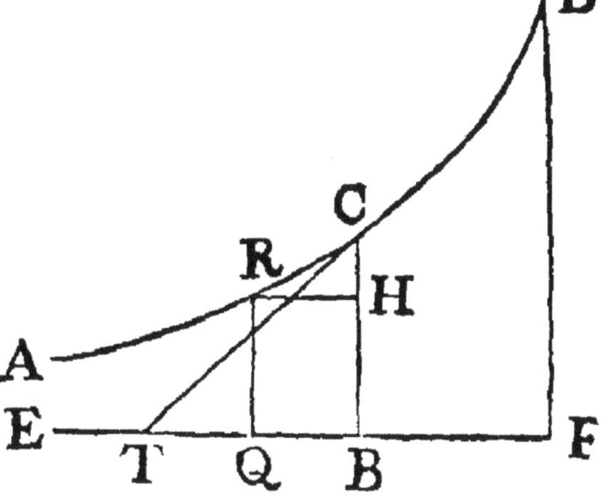

LET A C D represent the Logarithmic Curve, F E its Asymptote, B C an Ordinate rightly apply'd

THROUGH the Point C, where the Ordinate meets the Curve, let the Tangent C T be drawn, to cut the Asymptote in T

AND inasmuch as from the Nature of the Curve, the Subtangent is always equal to itself, and to a given right Line, put B T $= a$, B C $= y$, F E $= x$, and because the Sides T B, B C, of the Triangle T B C, in the evanescent State, are similar to the Velocities of the nascent Augments of the Ordinate and Abscisse, it will be as $y \quad x \quad y \quad a$, whence $y = \frac{a y}{x}$ consequently $\frac{a y}{x} \times x = a y$ will be the Fluxion of the Area, whence $a y$, the Fluent, will be the Area itself, or Value of the Space A C B E Whence it follows,

First, THAT the Logarithmic Space A C B E, though infinitely extended, is to the Triangle T B C, form'd by the Tangent T C, Subtangent T B, and Ordinate B C, as 2 to 1, for $a y$, the Value of the Logarithmic Space, is equal to the Rectangle made of the Subtangent a, or T C, and the Ordinate y, or B C, the Double of the Triangle T B C

Secondly, THAT any Space, as B C R Q, comprehended between any two Ordinates B C, Q R, will be equal to the Rectangle

Rectangle made of the Subtangent TC, and CH, the Difference between the Ordinates QR and BC.

For the Space ARQE is equal to TB × RQ, and the Space ACBE is equal to TB × BC; and consequently the Space CBQR, or Difference of the Spaces ACBE, and ARQF, must be equal to $\overline{TB} \times \overline{BC} - \overline{TB} \times \overline{RQ} = TB \times \overline{BC - RQ} = TB \times CH$, for BH = QR. And consequently,

Thirdly, That the Spaces comprehended between any two Ordinates, are as the Differences of those Ordinates themselves.

EXAMPLE VIII

To find the Space inclosed by the common Archimedian *Spiral Line*

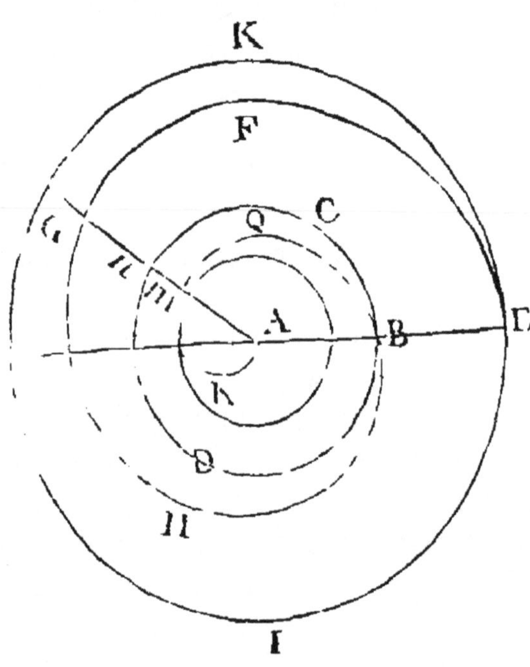

The Generation of the *Archimedian* Spiral Line may be conceived after the manner following

If while the Line AB revolves about the immoveable Point A, the Point B moves towards A in such a manner, that while the whole Line AB makes one entire Revolution, and describes a Circle, the Point B moves through the whole Line BA with an equal and uniform Motion I say, that the Point B will, by this Motion, describe the

the Line A K M Q B, which is called the *Archimedian* Spiral Line, as will the generating Line A B describe the Spiral Space B Q M K A B in the same time, and this is called the first Spiral Space. Or, which is the same thing,

If the Point B, set out from A at the same time that the Line A B begins to revolve about the Point A, and move towards B with the same uniform Law of Velocity, as in the former Case, it will describe the Spiral Line A K M Q B in the same time, and if after that the same Point B be imagined to flow with the same uniform Law of Velocity along the infinite Line A B E, and in such a manner, that while the whole Line A E, the Double of A B, shall describe the Circle E K I, the Point E shall describe the Periphery I K G I, and the Point B shall have moved from B to E, the Point B, by this Compound Motion, will describe the Spiral Portion B H G F E, then the Space B H G F E B, is called the second Spiral Space. And after the same manner, by imagining the Point B to move in the same Line, according to the same Law, may an infinite Number of Spiral Spaces be generated

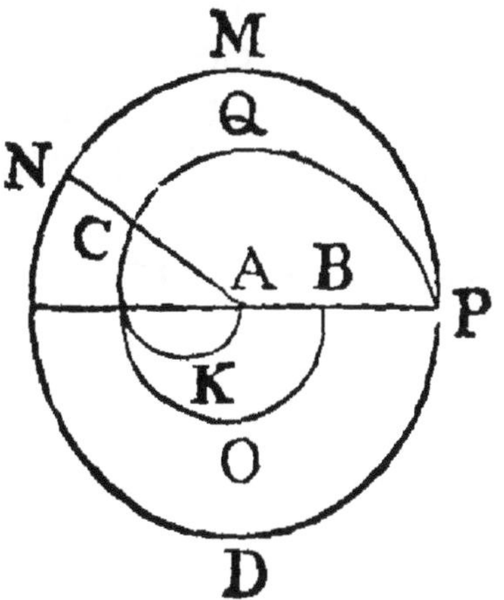

Let therefore PQCKAP represent the common Spiral Space, and PMNDP, the Circle described [illegible] Ray A P.

[illegible] $AP = AN = r$, the Circumference of the Circle [illegible] DP $= c$, the Arch P D N [illegible] the Ray $AC = y$, and because, from the Property of the Curve, as c [illegible] x [illegible] r [illegible] y, therefore $y = \frac{rx}{c}$, and inasmuch as the Velocity of the Points N and C are equable, and uniform (that is, the Velocity of the Point N in the Direction N M P, and the Velocity of the Point C in the Direction C Q P, therefore the Fluxions of the Circumference, and the Spiral Line, shall be proportional to each other, as the Radii A N and A C,

 where-

wherefore as $r\ y\ \ \dot{x}\ \frac{y\dot{x}}{r}$, the Fluxion of the Spiral AKC, whence the Fluxion of the Area will be $\frac{yy\dot{x}}{2r} = \frac{xxrr\dot{x}}{2ccr}$ (by ſubſtituting $\frac{xxrr}{cc}$ in the room of yy) and the Area itſelf will be $\frac{rrx^3}{6ccr} = \frac{rx^3}{6cc}$, and conſequently the Area of the whole Spiral Space will be $\frac{rc^3}{6c^2} = \frac{rc}{6}$, for when the generating Line AN has made one entire Revolution, x becomes equal to c. But it has been already ſhewn in *Example* III that $\frac{rc}{2}$ is the Area of the Circle PMNDP, whence it follows, that the Area of the Circle generated by the Ray AP, is to the firſt Spiral Space PQCKAP, as 6 to 2, or as 3 to 1, and conſequently the Spiral Space is $\frac{1}{3}$ of the circumſcribing Circle

AND univerſally if n repreſents the Exponent of the Power of the Velocity of the Point P, according to the Direction PM, and m the Exponent of the Power of the Velocity, according to the Direction PA, then as $c^n\ \ x^n\ \ r^m . y^m$, whence $y^m = \frac{r^m x^n}{c^n}$, and $y = \frac{r x^{\frac{n}{m}}}{c^{\frac{n}{m}}}$, and $yy = \frac{r^2 x^{\frac{2n}{m}}}{c^{\frac{2n}{m}}}$, whence the Fluxion of the Area will be $\frac{r^2 x^{\frac{2n}{m}} \dot{x}}{2c^{\frac{2n}{m}}}$, and conſequently the Area itſelf will be $\frac{m}{2n+m} \times \frac{r x^{\frac{2n}{m}+1}}{2c^{\frac{2n}{m}}} = \frac{m}{2n+m} \times \frac{rc}{2}$, for when the Point P, according to the Direction PM,

has

has made one entire Revolution, x becomes equal to c, and because $\frac{rc}{2}$ expresses the Area of the circumscribing Circle, it follows

THAT the Spiral Space is to the circumscribed Circle as m to $m+2n$, that is, the first Spiral Space is to the correspon-ding circular Space, as the Exponent of the generating Ray to the Exponent of the same Ray encreased by twice the Exponent of the Circumference

IF $m=1$, and $n=1$, then the Area of the Spiral Space is $\frac{1}{1+2}=\frac{1}{3}$ of the circumscribed Circle, as was before found

IF $m=2$, and $n=3$; that is, if the Velocity of the Point P, according to the Direction PA, be to the Velocity of the same Point B, according to the Direction PM, as the Squares of the Spaces run over, in the Direction PA, to the Cubes of the Spaces described according to the Direction PM, then the first Spiral Space will be to the circumscribing Circle as 2 to $2+6$, or as 1 to 4, and consequently the Spiral Space will be $\frac{1}{4}$ of the circumscribing Circle Whence to find a Spiral Space that shall be to the circumscribing Circle in any given Ratio, as suppose of p to q, we must say, as $q \;\; p \;\; m+2n \;\; m$; whence as $q-p \;\; p \;\; (m+2n-m=) \;\; 2n \;\; m$, and consequently as $\frac{q-p}{2} \;\; p \;\; n \;\; m$, whence it follows, that if p be taken for the Exponent of the Radius, $\frac{q-p}{2}$ must be the Exponent of the Circumference.

IMAGINE the Spiral Line AKMB (*See the following Figure*) to be continued from B to R, and H to E, then is BE $=$ AB; and to find the Space contained between the second Spiral Line BRHE and BE, because $AN=r$, $BDPN=c$,

put

put N H $=y$, and B D H $=x$, then is $\frac{r\dot{x}+y\dot{x}}{r}$ equal to the

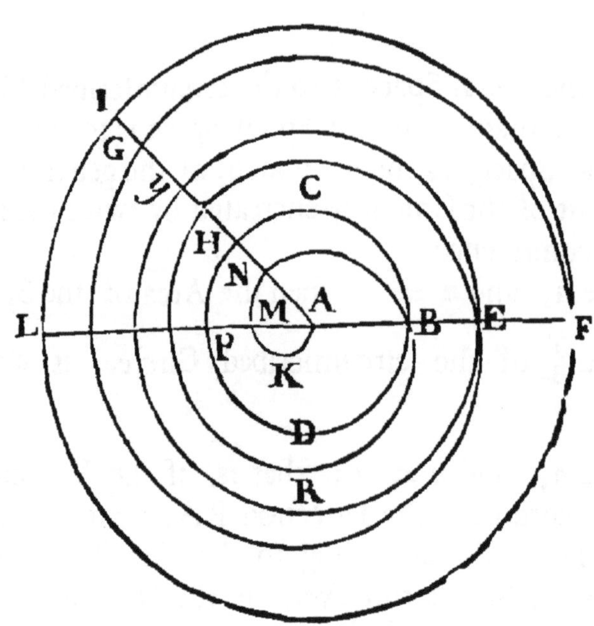

Fluxion of B H, and consequently the Fluxion of the Area is $\frac{r+y}{2}\times\frac{r\dot{x}+y\dot{x}}{r}=\frac{rr\dot{x}+2ry\dot{x}+yy\dot{x}}{2r}$; but because, from the Nature of the Spiral it will be as $c\cdot c+x \cdot r \cdot r+y$, therefore $cr+cy=cr+rx$, and $cy=rx$, whence $y=\frac{rx}{c}$. Substituting this Value therefore in the room of y, in the former Expression $\frac{rr\dot{x}+2ry\dot{x}+yy\dot{x}}{2r}$, and we shall have $\frac{ccr\dot{x}+2crx\dot{x}+rxx\dot{x}}{2cc}$, for the Fluxion of the Space B R H N, whose Fluent $\frac{ccrx+crxx+\frac{1}{3}rxxx}{2cc}$, will be the Value of the Space itself

itself, but when the Ray I A, by revolving about the Point A, arrives at, or is coincident with the Ray A F, the Point N will arrive at, or coincide with the Point B, consequently x will become equal to c, and we shall have $\frac{ccrc + crcc + \frac{1}{3}rccc}{2cc} = 1 \times 1 \times \frac{1}{3} \times \frac{rc}{2} = \frac{1}{3} \times \frac{rc}{2}$ for the Area of the Space B R H E B, and universally if n be put for the Power of c and x, and m for the Power of r and y, it will be as c^n $c^n + x^n$ r^m $r^m + y^m$, whence $c^n r^m + c^n y^m = c^n r^m + r^m x^n$, and $c^n y^m = r^m x^n$, and $y^m = \frac{r^m x^n}{c^n}$, and $y = \frac{r x^{\frac{n}{m}}}{c^{\frac{n}{m}}}$

Substituting therefore this Value of y in the fluxionary Expression $\frac{rr\dot{x} + 2ry\dot{x} + yy\dot{x}}{2r}$, and we shall have $\frac{rc^{\frac{2n}{m}}\dot{x} + 2rc^{\frac{n}{m}}\dot{x} + rx^{\frac{2n}{m}}\dot{x}}{2r^{\frac{2n}{m}}}$, for the Fluxion of 2d Spiral Space B R H, whose Fluent $\frac{rc^{\frac{2n}{m}}x + \frac{2m}{m+n}rc^{\frac{n}{m}}x^{\frac{n}{m}+1} + \frac{m}{m+2n}rx^{\frac{2n}{m}+1}}{2c^{\frac{n}{m}}}$ will be the Area of the same Spiral Space; but when the Point N, by flowing, arrives at B, x becomes equal to c, and we shall have $\frac{rc^{\frac{2n}{m}+1} + \frac{2m}{m+n}rc^{\frac{2n}{m}+1} + \frac{m}{m+2n}rc^{\frac{2n}{m}+1}}{2c^{\frac{2n}{m}}}$ equal to

$\frac{rc + \frac{2m}{m+n}rc + \frac{m}{m+2n}rc}{2}$ (by dividing by $c^{\frac{2n}{m}}$) equal to $\frac{4mm + 8mn + 2nn}{mm + 3mn + 2nn} \times \frac{rc}{2}$, by reducing all the Fractions

ons to one Denominator, for the Area of the ſecond Spiral Space B R H E B, which is a general Theorem for finding the Areas of an infinite Variety of ſecond Spiral Spaces

IF $m=1$, and $n=1$, as in the *Archimedian* Spiral Line, then the ſecond Spiral Space B R H E B, is $\frac{7}{3}$ of $\frac{rc}{2}$, or of the Area of the Circle B D N C B, and to $\frac{7}{12}$ of the circumſcribing Circle E Y E, inaſmuch as the Circle E Y E is quadruple of the Circle B D N C B.

AGAIN, becauſe the firſt Spiral Space A K M B A is $\frac{1}{3}$ of its circumſcribing Circle B D N C B, and the Circle is $\frac{1}{4}$ of the Circle E y E circumſcribing the ſecond Spiral Space, therefore the firſt Spiral Space is $\frac{1}{3}$ of $\frac{1}{4}$, or $\frac{1}{12}$ of the Circle E y E

THE ſecond Spiral Space is $\frac{7}{12}$ of its conterminating Circle, and the firſt Spiral Space is $\frac{1}{12}$; therefore their Difference, or the Exceſs of the ſecond Spiral Space above the firſt is $\frac{6}{12}$, and conſequently the Exceſs of the ſecond Spiral Space above the firſt, is to the firſt Spiral Space as 6 to 1.

TO find the Area of the third Spiral Space, put y G $=y$, and becauſe as $r : \dot{x} :: 2r+y : \frac{2r\dot{x}+y\dot{x}}{r}$. Therefore $\frac{2r+y}{2}\times\frac{2r\dot{x}+y\dot{x}}{r}=\frac{4rr\dot{x}+4ry\dot{x}+yy\dot{x}}{2r}$ will be the Fluxion of the Area $=\frac{4rc^{\frac{2n}{m}}\dot{x}+4rc^{\frac{n}{m}}x^{\frac{n}{m}}\dot{x}+rx^{\frac{2n}{m}}\dot{x}}{2c^{\frac{2n}{m}}}$ (by ſubſtituting $\frac{2rx^{\frac{n}{m}}}{2c^{\frac{n}{m}}}$ in the room of y, to which it is equal) conſequently the flowing Quantity itſelf will be $\frac{4rc^{\frac{2n}{m}}x+\frac{4m}{m+n}rc^{\frac{n}{m}}x^{\frac{n}{m}+1}+\frac{m}{m+2n}rx^{\frac{2n}{m}+1}}{2c^{\frac{2n}{m}}}$. But when the

Line

Line A I, revolving about the Point A, arrives at, or coincides with the Line A F, the Point G in the Spiral Line will arrive at, or coincide with the Point F, at which Time x will become equal to c, and consequently the whole Spiral Space will be equal to $\dfrac{4rc^{\frac{2n}{m}+1}+\frac{4m}{m+n}rc^{\frac{2n}{m}+1}+\frac{m}{m+2n}rc^{\frac{2n}{m}+1}}{2c^{\frac{2m}{m}}}$,

whence, by dividing by $c^{\frac{2n}{m}}$, we shall have

$$\frac{4rc+\frac{4m}{m+n}rc+\frac{m}{m+2n}rc}{2}=\frac{9mm+21mn+8nn}{mm+3mn+2nn}$$

$\times\frac{rc}{2}$, for the Area of the third Spiral Space; and when $m=1$ and $n=1$, it will be equal to $\frac{9+21+8}{1+3+2}=\frac{38}{6}=\frac{19}{3}$ of $\frac{rc}{2}$ $=\frac{19}{27}$ of the circumscribing Circle; and after the same manner may the Value of the fourth, fifth, &c. Spiral Spaces be investigated

Whence it appears, that the Value of the first, second, and third Spaces in the common, or *Archimedian* Spiral, are as the Numbers $\frac{1}{3}$, $\frac{7}{12}$, $\frac{19}{27}$, that is, as a Series of Fractional Numbers, whose Numerators are the Differences of the Cubes of a Series of Numbers in Arithmetical Proportion, beginning from Unity and Denominators, the Multiples of the Squares of the same Arithmetical Series arising from a continual Multiplication of the Number 3 Thus the Value of the fifth Spiral Space will be expressed by the fractional Number $\frac{61}{75}$, whose Numerator is equal to the Difference of the Numbers 64 and 125, the Cubes of the Numbers 4 and 5, and Denominator 75 equal to the Product arising from the Multiplication of 25, the Square of 5 (the Number denoting the Space) by the Number

Number 3. And after this manner may the Value of any Space be determined.

AGAIN, the same things being supposed as before, put $AB = y$, and it will be as $r \; y : x \; \frac{yx}{r}$, whence $\frac{xy\dot{y}}{r}$ will be the Fluxion of the extream Space, but as $c : x \;.\; r \; y$, therefore $x = \frac{cy}{r}$, whence $\frac{cyy\dot{y}}{rr}$ will be the Fluxion of the Area; whence $\frac{cy^3}{3r^2}$, will be the Area itself BDC, and $\frac{crrr}{3rr} = \frac{cr}{3} = \frac{1}{3}cr$, will be the Area of the entire Space, for when x, by flowing, becomes equal to c, y becomes equal to r, and consequently the extream Space is to the whole Circle as 2 to 3, whence the inner Space will be as 1 to 3, as was before shewn.

AGAIN, suppose the Property of the Spiral such that as $\overline{BDPNCB}^n \; \overline{BDN}^n \; AN^m \; HN^m$, as before, put the Circle $BDPNCB = c$, $BH = x$, $HN = y$, then $AN = r - y$, and as $r \; r - y \; \dot{x} \; \frac{r\dot{x} - y\dot{x}}{y}$, the Fluxion of the Absciffe, whence $\frac{r-y}{2} \times \frac{r\dot{x} - y\dot{x}}{r} = \frac{rr\dot{x} - 2ry\dot{x} + yy\dot{x}}{2r}$, will be the Fluxion of the Area, but as $c^m \; x^m \; r^m \; y^m$, therefore $x^n = \frac{c^n y^m}{r^m}$, and $x = \frac{cy^{\frac{m}{n}}}{r^{\frac{m}{n}}}$, and $\dot{x} = \frac{\frac{m}{n} cy^{\frac{m}{n}-1}\dot{y}}{r^{\frac{m}{n}}} = \frac{mcy^{\frac{m}{n}-1}\dot{y}}{nr^{\frac{m}{n}}}$, and substituting this in the room of $\dot{x}$, we

shall

shall have $\frac{rr-2ry+yy}{2r}\times\frac{mcy^{\frac{m-n}{n}}\dot{y}}{nr^{\frac{m}{n}}}=\frac{mcrry^{\frac{m}{n}-1}\dot{y}}{2nr^{\frac{m}{n}+1}}$

$$-\frac{2mcry^{\frac{m}{n}}\dot{y}+mcy^{\frac{m}{n}+1}\dot{y}}{2nr^{\frac{m}{n}+1}}=\frac{mcy^{\frac{m}{n}-1}\dot{y}}{2nr^{\frac{m}{n}-1}}-$$

$-\frac{mcy^{\frac{m}{n}}\dot{y}}{nr^{\frac{m}{n}}}+\frac{mcy^{\frac{m}{n}+1}\dot{y}}{2nr^{\frac{m}{n}+1}}$, for the Fluxion of the Space, whose Fluent $\frac{n}{m}\times\frac{mcy^{\frac{m}{n}}}{2nr^{\frac{m}{n}-1}}-\frac{n}{m+n}\times\frac{mcy^{\frac{m}{n}+1}}{nr^{\frac{m}{n}}}+\frac{n}{m+2n}$ $\times\frac{mcy^{\frac{m}{n}+2}}{2nr^{\frac{m}{n}+1}}=\frac{cy^{\frac{m}{n}}}{2r^{\frac{m}{n}-1}}-\frac{m}{m+n}\frac{cy^{\frac{m}{n}+1}}{r^{\frac{m}{n}}}+\frac{mcy^{\frac{m}{n}+2}}{2m+4nr^{\frac{m}{n}+1}}$, which when y becomes r, gives $\frac{cr}{2}-\frac{m}{m+n}cr+\frac{m}{2m+4n}$ cr, or $\frac{1}{2}-\frac{m}{m+n}+\frac{m}{2m+4n}cr=\frac{nm}{mm+3mn+2nn}rc$, for the whole Space.

Again, because as $c^n : x^n :: r^m : y^m$, therefore $y^m=\frac{x^n r^m}{c^n}$ and $y=\frac{rx^{\frac{n}{m}}}{c^{\frac{n}{m}}}$, and $yy=\frac{rrx^{\frac{2n}{m}}}{c^{\frac{2n}{m}}}$. Now if we substitute these Values in the room of y, and yy in the fluxionary Equation, $\frac{rr\dot{x}-2ry\dot{x}+yy\dot{x}}{2r}$, we shall have $\frac{r\dot{x}}{2}-\frac{rx^{\frac{n}{m}}\dot{x}}{c^{\frac{n}{m}}}+\frac{rx^{\frac{2n}{m}}\dot{x}}{2c^{\frac{2n}{m}}}$;

whence the Fluent will be $\frac{rx}{2} - \frac{mrx^{\frac{n}{m}+1}}{\overline{n+m}\,c^{\frac{n}{m}}} + \frac{mrx^{\frac{2n}{m}+1}}{\overline{4n+2m}\,c^{\frac{2n}{m}}}$ $= \frac{rc}{2} - \frac{mrc}{n+m} + \frac{mrc}{4m+2n} = \frac{1}{2} - \frac{m}{n+m} + \frac{m}{4n+2m}\,rc$ $= \frac{nn}{mm+3mn+2nn}\,rc$, the same as was before determined, for when y becomes equal to r, x becomes equal to c; whence the Space is to the conterminate Circle as $2nn$ to $mm+3mn+2nn$.

AGAIN, because as $r : r-y :: x : \frac{rx-yx}{r} = BC$, we shall have $\frac{rx\dot{y}-xy\dot{y}}{r}$ for the Fluxion of the Space BCNB, but $x = \frac{cy^{\frac{m}{n}}}{r^{\frac{m}{n}}}$ as has been already shewn, therefore $\frac{rx\dot{y}-xy\dot{y}}{r}$ (by substituting the Value of x) will be equal to $\frac{cy^{\frac{m}{n}}\dot{y}}{r^{\frac{m}{n}}}$ $- \frac{cy^{\frac{m}{n}+1}\dot{y}}{r^{\frac{m}{n}+1}}$, whence the Fluent will be $\frac{ncy^{\frac{m}{n}+1}}{\overline{m+n}\,r^{\frac{m}{n}}} - \frac{ncy^{\frac{m}{n}+2}}{\overline{m+2n}\,r^{\frac{m}{n}+1}}$ equal to $\frac{ncr}{m+n} - \frac{ncr}{m+2n} = \frac{n}{m+n} - \frac{n}{m+2n}\,cr$ equal to $\frac{nn}{mm+3mn+2nn}\,cr$ (when y becomes equal to r) for the whole Spiral Space, the same as has been determined from the preceding Investigations.

EXAM-

EXAMPLE IX.

To find the Space enclosed by the Logarithmic Spiral

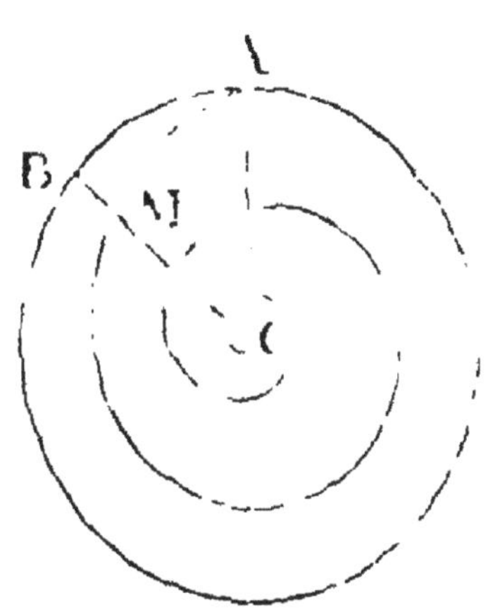

THE Logarithmic Spiral may be conceived to be generated after the manner following

IF while the Line CA (revolving about the immoveable Point C) describes equal Spaces in equal Times, the Point A be carried towards C with such a Velocity, that the Line CM decreases, or, which is the same thing, the several Distances of the Point A, from the Point C, are, in a direct Proportion, Geometrically; the Point A, by this compound Motion will describe the Proportional or Logarithmic Spiral, while the Ordinate CM will describe the Logarithmic Spiral Space CMAC

LET ABMC represent the Logarithmic Spiral, and put $AC = c$, $CB = y$,

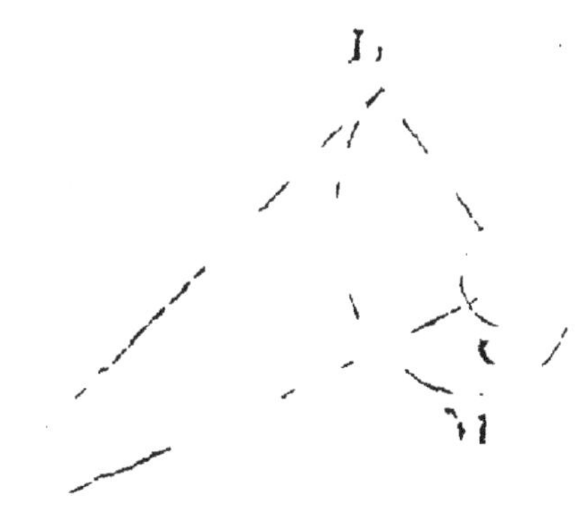

and $\dot{x}$ for the Fluxion of the Absciss, then will $\frac{y\dot{x}}{2}$ be the Fluxion of the Area.

BUT because, from the Nature of the Curve, the Angle CBT, formed by the Ordinate CB, and the Tangent TB is in all Points of the Curve the same, if CT be drawn perpendicular to CB, the Ratio of the Ordinate CB, to the Subtangent C T will be constantly the same. Let these therefore be represented by n and m, then as $y \quad x \quad m \quad n$, and $x = \frac{ny}{m}$, and consequently $\frac{nyy}{2m}$, will be the Fluxion of the Area, whence $\frac{nyy}{4m}$ will be the Fluent of the Space A B C A, and $\frac{naa}{4m}$ equal to the whole Logarithmic Space, for when the Point B, by flowing, arrives at A, y becomes equal to a.

PUT C T, the Subtangent, equal to t, then, because as $y \quad x \quad y \quad t$, therefore $yt = xy$, and $yt = xy$, which, because yx is double to the Space contained between the Ordinate y, and the Spiral, and ty equal to the Triangle formed by the Ordinate, Tangent, and Subtangent, it follows, that the Spiral Space is $\frac{1}{2}$ of the Triangle B C T.

EXAMPLE X.

To find the Value of a Parabolic Spiral Space

LET A B F represent an Arch of a Circle, E B the Radius, and A C D a Portion of a Curve generated in such a manner, that having drawn the Ordinate E C, and produced it 'till it meet the Circumference of the Curve in B, the Ratio of the Arch A B, and the Square of the intercepted Part of the Radius B C, may be a constant Quantity, and always equal to a given right Line

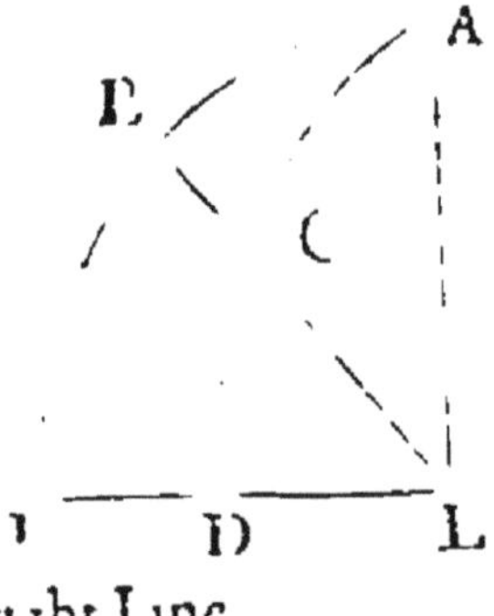

PUT E A = E B = r, E C = y, then B C = $r - y$, and the Arch A B = x, whence $ax = rr - 2ry + yy$,

and

and $x = \frac{rr - 2ry + yy}{a}$, and $\dot{x} = \frac{-2r\dot{y} + 2y\dot{y}}{a}$, but as r y $\frac{2y\dot{y} - 2r\dot{y}}{a}$ $\frac{2yy\dot{y} - 2ry\dot{y}}{ra}$ equal to the Fluxion of the Spiral Arch A C D This therefore being multiplied by $\frac{y}{2}$, will give $\frac{y^3\dot{y} - ry^2\dot{y}}{ra}$, for the Fluxion of the Area, whence $+\frac{y^4}{4ra} - \frac{y^3}{3a}$ will be the Area of the Space ABC, and $\frac{r^3}{4a} - \frac{r^3}{3a} = \frac{3ar^3 - 4ar^3}{12aa} = \frac{r^3}{12a}$ for the whole Spiral Space, for when C, by flowing, arrives at A, y becomes equal to r.

But $\frac{r\dot{x} + y\dot{x}}{r} \times \frac{r - y}{2} = \frac{rr\dot{x} - yy\dot{x}}{2r}$, the Fluxion of the Trilinear Space B A C, and putting $\frac{2y\dot{y} - 2r\dot{y}}{a}$ in the room of $\dot{x}$, we shall have $\frac{rry\dot{y} - y^3\dot{y} - r^3\dot{y} + ryy\dot{y}}{ra}$ for the Fluxion of the same Space, whose Fluent $\frac{ryy}{2a} - \frac{rry}{a} - \frac{y^4}{4ar} + \frac{y^3}{3a}$ will give the Value of the same Space B A C, but when the Point C coincides with the Point A, y becomes equal to r, and we shall have $\frac{r^3}{2a} - \frac{r^3}{a} - \frac{r^3}{4a} + \frac{r^3}{3a} = \frac{r^3}{3a} + \frac{2r^3}{4a} - \frac{5r^3}{4a} = \frac{r^3}{3a} - \frac{3r^3}{4a} = \frac{5r^3}{12a}$, but if $\frac{rr}{a} = c$,

then

then $ca = rr$, and $a = \frac{rr}{c}$, whence putting $\frac{rr}{c}$ in the room of a, we ſhall have $\frac{5r^3}{12} \times \frac{c}{rr} = \frac{5cr}{12}$

WHENCE the Spiral Space, the Supplemental Space, and the Circle are as the Numbers 1, 5, 6

EXAMPLE XI.

To find the Area of the Lunula *of* Hippocrates

IF about any Point O, as a Centre, a Semi circle, as A D G, be drawn, and if about E, the Extremity of the Diameter D E, another Quadrant, as A F G, with the Radius E A be drawn, the Space A D G F A is called the *Lunula* of *Hippocrates*

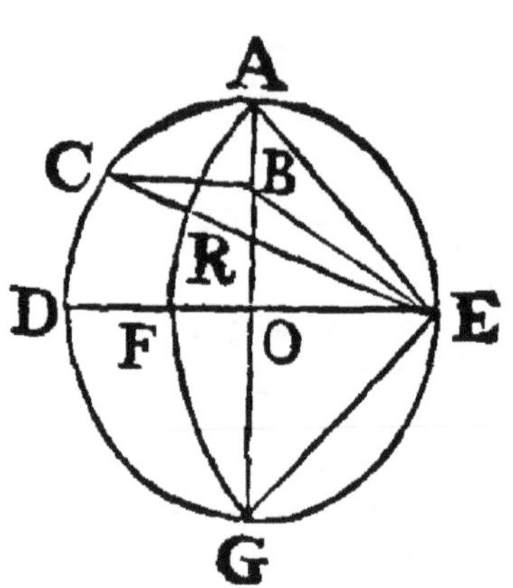

PUT therefore O A = O E = r, the Circumference A D G F = c; then will E A = $\sqrt{2rr}$, or $r \times \sqrt{2}$

BUT the Area of the Circle ADGE is $\frac{cr}{2}$, whence the Area of the Circle A F G E will be cr (by the 31ſt of the 6th of *Euclid*) but the Sector A F G E is $\frac{1}{4}$ of the Circle deſcribed with the Radius E A, whence the Sector A E G F A is equal to the Semicircle A D G O A Taking away therefore from each the Segment A F G O, and we ſhall have the *Lunula* A D G F A equal to the Triangle A E G Whence it follows,

THAT if any Ordinate E C be drawn, that the Triangle A E B is equal to the Segment of the *Lunula* A CR, as is the Triangle E B G equal to the Segment C G R.

2 EXAM-

EXAMPLE XII.

LET A C D represent such a Curve, that having drawn any Ordinate, as B C, putting $BC = y$, $AB = x$, $AD = a$, and $BD = a - x$, we shall have

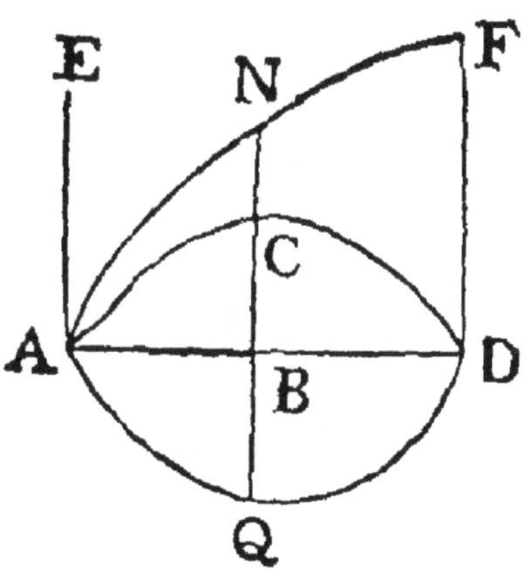

as $a^m \quad x^m \quad \overline{a-x}^n \quad y$, or, which is the same, as $x^m \quad y^n \quad a^m \quad \overline{a-x}^n$, and let it be required to find the Area, because $a^m \quad x^m \quad \overline{a-x}^n \quad y^n$, therefore $y^n = x^m \times \frac{\overline{a-x}^n}{a^m}$, whence $y = x^{\frac{m}{n}} \times \frac{a-x}{a^{\frac{m}{n}}}$. This therefore being multiplied by $\dot{x}$ will give $\frac{\overline{a-x} \times x^{\frac{m}{n}} \dot{x}}{a^{\frac{m}{n}}}$ for the Fluxion of the Area, whence the Fluent will be $\frac{n\,\overline{a-x} \times x^{\frac{m}{n}+1}}{\overline{m+n}\, a^{\frac{m}{n}}} = \frac{n a x^{\frac{m}{n}+1}}{\overline{m+n}\, a^{\frac{m}{n}}}$

$$- \frac{n x^{\frac{m}{n}+2}}{\overline{m+2n}\, a^{\frac{m}{n}}} = \frac{n a a^{\frac{m}{n}+1}}{\overline{m+n}\, a^{\frac{m}{n}}} - \frac{n a^{\frac{m}{n}+2}}{\overline{m+2n}\, a^{\frac{m}{n}}} = \frac{n a a}{m+n}$$

$$- \frac{n a a}{m+2n} = \frac{n n}{m m + 3 m n + 2 n n} a a,$$ for the whole Area A C B A, for while A B flows into, or becomes A D, x becomes equal to a, whence the Space is to the Square made upon A D as nn to $mm + 3mn + 2nn$.

If $m = 2$, and $n = 1$, then $y = \frac{ax^2 - x^3}{aa}$, and the Area will be $\frac{1}{12} aa$

Imagine the Ordinate B C in a flowing State, and the Point C to move 'till it arrive at, or coincide with the Point N, then putting B N $= z$, we shall have as $a : z :: a - x : y$, whence the Equation expressing the Nature of the Curve A N F, will be $ay = \overline{a - x} \times z$, and let it be required to find the Area of the Curvilinear Space A N F D, and the Ratio it has to the Space A C D.

Because $ay = \overline{a - x} \times z$, therefore $y = \frac{a - x}{a} \times z$, but it has been shewn that $y = \frac{a - x}{a^{\frac{m}{n}}} \times x^{\frac{m}{n}}$, therefore $\frac{a - x}{a}$ $\times z = \frac{a - x}{a^{\frac{m}{n}}} \times x^{\frac{m}{n}}$, whence $\frac{z}{a} = \frac{x^{\frac{m}{n}}}{a^{\frac{m}{n}}}$, and $z = \frac{x^{\frac{m}{n}}}{a^{\frac{m}{n} - 1}}$, and $z^n = \frac{x^m}{a^{m - n}} = x^m a^{n - m}$, which is a general Equation expressing the Nature of all sorts of Parabolas, whence the Space A N F D A shall be to the Square of A D as n to $m + n$, whence the Parabolic Space is to the Curvilinear Space A C D A, as $mm + 3mn + 2nn$ is to $mn + nn$, or as $m + 2n$ is to n

It is evident, that if in the Equation expressing the Nature of the Parabola, m be greater than n, we shall have $x^m = \frac{a^m z^n}{a^n}$, and the Parabola will have for its Axis A E, and the Point A will be the Vertex, but if n be greater than m, $z^n = \frac{a^n x^m}{a^m}$, and the Parabola will have the Line A D for its Axis, and the Point A for its Vertex.

IMAGINE the same Ordinate BC to flow according to the Direction BQ, 'till the Point B arrives at, or coincides with the Point Q; then putting BQ = z, let it be as a x y z, and supposing the same Law to obtain in every Point of the Curve, let it be required to find the Area

BECAUSE from the Nature of the Curve AQD, $y = \frac{az}{x}$, whence $y^n = \frac{a^n z^n}{x^n}$, and because in the Curve AQD $y^n = \frac{\overline{a-x}^n \times x^m}{a^m}$, therefore $\frac{a^n z^n}{x^n} = \frac{\overline{a-x}^n \times a^m}{a^m}$, whence $a^{m+n} z^n = \overline{a-x}^n \times x^{m+n}$, and consequently as a^{m+n} x^{m+n} $\overline{a-x}^n$ z^n, whence it follows, that the Curve is of the same Nature with the former Curve ACD

To find the Relation that this Curve has to the Curve ACD, multiply $z = \frac{\overline{a-x} \times x^{\frac{m+n}{n}}}{a^{\frac{m+n}{n}}}$ by x, and we shall have $zx = \frac{\overline{a-x} \times x^{\frac{m+n}{n}} x}{a^{\frac{m+n}{n}}} = \frac{a x^{\frac{m+n}{n}} x - x^{\frac{m+n}{n}+1} x}{a^{\frac{m+n}{n}}}$ for the Fluxion of the Area, and $\frac{n a x^{\frac{m+n}{n}+1}}{\overline{m+2n}\, a^{\frac{m+n}{n}}} - \frac{n x^{\frac{m+n}{n}+2}}{\overline{m+3n}\, a^{\frac{m+n}{n}}}$ for the Space ABQ $= \frac{naa}{m+2n} - \frac{naa}{m+3n} = \overline{\frac{n}{m+2n} - \frac{n}{m+3n}} \times aa = \frac{nn}{mm+5mn+6nn} \times aa$, for the Space ABDQA

For when A B flows into, or becomes equal to A D, x will become equal to a, whence the Space A B D Q A is to the Space A C D B A as $mm + 3mn + 2nn$ to $mm + 5mn + 6nn$, or as $m + n$ is to $m + 3n$.

EXAMPLE XIII.

To find the Space inclosed by the Cycloid A N F D

The Generation of the Cycloid may be conceived after this manner.

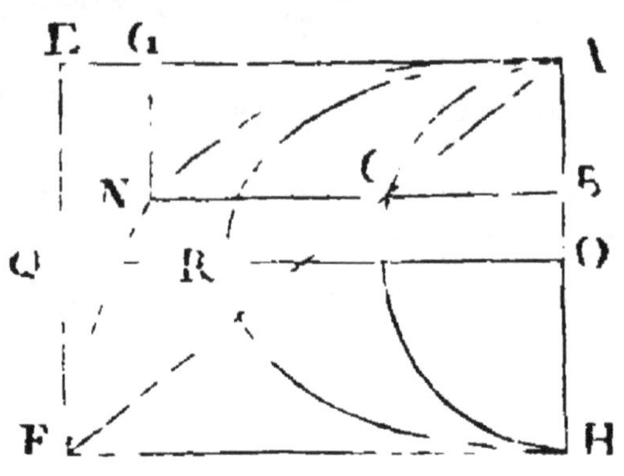

If the Semicircle ACH be conceived to roll along the Line H F, while the Centre O describes the Line O Q, the Vertical Point A will describe the Curve Line A N F, which is called a Cycloid, whose Diameter is A H, the same with that of the generating Circle, and its Base H F, equal to the Semiperiphery A C H.

Through any Point B of the Diameter A H, draw the Ordinate B N, cutting the Periphery of the Circle in C, also the Line G N parallel to A H.

Put A H $= 2r$, and because, from the Nature of the Circle, $2rx - xx = yy$, therefore $2\dot{y}y = 2r\dot{x} - 2x\dot{x}$, whence $\dot{y}y = r\dot{x} - x\dot{x}$, and $\dot{y} = \dfrac{r\dot{x} - x\dot{x}}{y}$, but because the Triangle A C B, in its nascent Form, is similar to the Triangle O B C, therefore as $y : r :: \dot{x} : \dfrac{r\dot{x}}{y}$, the Fluxion of the Arch A C, which is always equal to C N, from the Generation of the Curve, wheresoever the Point C be taken, wherefore $\frac{r\dot{x} - x\dot{x}}{y} + \frac{r\dot{x}}{y} = \frac{2r\dot{x} - x\dot{x}}{y}$, will be the Fluxion of the Ordinate B N equal to $\frac{2r\dot{x} - x\dot{x}}{\overline{2rx - xx}^{\frac{1}{2}}}$ (by substituting $\overline{2rx - xx}^{\frac{1}{2}}$ in the room of y, to which it is equal, from the Property of the Circle, whence $\frac{2r\dot{x} - x\dot{x}}{\overline{2rx - xx}^{\frac{1}{2}}} \times x$ $= \frac{2rx\dot{x} - xx\dot{x}}{\overline{2rx - xx}^{\frac{1}{2}}} = \dot{x} \times \overline{2rx - xx} \times \overline{2rx - xx}^{-\frac{1}{2}} = \dot{x}$ $\times \overline{2rx - xx}^{\frac{1}{2}}$, will be the Fluxion of the Area of the circular Segment A C B. Whence it follows, that the circular Segment A C B, and the Cycloidal Supplemental Segment A G N are equal, and consequently the whole Supplemental or Exterior Space A N F E A, and the generating Semicircle A C H are equal. But the Parallelogram A H F E, equal to A H × H F, is equal to A H multiplied by the Arch A C H, equal to four times the Area of the Semicircle A C H A, therefore whereas the Supplemental Space A N F E A is equal to the Semicircular Space A C H, the Cycloidal Space A N F H must be equal to three times the Semicircular Space A C H A. Whence it follows,

THAT the Cycloidal Space is $\frac{3}{4}$ of the circumscribing Parallelogram, and consequently if an Ellipsis be described about the Diameter A H, whose longest Diameter shall be double to the Diameter A H, that the Semi-Circle, the Semi Ellipsis and Semi Cycloid will be as the Numbers 1, 2 and 3, and consequently the Spaces A C H A, A R H C A, A N F H R A, A F F N A, will be equal to each other.

AGAIN, if from the Point A the right Line A I be drawn, the Space A N F C A will be equal to the generating Semicircle, and to the external Space A N F E A. For the Triangle

gle A F E is $\frac{1}{2}$ of the Parallelogram A H F E, and the external Space A E F N A is $\frac{1}{4}$; whence it follows, that the Space A N F C A ſhall be $\frac{1}{4}$ alſo.

EXAMPLE XIV.

To find the Area of the Ciſſoid

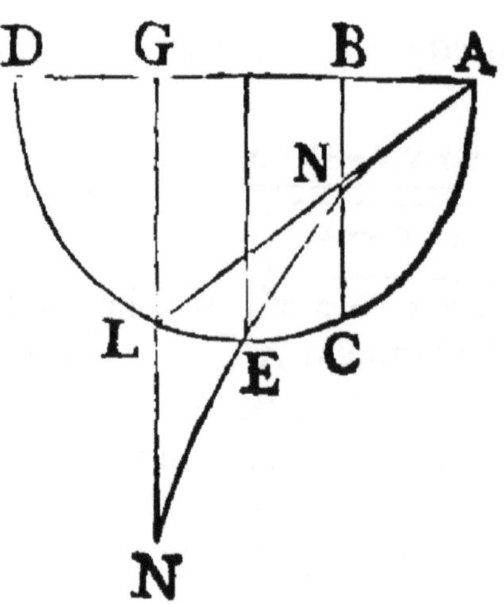

THE Ciſſoid may be conſtructed after this manner

IF through the Extream Point L of L G, the Sine of the Arch D L, a right Line, as A N L, be drawn, it will interſect the Sine B C of the equal Arch A C in the Point N; and if after this manner an infinite Number of Points N be found, through which if a Curve Line be drawn, it will be the Ciſſoid; whence it follows, that as D B B C A B B N

FOR becauſe the Arches D L and A C are equal, the right Lines L G, C B, and the verſed Sines A G, D B, are alſo equal, and the Triangles A B N and A G L are ſimilar, it will be as A G . G L · A B B N, but A G = D B, and G L = B C, therefore as D B B C A B B N Wherefore in the adjacent Figure let A N E G repreſent a Ciſſoid, D F its Aſymptote, A E D the generating Semicircle, and let it be required to find the Space A N E G F D contained between the Diameter A D, the Aſymptote D F, and the Curve A E G.

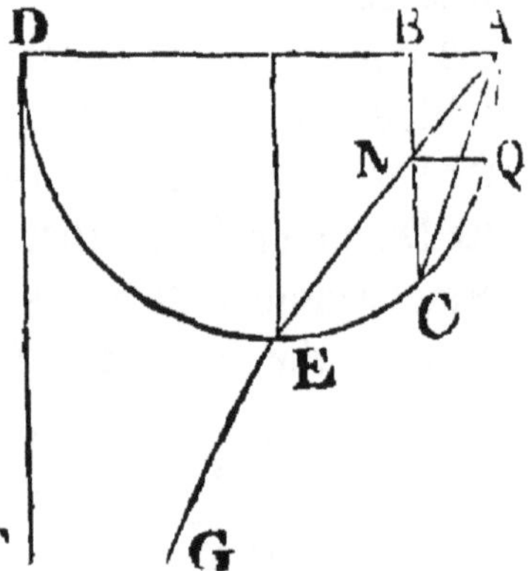

HAVING

HAVING drawn any Ordinate, as B N C, cutting the Cissoid in N, put $AD = 2r$, $AB = x$, $BC = y$, then will $DB = 2r - x$, and because, from the Nature of the Curve, as BC : BA :: BA . BN, it will be as $y : x :: x . \frac{xx}{y} = BN$; whence $\frac{x\dot{x}x}{y} = \frac{x\dot{x}x}{\overline{2rx - xx}|^{\frac{1}{2}}}$ (putting for y, its Equal, $\overline{2rx - xx}|^{\frac{1}{2}}$) will be the Fluxion of the Area, but $\frac{x\dot{x}x}{\overline{2rx - xx}|^{\frac{1}{2}}} = \frac{2rx\dot{x}}{\overline{2rx - xx}|^{\frac{1}{2}}} - \frac{\overline{2rx - xx}\,\dot{x}}{\overline{2rx - xx}|^{\frac{1}{2}}}$ (because $2rx - \overline{2rx - xx} = xx$) $= \frac{2rx\dot{x}}{\overline{2rx - xx}|^{\frac{1}{2}}} - \dot{x} \times \overline{2rx - xx}|^{\frac{1}{2}}$ (because $\frac{\overline{2rx - xx}}{\overline{2rx - xx}|^{\frac{1}{2}}} = \overline{2rx - xx} - \overline{2rx - xx}|^{\frac{1}{2}} =$ $= \overline{2rx - xx}|^{\frac{1}{2}}$) equal to the Expression $\frac{2rx\dot{x}}{\overline{2rx - xx}|^{\frac{1}{2}}}$ minus the Semi-Segment A Q C B (for the Expression $\dot{x} \times \overline{2rx - xx}$ = the Semi-Segment A Q C B) but the Expression $\frac{2rx\dot{x}}{\overline{2rx - xx}|^{\frac{1}{2}}}$ is equal to four times the Segment A Q C A. For having drawn the Chord A C, it will be, from the Property of the Circle, as $2r : AC :: AC : x$, whence $AC = \overline{2rx}|^{\frac{1}{2}}$, and $r\dot{x} \times \overline{2rx}|^{-\frac{1}{2}}$ is equal to the Fluxion of A C.

BUT as $\overline{2rx - xx} : \dot{x} :: \frac{r\dot{x}}{\overline{2rx}|^{\frac{1}{2}}} : \frac{rx\dot{x}}{\overline{2rx}|^{\frac{1}{2}} \times \overline{2rx - xx}|^{\frac{1}{2}}}$, which being multiplied by $\frac{\overline{2rx}|^{\frac{1}{2}}}{2}$ will give $\frac{rx\dot{x}}{2 \times \overline{2rx - xx}|^{\frac{1}{2}}}$ for

for the Fluxion of the Segment A Q C A, and consequently $\frac{2rx\dot{x}}{2\times\overline{2rx-xx}|^{\frac{1}{2}}}\times 4$, will give $\frac{2rx\dot{x}}{\overline{2rx-xx}|^{\frac{1}{2}}}$, whence it is manifest, that the Quantity $\frac{2rx\dot{x}}{\overline{2rx-xx}|^{\frac{1}{2}}}$ is equal to four times $\frac{rx\dot{x}}{2\times\overline{2rx-xx}}$, the Fluxion of the Segment A Q C A

BUT when A B, by flowing, becomes equal to A D, the Points B, D and C will coincide, and the Segment A Q C will become equal to the generating Semicircle A E D, whence it follows, that the Cissoidal Space is equal to four times the Semicircular Space A C E D A minus, the same Semicircular Space A C E D A, equal to thrice the Area of the generating Semicircle.

EXAMPLE XV

Let it be required to find the Space inclosed between the Conchoid and its Asymptote

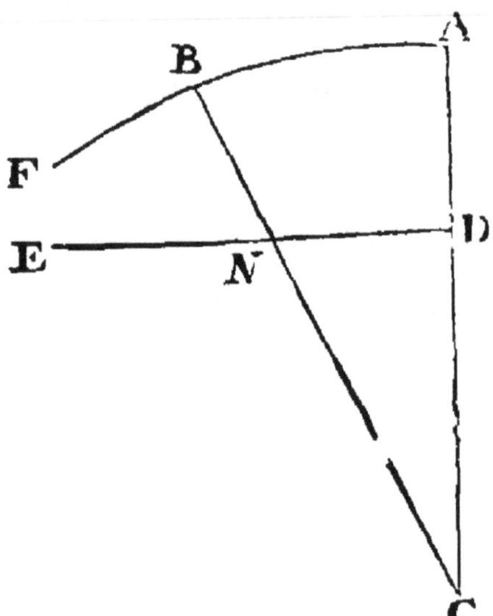

THE Conchoid is generated after this manner

IMAGINE the Line B C to move about the Point C in such a manner, that the Segment B N, intercepted between the right Line E D, drawn at right Angles to the Line A D C, and the Extremity B, may be always equal to itself, the Point B, by this Motion, will describe the Curve F B A, which is called the Conchoid of *Nicomedes*

LET

LET ABF represent a Conchoid, C its Pole, D E its Asymptote.

PUT $CD = a$, $DA = b$, $CN = x$, $NB = y$, and because, from the Nature of the Curve, $CN \times NB = CD \times DA$, we shall have $xy = ab$, whence $y = \frac{ab}{x}$, and $CB = y + x$ $= \frac{ab}{x} + x = \frac{ab + xx}{x}$, but as $\overline{xx - aa}^{\frac{1}{2}}$ a $\dot{x}$ $\frac{a\dot{x}}{\overline{xx - aa}^{\frac{1}{2}}}$; and again because as x $\frac{ab + xx}{x}$ $\frac{a\dot{x}}{\overline{xx - aa}^{\frac{1}{2}}}$ $\frac{aabx + axx\dot{x}}{x \times \overline{xx - aa}^{\frac{1}{2}}}$, therefore $\frac{aab\dot{x} + axx\dot{x}}{x^2 \times \overline{xx - aa}^{\frac{1}{2}}}$ will be the Fluxion of the Absciffe. This therefore being multiplied by $\frac{1}{2}CB$ $= \frac{xx + ab}{2x}$, will give $\frac{aabxx\dot{x} + ax^4\dot{x} + a^3b^2\dot{x} + a^2bx^2\dot{x}}{2x^3 \times \overline{xx - aa}^{\frac{1}{2}}}$ $= \frac{ax\dot{x}}{2 \times \overline{xx - aa}^{\frac{1}{2}}} + \frac{aab\dot{x}}{2x \times \overline{xx - aa}^{\frac{1}{2}}} + \frac{a^3bb\dot{x}}{2x^3 \times \overline{xx - aa}^{\frac{1}{2}}}$ for the Fluxion of the Space CAB, but the first Member $\frac{ax\dot{x}}{2 \times \overline{xx - aa}^{\frac{1}{2}}}$ is the Fluxion of the Space CDN, whence the Fluent Quantity of the remaining Quantities $\frac{aab\dot{x}}{x \times \overline{xx - aa}^{\frac{1}{2}}}$ $+ \frac{a^3b^2\dot{x}}{2x^3 \times \overline{xx - aa}^{\frac{1}{2}}}$ will give the Space B A D N.

FOR the obtaining of which, having described the Quadrant ADE (*See the following Figure*) whose Radius is equal to CD in the former Figure, take $CB = \frac{aa}{x}$, and

through

through the Point B draw the Ordinate B D; whence by the Property of the Circle, we ſhall have $BD = \frac{a}{x} \times \overline{xx - aa}|^{\frac{1}{2}}$; whence the Fluxions of C B and B D will be $\frac{aa\dot{x}}{xx}$ and $\frac{a^3 \dot{x}}{xx \times \sqrt{xx - aa}}$; but the Fluxion

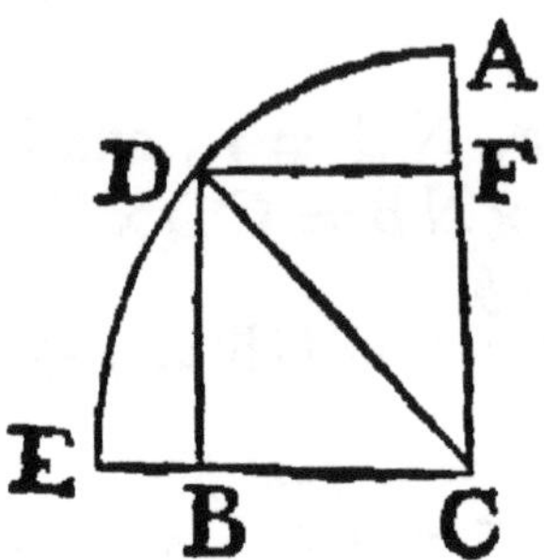

of the Arch A D $= -\frac{aa\dot{x}}{x \times \overline{xx - aa}|^{\frac{1}{2}}}$, the Fluent of which will give the Arch D E, where it is to be obſerved, that the Sign — ſhews, that while x diminiſhes $\frac{aa}{x}$ augments, and that for the Fluent we muſt take the Arch D E, and not the Arch A E, inaſmuch as it is neceſſary here to have the Fluent of all the Fluxions $\frac{aab\dot{x}}{x \times \overline{xx - aa}|^{\frac{1}{2}}}$, beginning from the Value of C N to the Value of C D, from whence it is evident, that if we multiply the Arch D E by a given Quantity b, we ſhall have the Fluents of the Quantity $\frac{aab\dot{x}}{2 \times \overline{xx - aa}|^{\frac{1}{2}}}$

Now the Fluxion of the Area is equal to $\frac{a^5 \dot{x}}{x^3 \times \overline{xx - aa}|^{\frac{1}{2}}}$, and conſequently the Fluent will be equal to the Segment of the Circle C F D E Multiplying then this Segment by bb, and dividing by aa, we ſhall have the Fluent of $\frac{a^3 bb\dot{x}}{2x^3 \times \overline{xx - aa}|^{\frac{1}{2}}}$, which anſwers to all the Values of x, from C N to C D. The Conchoidal Space B A D N is therefore equal to the Circular

lar Arch D E multiplied by the given right Line D A, equal to b, and to the Segment of the Circle C F D E, multiplied by bb, and divided by $2aa$

IF B N be equal to A D, as in the Conchoid of *Nicomedes*, putting $CN = x$, $CB = z = a - x$, we shall have

$$\frac{a^3 \dot{x}}{2x \times \overline{xx - aa}^{\frac{1}{2}}} + \frac{aa\dot{x}}{2\overline{x - aa}^{\frac{1}{2}}} + \frac{ax\dot{x}}{2 \times \overline{xx - aa}^{\frac{1}{2}}}$$ for the Fluxion of the Space A B C, the last Member of which is the Fluxion of the Space C N D

Now to find the Fluent of the Expression $\frac{a^3 \dot{x}}{2x \times \overline{xx - aa}^{\frac{1}{2}}}$, suppose $CE = a$, then will $CB = \frac{aa}{x}$, for having drawn the Radius C D, and the Ordinate D B, we shall have D B equal to $\frac{a}{x} \times \overline{xx - aa}^{\frac{1}{2}}$, and $\frac{aa\dot{x}}{xx}$ for the Fluxion of C B.

but as $\frac{a}{x} \times \overline{xx - aa}$: a :: $\frac{aa\dot{x}}{xx}$: $\frac{aa\dot{x}}{x \times \overline{xx - aa}}$, and multiplying this by $\frac{a}{2}$, we shall have $\frac{a^3 \dot{x}}{2x \times \overline{xx - aa}^{\frac{1}{2}}}$ for the Fluxion of the Sector A C D, whose Fluent is equal to the Sector C D E

To find the Fluent of the other Member $\frac{aa\dot{x}}{\overline{xx - aa}^{\frac{1}{2}}}$, we must describe an Equilateral Hyperbola A C E, whose Centre is D, and Semi-transverse Diameter $AD = a$, and drawing the Ordinate B C, and from

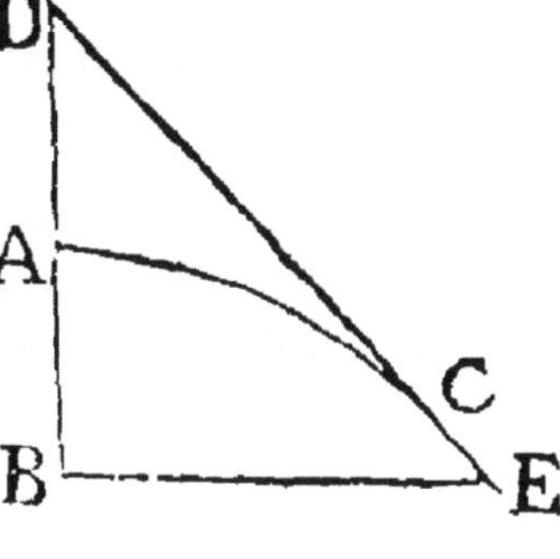

the Point C drawing the Line DC I say, that $\frac{aa\dot{x}}{2\times\overline{xx-aa}}$ is the Fluxion of the Line D C, whose Fluent is the Space A D C, whence the Double of this Space will be the Fluent of $\frac{aa\dot{x}}{\overline{xx-aa}^{\frac{3}{2}}}$.

And as a Proof of this, let D B $= x$, B C $= y$, then, from the Nature of the Hyperbola, $yy = aa - xx$, and $y = \frac{xx}{\overline{xx-aa}^{\frac{1}{2}}}$, but the Fluxion of the Curve A C is equal to

$$xx + yy = \frac{2xxxx - aaxx}{xx-aa}, \text{ and } DC = \overline{2xx-aa}^{\frac{1}{2}},$$

whose Fluxion $\frac{2x\dot{x}}{2\overline{xx-aa}^{\frac{1}{2}}}$; whence we shall have

$$\frac{2xxx\dot{x} - aax\dot{x}}{xx-aa} - \frac{4xxx\dot{x}}{2xx-aa} = \frac{a^4\dot{x}}{2xx-aa\times xx-aa}$$

for the Fluxion of the Ordinate, and multiplying this Quantity by $\frac{1}{2}$ DC $= \frac{1}{2}\overline{2xx-aa}^{\frac{1}{2}}$, we shall have $\frac{aa\dot{x}}{2\times\overline{xx-aa}^{\frac{3}{2}}}$ for the Fluxion of the Line D C, whose Fluent will be the Space A D C

It is evident then, that the Conchoidal Space, tho' infinitely extended, is a finite Magnitude, and that the same holds good in a Cissoidal Space.

SECT. III.

Containing the Use of FLUXIONS *in finding the Values of the Surfaces of* Solids *generated by the Rotation of* Plane Surfaces *about their Axes*

PROPOSITION V.

IF the Surface AFCB be revolved about AB as an Axis, I say, that the Fluxion of the Surface generated by the Curve Line AC, is to the Fluxion of the Cylindric Surface, generated by the right Line FC, as the Rectangle under the Periphery described by the Radius BC, and the Fluxion of the Curve Line AC, to the Rectangle under the Periphery described by the same Ordinate BC, and the Fluxion of the Absciss AB.

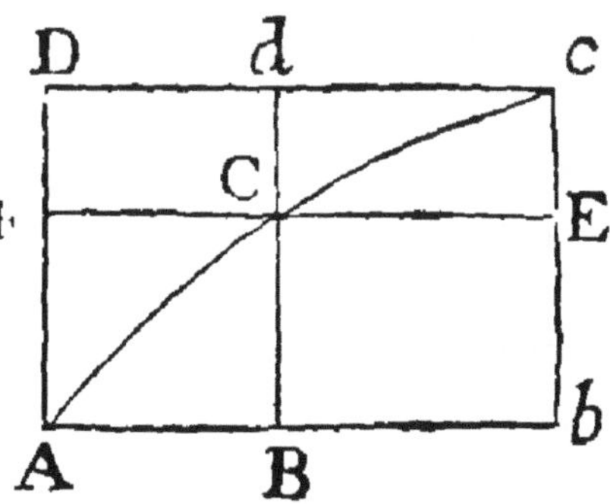

IMAGINE the Ordinate BC in a flowing State, and let C*c* and B*b* (= CF) represent the nascent Augment of the Curve Line AC, and Absciss AB, generated in the same very small Particle of Time. Now if the Surface AD*cb* be conceived to revolve about AB*b* as an Axis, then will the Surfaces generated by these nascent Augments C*c* and *dc* (= B*b*) be the nascent Augments of the Surfaces generated by the nascent Curve Line AC, and the Absciss AB, in the same very small Particle of Time; but the Surface generated by the nascent Augment C*c*, is to the Surface generated by the nascent Augment *dc* = CE = B*b*, as the Rectangle made of the nascent Augment C*c* and the Periphery of the Circle described by the Radius BC to the Rectangle made of the nascent Augment *dc* = CE = B*b*, and the Periphery of the Circle described by the Ordinate BC; but by *Section* III. *Part* I. the nascent of the Curve Line A C is to the Fluxion of the Absciffe A B, as the nascent Augment Cc is to the nascent Augment dc = C E = Bb, therefore the Fluxion of the Surface, generated by the Curve Line A C, is to the Fluxion of the Cylindric Surface, generated by the Right Line F C = A B, as the Rectangle made of the Periphery described by the Ordinate B C, and the Fluxion of the Curve Line A C to the Rectangle made of the Periphery described by the same Ordinate B C, and the Fluxion of the Absciffe A B.

AND since the Fluxion of the Cylindric Surface, generated by the Right Line F C, is a fixed and constant Quantity, the Fluxion of the Surface, generated by the Curve Line A C, will be every where as the Circumference of the generating Circle, and the Fluxion of the Curve conjunctly. Whence it follows,

THAT the Product arising from the Multiplication of the Value of the Circumference of the Circle generated by the Rotation of any Ordinate about the Axis of the Curve into the Fluxion of the Curve Line, will give the Fluxion of the Surface generated by the Rotation of the Curve, whose Fluent will give the Value of the Surface itself. Wherefore

IF ACE represent a Curve, A D its Axis, D E and B C Ordinates rightly applied, and we put A D = a, D E = r, the Circumference of the Circle generated by the Point E = c, A B = x, and B C = y, we shall have $\frac{cy}{r}$ for the Circumference of the Circle generated by C, the extream Point of the Ordinate B C for as $r : c :: y : \frac{cy}{r}$.

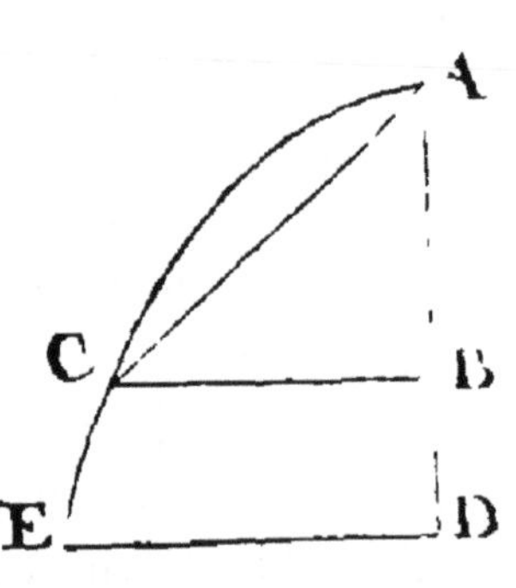

JOIN the Points C and A by the Right Line C A, and imagine the Ordinate B C to return back again 'till the Point B, C and A coincide, then will the Triangle, formed by the Lines A B, B C, and the Curve Line A C, in its evanescent Form, be similar to the right-angled Triangle A B C.

BUT by the 47th of *Euclid* I. $\overline{AC}^2 = \overline{AB}^2 + \overline{BC}^2$, that is, $AC^2 = xx + yy$, and putting $z = AC$, we shall have $zz = xx + yy$, and by *Section* III *Part* I $zz = xx + yy$, whence $\dot{z} = \overline{\dot{x}\dot{x} + \dot{y}\dot{y}}^{\frac{1}{2}}$ will be the Fluxion of the Curve Line A C. This therefore being multiplied by $\frac{cy}{r}$, the Circumference of the Circle generated by the Point C, will give $\frac{cy}{r} \times \overline{\dot{x}\dot{x} + \dot{y}\dot{y}}^{\frac{1}{2}}$ for the Fluxion of the Surfaces generated by the Curve Line A C about the Abscisse A B, as an Axis.

NOW if in the room of xx be substituted its Value deduced from the Equation expressing the Nature of the Curve, the Fluent arising from this last Fluxion will give the Value of the Surfaces itself.

EXAMPLE I.

Let it be required to find the Value of the Superficies of a Prism.

LET us suppose the Prism to have a square Base, and put $AB = a$, and r for one of the Sides of the Square of the Base, then will $4r$ be the Perimeter of the Base, and $4ra$ will be the Fluxion of the Superficies. But inasmuch as the Prism is generated by the uniform Motion of the Square A, according to the Direction A B, and that the Sides of the generating Square are constant and permanent Quantities, therefore $4ra$ will give the Superficies itself.

NOW if in the room of $4r$, we substitute the Perimeter of the Base of any Sort of Prism, we shall have an Expression whereby the Superficies of the Prism may be found.

WHENCE

WHENCE it follows, that the Surface of any Prism is equal to a Parallelogram, whose Height is equal to that of the Prism, and its Base equal to the Prism's Perimeter.

AGAIN, if we suppose the Base A to be a Circle, then will the Solid generated thereby be a Cylinder, wherefore if we put C for the Circumference of the Base, then ac will be the Superficies

WHENCE it follows, that the Surface of a Cylinder is equal to a Parallelogram, whose Height is equal to the Height of the Cylinder, and Base equal to the Circumference of the Base of the Cylinder Whence it follows,

THAT the Surface of the circumscribing Prism is to the Surface of the inscribed Cylinder, as four times the Diameter of the Cylindrical Base is to its Circumference.

AND after the same manner may the Surface of any right Solid (that is, such a Solid whose Surface stands at right Angles to its Base) be found, whether the Base be Elliptical, Parabolical, Hyperbolical, or any Sort of Curve Line whatsoever.

EXAMPLE II

Let it be required to find the Surface of a Pyramid

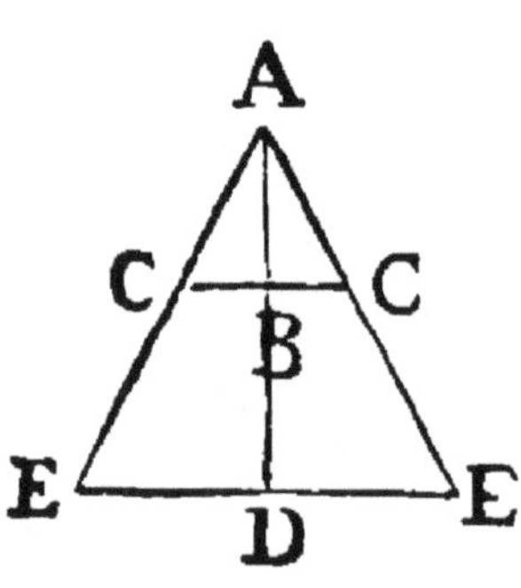

LET the Pyramid be supposed to have a Square Base, and let the Triangle A E E represent one of the Faces.

PUT AD $= a$, EE $= b$, AB $= x$, and CC $= y$, then will $y\dot{x}$ be the Fluxion of the Area, but because the Triangles ACC and AEE are similar, it will be as $x : y :: a : b$, whence $y = \frac{bx}{a}$, and substituting this Value of y, in the Expression

$y\dot{x}$,

$y\dot{x}$, in the room of y, we shall have $\frac{bx\dot{x}}{a}$, for the Fluxion of the Space ACC, whose Fluent $\frac{bxx}{2a}$, equal to $\frac{yx}{2}$ (by substituting y in the room of $\frac{bx}{a}$, to which it is equal from the Property of the Triangle) will be the Area of the same Space. Now if we imagine the Line C B C in a flowing State, and to move 'till it arrives at, or is coincident with E D E, then A B will become equal to A D, x will become equal to a, y will become equal to r, and we shall have $\frac{ar}{2}$ for the Area of the whole Triangle E B E, whose Quadruple $\frac{4ra}{2} = 2ra$, will be the Area of the whole Superficies of the Pyramid.

Now if we put the whole Perimeter of the Pyramid $4r = p$, we shall have $\frac{pa}{2}$ for the whole Surface.

Whence to find the Surface of any Pyramid, we must multiply the Perimeter of the Base by the Side, and half the Product will be the Superficies.

Again, if we put c for the Circumference of a right Cone, and a for its Side, we shall have $\frac{ca}{2}$ for the Surface, as will appear by the following Example.

EXAM-

EXAMPLE III.

Let it be required to find the Surface of a Right Cone

IF the right angled Triangle ADE be revolved about the Line AD as an Axis, then will the Side AE describe a Conical Superficies, as will the Triangle ADE at the same time generate a right Cone, whose Axis will be AD, and its Section through the the Vertex will be the Triangle EAE.

PUT $AD = a$, $DE = r$, $BC = y$, $AB = x$, $AE = z$, and c for the Circumference of the Circle generated by the Point E, whence $\frac{cy}{r}$ will be the Circumference of the Circle described by the Point C (for as $r : c :: y : \frac{cy}{r}$), whence we shall have $z \times \frac{cy}{r}$ for the Fluxion of the Surface, equal $\frac{cy}{r} \times \overline{xx+yy}^{\frac{1}{2}}$; because $z = \overline{xx+yy}^{\frac{1}{2}}$ by the foregoing Proposition. Again, because as $x : y :: a : r$, therefore $x = \frac{ay}{r}$, whence $x = \frac{ay}{r}$, and $xx = \frac{aayy}{rr}$. Substituting therefore this Quantity in the general Equation $z = \overline{xx+yy}^{\frac{1}{2}}$ in the room of xx, and we shall have $z \times \frac{cy}{r} = \frac{cy}{r} \times \overline{\frac{aayy}{rr}+yy}^{\frac{1}{2}} = \frac{cy}{r} \times \frac{\overline{aayy+rryy}^{\frac{1}{2}}}{\overline{rr}^{\frac{1}{2}}}$

=

$= \frac{cy}{r} \times \frac{\overline{yy}^{\frac{1}{2}}}{rr^{\frac{1}{2}}} \times \overline{aa+rr}^{\frac{1}{2}} = \frac{cy}{r} \times \frac{y}{r} \times \overline{aa+rr}^{\frac{1}{2}} = \frac{cyy}{rr}$ $\times \overline{aa+rr}^{\frac{1}{2}}$ for the Fluxion of the Surface, whose Fluent $\frac{cyy}{2rr} \times \overline{aa+rr}^{\frac{1}{2}}$, will give the Surface of the Cone CAC, but when B C, by flowing, becomes equal to D E, then y becomes equal to r, consequently we shall have $\frac{c}{2} \times \overline{aa+rr}$ for the Surface of the whole Cone E A E, but $\overline{rr+aa}^{\frac{1}{2}} = z$ = A E (by the 47th of *Euclid* I.) Wherefore $\frac{cz}{2}$ will be the whole Surface, the same as was deduced in the former Example.

AGAIN, if we put A E $= z$, A C $= x$, y for the Circumference of the Circle generated by the Point C, and c for the Circumference of the Circle generated by the Point E, and S for the whole Surface, we shall have $yx = S$ for the Fluxion of the Surface, but because of the Similitude of the Triangles A B C and A D E, as A C : A E :: B C : D E; and so is the Circumference of the Circle generated by B C, to the Circumference of the Circle generated by D E. Wherefore as $x : y :: z : c$, whence $y = \frac{cx}{z}$. Substituting this Quantity therefore in the room of y, in the Equation $S = yx$, and we shall have $S = \frac{cxx}{z}$ for the Fluxion of the Surface, whose Fluent $S = \frac{cxx}{2z}$ will give the Surface of the Cone described about A B, but when A C flows into, and becomes equal to A E, then x becomes equal to z, and we shall have $S = \frac{czz}{2z} = \frac{cz}{2}$ for the whole Surface, as was before found. Whence it follows,

First, THAT the Surface of a Cone is equal to a Triangle, whose Height is equal to the Side of the Cone, and whose Base is equal to the Circumference of the Base of the Cone.

Secondly, THAT the Surface of the Cone is to the Surface of a Cylinder, whose Base is the same with the Base of the Cone, and whose Height is equal to the Side of the Cone as 1 to 2.

Thirdly, THAT the Surface of a Cylinder, whose Height is equal to the Radius of its Circular Base, is to the Surface of the same Circle as 2 to 1, for the Surface of the Cylinder is cr, but the Surface of the Base is $\frac{cr}{2}$, and as cr : $\frac{cr}{2}$ :: 2 : 1. In like manner any Portion of a Cylindrical Surface, cut by a Plane passing through the Axis, which hath for its Base the Arch of the Sector of the Base, and for its Altitude the Radius of the generating Circle, will be to the Area of the Sector of the Base as 2 to 1.

Fourthly, THAT the Cylindric, Conic and Circular Spaces are as 2, $\sqrt{2}$ and 1, and by Consequence they are continual Proportionals.

Fifthly, THAT the Surface of any Cone is to the Surface of its Base, as the Side of the Cone is to the Radius of its Circular Base, for the Surface of the Cone is $\frac{za}{2}$, and the Surface of the Base is $\frac{cr}{2}$, but as $\frac{zc}{2}$: $\frac{cr}{2}$ :: z : r.

Sixthly, THAT the Surfaces of two right Cones are to each other in a Ratio compounded of their Sides, and the Radii of their Bases, for let z and b represent the Sides of two Cones, and c and d the Circumferences of their Bases, then will their Surfaces be $\frac{zc}{2}$ and $\frac{bd}{2}$. Now the Semi-diameters of Circles are to each other as their Circumferences, whence the Surfaces of the Cones will be to each other in a Ratio compounded of their Sides, and their respective Radii.

Seventhly, If the Surfaces of the Cones are parallel to each other, that is, if their generating or describing Triangles are similar, then their Surfaces will be in a duplicate Ratio, or as the Squares of the Semi-diameters of their Bases.

EXAMPLE IV.

Let it be required to find the Surface of a Sphere.

If the Semi-circle ACFDE be carried about its Diameter AD, as an Axis, 'till it return to the Place from whence it began to move, the Semi-circumference ACFD will describe the Surface of a Sphere, as will at the same time the Semi-circle ACFDE describe a Sphere, whose Axis will be the Line AD.

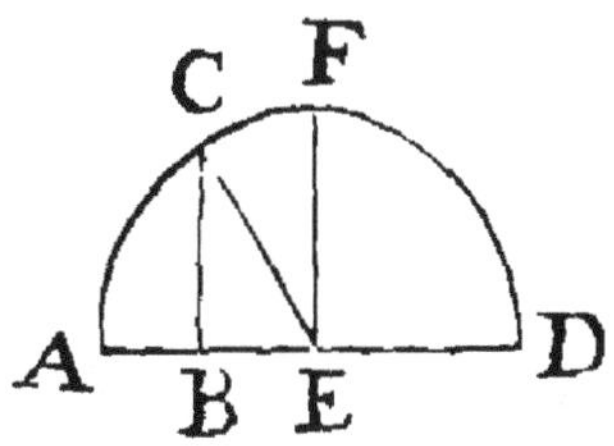

Put $AE = r$, $AB = x$, $BC = y$, the Circumference of the Circle generated by the Point $F = c$, then will $\frac{cy}{r}$ be the Circumference generated by the Point C (for as $r : c :: y : \frac{cy}{r}$) whence $\frac{cy}{r} \times \overline{\dot x\dot x + \dot y\dot y}^{\frac{1}{2}}$, will be the Fluxion of the Surface, but because, from the Nature of the Circle, $yy = 2rx - xx$, therefore $2y\dot y = 2r\dot x - 2x\dot x$, whence $y\dot y = r\dot x - x\dot x$, and $\dot y = \frac{r\dot x - x\dot x}{y}$, consequently $\dot y\dot y = \frac{rr\dot x\dot x - 2rx\dot x\dot x + xx\dot x\dot x}{yy}$ $= \frac{rr\dot x\dot x - 2rx\dot x\dot x + xx\dot x\dot x}{2rx - xx}$ (by putting $2rx - xx$ in in the room of $\dot{y}y$, to which it is equal) and substituting this last Quantity in the general Equation $\frac{cy}{r} \times \overline{\dot{x}\dot{x}+\dot{y}\dot{y}}^{\frac{1}{2}}$ instead of $\dot{y}y$, we shall have $\frac{cy}{r} \times \overline{\frac{rr\dot{x}\dot{x}}{2rx-xx}}^{\frac{1}{2}} = \frac{cy}{r} \times \overline{\frac{rr\dot{x}\dot{x}}{y}}^{\frac{1}{2}}$ (by substituting y in the room of $\overline{2rx-xx}^{\frac{1}{2}}$) $= \frac{cy}{r} \times \frac{r\dot{x}}{y} = \frac{cyr\dot{x}}{yr} = c\dot{x}$, for the Fluxion of the Surface generated by the Arch A C, whose Fluent cx will give the Surface itself, but when A B flows into, and becomes equal to A D, x will become equal to $2r$, whence we shall have $2cr$ for the Surface of the whole Sphere

Because, from the Property of the Circle, the Ordinate is to the Radius as the Subtangent is to the Tangent, and because by *Proposition* II, of *Section* I, *Part* III, the Subtangent is to the Tangent as the Fluxion of the Absciffe is to the Fluxion of the Curve Line, therefore as B C : C E :: $\dot{x}$: $\dot{z}$, that is, as $y : r :: \dot{x} : \dot{z}$, whence $\dot{z} = \frac{r\dot{x}}{y}$, and multiplying this Quantity by $\frac{cy}{r}$, the Circumference of the Circle generated by the Point C, we shall have $\frac{cyr\dot{x}}{yr} = c\dot{x}$, for the Fluxion of the Superficies generated by the Arch A C, whence cx, the Fluent of this Fluxion, will be the Superficies itself, and $2cr$ will be the Superficies of the whole Sphere, for when A B, by flowing, becomes equal to A D, x becomes equal to $2r$

But if the Diameter A B be supposed equal to Unity, then $\dot{z} = \frac{\dot{x}}{2y}$, which being multiplied by $2cy$, the Area of the Circle

Circle generated by the Point C, will give $\frac{2cyx}{2y} = cx$, for the Fluxion of the Surface generated by the Arch A C, whence cx will be the Surface itself, and if we put d for the Diameter A D of the generating Circle, we shall have dc for the whole Surface, as before, for when the Point B by flowing arrives at D, then x becomes equal to d, and putting $d = 2r$, we shall have $2cr$ for the whole Surface, the same as has been already determined Whence it follows,

First, THAT the Surface of any Sphere is equal to four times the Area of its greatest Circle, for $2cr$ is to $\frac{1}{2}cr$ as 2 to $\frac{1}{2}$, or as 4 to 1

Secondly, THAT the Superficies of any Segment of a Sphere is to the entire Superficies of the Sphere, as the Altitude of the Segment is to the Diameter of the Sphere; for put the whole Diameter equal to Unity, then as cx $1c$ x 1, whence it follows, that any Portion of a Sphere cut off by two parallel Planes is to the whole Surface, as the intercepted Part of the Diameter is to the whole Diameter

Thirdly, THAT the Surface of a Sphere is equal to the Surface of a Cylinder, that has for its Base the Circumference of the great Circle of the Sphere and for its Height the Diameter of the Sphere, for if the Height of the Cylinder be put equal to $2r$, then its Surface will be $2rc$

Fourthly, THAT the Surface of a Cone is to the Surface of a Sphere, having the same Radius with the Base of the Cone, as the Side of the Cone is to four times the Radius, for if s be put for the Side of the Cone, then as $\frac{1}{2}sc$ $2cr$ $\frac{1}{2}s$ $2r$, or as s to $4r$.

Fifthly, THAT the Portion of the Surface of any Sphere cut off by two great Circles, which have for their common Intersection the Diameter of the Sphere, is to the whole Surface of the Sphere, as the Angle of Inclination of these two great Circles is to four right Angles.

Sixthly, THAT the Surface of the Cylinder circumscribing the Sphere, whose Height is equal to the Diameter of the Sphere, is quadruple of its Base, which is equal to the great Circle, for the Cylindric Surface is $2cr$, and the Base is $\frac{1}{2}cr$, and as $2cr\ \frac{1}{2}cr\ \ 4 . 1$

Seventhly, THAT the Surface of the circumscribing Cylinder, exclusive of its Bases, is equal to the Surface of the inscribed Sphere, for each are equal to $2cr$; but the Surface of the Cylinder, with its Bases, is to the Surface of the same Sphere as 3 to 2; for each of the circular Bases being $\frac{1}{2}cr$, the whole Surface will be $3cr$, which is to $2cr$ as 3 to 2; whence it follows, that the Sum of the Surfaces of the Bases is equal to the Surface of the inscribed Hemisphere.

EXAMPLE V

Let it be required to find the Surface of a Spheroid, generated by the Rotation of the Semi Ellipsis D A F *about the Axis* D F

PUT $AE = a$, $DE = b$, $AB = x$, and $BC = y$ Now because, from the Nature of the Ellipsis, as $aa\ \ bb\ \ 2ax - xx . yy$, therefore $yy = \frac{bb}{aa} \times \overline{2ax - xx}$, whence $\overline{2ax - xx}$ equal to $yy \times \frac{aa}{bb}$, and $2a\dot{x} - 2x\dot{x} = 2y\dot{y} \times \frac{aa}{bb}$, and $a\dot{x} - x\dot{x} = y\dot{y} \times \frac{aa}{bb}$, and

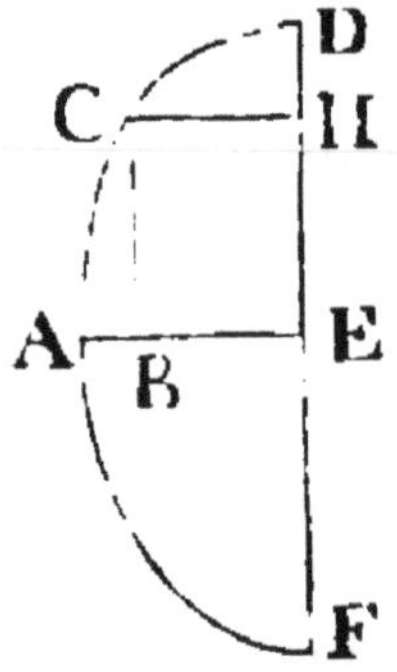

$$\dot{x} = \frac{aay\dot{y}}{bba - bbx}; \text{ whence } x\dot{x} = \frac{a^4yy\dot{y}\dot{y}}{b^4aa - 2b^4ax + b^4xx}$$

$$= \frac{a^4yy\dot{y}\dot{y}}{b^4aa - bb \times bb \times \overline{2ax - xx}},$$ but because, from the Property of the Curve, $bb \times \overline{2ax - xx} = aayy$, if we substitute

ſtitute this Value in the former Expreſſion in the room of $\overline{bb}\times\overline{2ax-xx}$, we ſhall have $xx=\dfrac{a^4yyyy}{\overline{b^4aa-bbyy}\,aa}$ equal, by dividing by aa, to $\dfrac{aayyyy}{b^4-bbyy}$, and putting this laſt Value of xx in the general Equation $z=\overline{xx+yy}^{\frac{1}{2}}$, we have $z=\overline{\dfrac{aayyyy}{b^4-bbyy}+yy}^{\frac{1}{2}}=\overline{\dfrac{a^2y^2y^2+b^4y^2-b^2y^2y^2}{b^4-b^2y^2}}^{\frac{1}{2}}$ $=\dfrac{y}{b}\times\overline{\dfrac{b^4+\overline{aa-bb}\times yy}{bb-yy}}^{\frac{1}{2}}$, and putting dd in the room of $bb-aa$, we ſhall have $z=\dfrac{y}{b}\times\overline{\dfrac{b^4-ddyy}{bb-yy}}^{\frac{1}{2}}$.

Again, becauſe C H is equal to $\dfrac{a}{b}\times\overline{bb-yy}^{\frac{1}{2}}$, therefore the Circumference of the Circle generated by the Point C, will be $\dfrac{ca}{rb}\times\overline{bb-yy}^{\frac{1}{2}}$ (where r is put for the Radius of a Circle, of which c ſtands for the Circumference) which being multiplied into $\dfrac{y}{b}\times\overline{\dfrac{b^4-ddyy}{bb-yy}}^{\frac{1}{2}}$, the Fluxion of the Arch A C, we ſhall have $\dfrac{ca}{r}\times\dfrac{y}{bb}\times\overline{b^4-ddyy}^{\frac{1}{2}}$, for the Fluxion of the Surface generated by the Arch of the Ellipſis A C, but the Square Root of $\overline{b^4-d^2y^2}$ is $b^2-\dfrac{d^2y^2}{2bb}-\dfrac{d^4y^4}{8b^6}$.

$-\frac{d^6y^6}{16b^{10}}-\frac{5d^8y^8}{128b^{14}}$, &c. This Series therefore being multiplied by $\frac{y}{bb}$, will give $y-\frac{d^2y^2y}{2b^4}-\frac{d^4y^4y}{8b^8}-\frac{d^6y^6y}{16b}$ $-\frac{5d^8y^8y}{128b^{16}}$, &c. whose Fluent $y-\frac{d^2y^3}{6b^4}-\frac{d^4y^5}{40b^8}-\frac{d^6y^7}{112b^{12}}$ $-\frac{5d^8y^9}{1152b^{16}}$, &c. being multiplied by $\frac{ca}{r}$, will give $\frac{ca}{r}\times y$ $-\frac{d^2y^3}{6b^4}-\frac{d^4y^5}{40b^8}-\frac{d^6y^7}{112b^{12}}-\frac{5d^8y^9}{1152b^{16}}$, &c. for the Surface generated by the Arch A C.

Now if we imagine the Ordinate B C to move according to the Direction A E, 'till it arrives at, or coincides with the Semi-transverse Diameter D E, then will y becomes equal to b, and we shall have $\frac{2ca}{r}\times b-\frac{d^2b^3}{6b^4}-\frac{d^4b^5}{40b^8}-\frac{d^6b^7}{112b^{12}}$ $-\frac{5d^8b^9}{1152b^{16}}=\frac{2ca}{r}\times b-\frac{d^2}{6b}-\frac{d^4}{40b^3}-\frac{d^6}{112b^5}-\frac{5d^8}{1152b^7}$ &c. equal (by putting $b=1$) to $\frac{2ca}{r}\times 1-\frac{1}{6}d^2-\frac{1}{40}d^4$ $-\frac{1}{112}d^6-\frac{5}{1152}d^8$, &c. $=\frac{2ca}{r}\times 1-\frac{1}{2\times 3}d^2-$ $-\frac{1\times 1}{2\times 4\times 5}d^4-\frac{1\times 1\times 3}{2\times 4\times 6\times 7}d^6-\frac{1\times 1\times 3\times 5}{2\times 4\times 6\times 8\times 9}d^8$, &c. for the Surface of the whole Spheroid.

EXAM

EXAMPLE VI.

Let it be required to find the Surface of a Parabolic Conoid, generated by the Rotation of the Semi Parabola A D E, *about its Axis* A D

FROM any Point B, let the Ordinate B C be drawn parallel to D E; then put A B $= x$, B C $= y$, D E $= r$, and the Circumference of the Circle generated by the Point E $= c$, whence $\frac{cy}{r}$ will be the Circumference generated by the Point C (for as $r : c :: y : \frac{cy}{r}$), but, from the Nature of

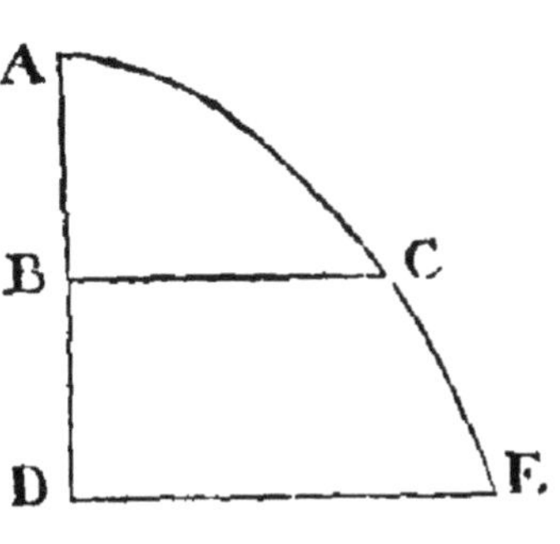

Curve, $ax = yy$, whence $a\dot{x} = 2y\dot{y}$, and $\dot{x} = \frac{2y\dot{y}}{a}$, consequently $\dot{x}\dot{x} = \frac{4y\dot{y}y\dot{y}}{aa}$. Substituting this Quantity therefore in the general Equation $\dot{z} = \overline{\dot{x}\dot{x} + \dot{y}\dot{y}}|^{\frac{1}{2}}$ in the room of $\dot{x}\dot{x}$, and we shall have $\dot{z} = \overline{\frac{4y\dot{y}y\dot{y}}{aa} + \dot{y}\dot{y}}|^{\frac{1}{2}} =$

$= \frac{\overline{4y\dot{y}y\dot{y} + aa\dot{y}\dot{y}}|^{\frac{1}{2}}}{\overline{aa}|^{\frac{1}{2}}}$, which being multiplied by $\frac{cy}{r}$, the Circumference generated by the Point C, will give $\frac{cy}{r}$

$\times \frac{\overline{4y\dot{y}y\dot{y} + aa\dot{y}\dot{y}}|^{\frac{1}{2}}}{\overline{aa}|^{\frac{1}{2}}} = \frac{cy}{r} \times \frac{\overline{\dot{y}\dot{y}}|^{\frac{1}{2}}}{\overline{aa}|^{\frac{1}{2}}} \times \overline{4yy + aa}|^{\frac{1}{2}} =$

$= \frac{cy\dot{y}}{ar} \times \overline{4yy+aa}^{\frac{1}{2}} = \frac{c}{r} \times \frac{y\dot{y}}{a} \times \overline{4yy+aa}^{\frac{1}{2}}$, for the Fluxion of the Surface generated by the Arch AC, but the Square Root of $\overline{4yy+aa}$, is $a + \frac{2yy}{a} - \frac{2y^4}{a^3} + \frac{4y^6}{a^5} - \frac{10y^8}{a^7} + \frac{28y^{10}}{a^9}$, &c. This therefore being multiplied by $\frac{y\dot{y}}{a}$, will give $y\dot{y} + \frac{2y^3\dot{y}}{aa} - \frac{2y^5\dot{y}}{a^4} + \frac{4y^7\dot{y}}{a^6} - \frac{10y^9\dot{y}}{a^8} + \frac{28y^{11}\dot{y}}{a^{10}}$, whose Fluent $\frac{yy}{2} + \frac{y^4}{2aa} - \frac{y^6}{3a^4} + \frac{y^8}{2a^6} - \frac{y^{10}}{a^8} + \frac{7y^{12}}{3a^{10}} \times \frac{c}{r}$, &c equal (by putting $a=1$) to $\frac{c}{r} \times \frac{yy}{2} + \frac{y^4}{2} - \frac{y^6}{3} + \frac{y^8}{2} - \frac{y^{10}}{1} + \frac{7y^{12}}{3}$, &c for the Surface generated by the Arch AC; but if we suppose DE $= b$, and imagine the Ordinate BC to move in the Direction AD, 'till it arrive at, or coincide with the Ordinate DE, then y will become equal to b, and we shall have $\frac{c}{r} \times \frac{1}{2}bb + \frac{1}{2}b^4 - \frac{1}{3}b^6 + \frac{1}{2}b^8 - b^{10} + \frac{7}{3}b^{12}$, for the Surface of the whole Parabolic Conoid.

EXAMPLE VII.

Let it be required to find the Surface of an Hyperbolic Conoid, formed by the Rotation of an Hyperbola about its conjugate Diameter EBF *(See the following Figure.)*

PUT AE $= a$, EF $= b$, BC $= x$, EB $= y$, and because, from the Nature of the Curve, $yy = \frac{bb}{aa} \times \overline{xx-aa}$, therefore

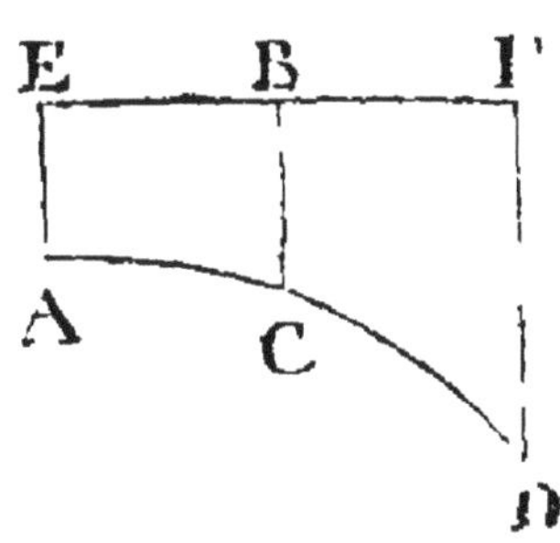

therefore $aayy = bbxx - bbaa$, and $xx = \frac{aayy+bbaa}{bb}$, and $x = \frac{\overline{aayy+bbaa}^{\frac{1}{2}}}{\overline{bb}^{\frac{1}{2}}} = \frac{a}{b}\times\overline{yy+bb}^{\frac{1}{2}}$

but $2y\dot{y} = \frac{bb}{aa}\times 2x\dot{x}$, whence $2x\dot{x}bb = 2y\dot{y}aa$, and $x\dot{x}bb = y\dot{y}aa$, whence $\dot{x} = \frac{aay\dot{y}}{bbx}$, and $\dot{x}\dot{x} = \frac{a^4yy\dot{y}\dot{y}}{b^4xx} = \frac{a^4yy\dot{y}\dot{y}}{b^4\times\frac{bb+yy}{bb}\times aa}$ (by substituting $\frac{yyaa+bbaa}{bb}$ in the room of xx), whence $\dot{x}\dot{x} = \frac{aayy\dot{y}\dot{y}}{bb\times\overline{bb+yy}}$, which being substituted in the general Equation $\dot{z} = \overline{\dot{x}\dot{x}+\dot{y}\dot{y}}^{\frac{1}{2}}$, in the room of $\dot{x}\dot{x}$, we shall have

$$\dot{z} = \frac{\overline{aayy\dot{y}\dot{y}+bbyy\dot{y}\dot{y}+b^4\dot{y}\dot{y}}^{\frac{1}{2}}}{\overline{bb\times\overline{bb+yy}}^{\frac{1}{2}}} = \frac{\overline{aayy+bbyy+b^4}^{\frac{1}{2}}}{\overline{bb\times\overline{bb+yy}}^{\frac{1}{2}}}\times\dot{y}$$

$$= \frac{\overline{aayy+bbyy+b^4}^{\frac{1}{2}}}{\overline{bb+yy}^{\frac{1}{2}}}\times\frac{\dot{y}}{b} = \frac{\dot{y}}{b}\times\frac{\overline{\overline{aa+bb}\times yy+b^4}^{\frac{1}{2}}}{\overline{bb+yy}^{\frac{1}{2}}}$$

= the Fluxion of the Curve Line AC.

Put FD $= r$, and the Circumference of the Circle generated by the Point D equal to c, then will the Circumference of the Circle generated by the Point C, be equal to $\frac{cx}{r}$, for (as (as r c $x : \frac{cx}{r}$) equal to $\frac{c}{r}x$; but $x = \frac{\overline{aayy + aabb}^{\frac{1}{2}}}{\overline{bb}^{\frac{1}{2}}}$ $= \frac{a}{b} \times \overline{yy + bb}^{\frac{1}{2}}$; whence $\frac{ca}{br} \times \overline{yy + bb}^{\frac{1}{2}}$, will be the Value of the Circumference of the Circle generated by the Point C, in the Terms of the Equation of the Curve This therefore being multiplied by $\frac{\dot{y}}{b} \times \frac{\overline{\overline{aa + bb} \times yy + b^4}^{\frac{1}{2}}}{\overline{bb + yy}^{\frac{1}{2}}}$, the Fluxion of the Curve Line A C, will give $\frac{ca\dot{y}}{rbb} \times \frac{\overline{\overline{aa + bb} \times yy + b^4}^{\frac{1}{2}}}{\overline{bb + yy}^{\frac{1}{2}}}$ $\times \frac{\overline{bb + yy}^{\frac{1}{2}}}{1} = \frac{ca\dot{y}}{rbb} \times \overline{\overline{aa + bb} \times yy + b^4}^{\frac{1}{2}}$, equal (by putting dd in the room of $\overline{aa + bb}$) to $\frac{ca\dot{y}}{rbb} \times \overline{ddyy + b^4}^{\frac{1}{2}}$ $= \frac{ca}{r} \times \frac{\dot{y}}{bb} \times \overline{ddyy + b^4}^{\frac{1}{2}}$, for the Fluxion of the Surface generated by the Rotation of the Arch A C about the Semi-conjugate Diameter E F, whose Fluent, or the Surface itself, will be found, after the manner taught in the preceding fifth Example, to be $\frac{ca}{r} \times y + \frac{d^2y^3}{6b^4} - \frac{d^4y^5}{40b^8} + \frac{d^6y^7}{112b^{12}} - \frac{5d^8y^9}{1152b^{16}}$, &c

EXAM-

EXAMPLE VIII

Let it be required to find the Surface of an Hyperbolic Conoid, generated by the Rotation of the Hyperbola A C E *about its Axis* A D.

LET E be the Center of the Hyperbola, and put A E, the Semi-transverse Diameter, equal to b, and A F, the Semi conjugate Diameter, equal to a, also B C $= x$, and E B $= y$ Now because, from the Nature of the Curve, $xx = \frac{aa}{bb} \times \overline{yy - bb}$, therefore $2 x \dot{x} = \frac{aa}{bb} \times 2 y \dot{y}$, whence $2 bb x \dot{x} = 2 aa y \dot{y}$, and $bb x \dot{x} = aa y \dot{y}$, and $\dot{x} = \frac{aa y \dot{y}}{bb x}$; whence $\dot{x}\dot{x} = \frac{a^4 y^2 \dot{y}^2}{b^4 x^2}$

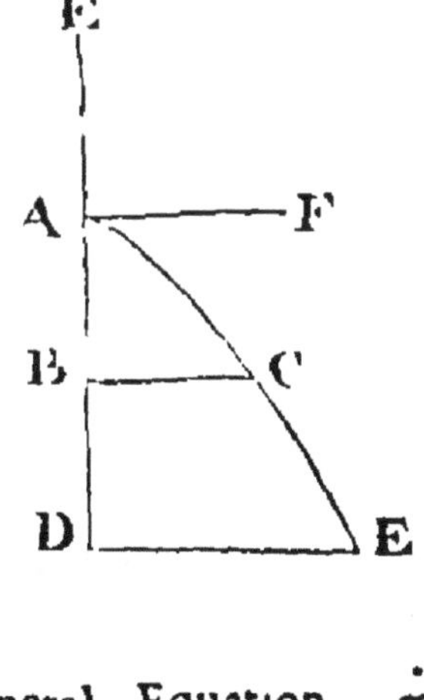

Substituting this therefore in the general Equation, $\dot{z} = \overline{\dot{x}\dot{x} + \dot{y}\dot{y}}^{\frac{1}{2}}$ in the room of $\dot{x}\dot{x}$, and we shall have $\overline{\frac{a^2 y^2 \dot{y}^2 b^2}{b^4 \times \overline{yy - bb}} + \dot{y}\dot{y}}^{\frac{1}{2}} = \frac{\overline{a^2 y^2 \dot{y}^2 b^2 + b^4 y^2 \dot{y}^2 - b^6 \dot{y}^2}^{\frac{1}{2}}}{b^4 \times \overline{yy - bb}^{\frac{1}{2}}} = \frac{\overline{a^2 y^2 + b^2 y^2 - b^6}^{\frac{1}{2}}}{b^2 \times \overline{yy - bb}^{\frac{1}{2}}} \times \dot{y} = \frac{\dot{y}}{b} \times \frac{\overline{ddyy - b^4}^{\frac{1}{2}}}{\overline{yy - bb}^{\frac{1}{2}}}$, by substituting dd in the room of $aa + bb$, for the Fluxion of the Curve

PUT A D $= r$, and the Circumference generated by the Point E $= c$, then will the Circumference generated by the Point

Point C be $= \frac{c\dot{x}}{r}$ (for as $c \cdot r \cdot \dot{x} \cdot \frac{c\dot{x}}{y}$) $= \frac{c}{r}\dot{x}$, but from the Nature of the Curve $xx = \frac{aa}{bb} \times \overline{yy - bb}$, therefore $x = \frac{a}{b} \times \overline{yy - bb}^{\frac{1}{2}}$, whence $\frac{c}{r}\dot{x}$ will be equal to $\frac{ca}{rb} \times \overline{yy - bb}^{\frac{1}{2}}$, the Circumference described by the Point C in the Terms of the Equation of the Curve. This therefore being multiplied $\frac{\dot{y}}{b} \times \frac{\overline{ddyy - b^4}^{\frac{1}{2}}}{\overline{yy - bb}^{\frac{1}{2}}}$, the Fluxion of the Curve Line A C, will give $\frac{ca}{rb} \times \overline{yy - bb}^{\frac{1}{2}} \times \frac{\dot{y}}{b} \times \frac{\overline{d^2y^2 - b^4}^{\frac{1}{2}}}{\overline{yy - bb}^{\frac{1}{2}}} = \frac{ca\dot{y}}{rbb} \times \overline{ddyy - b^4}^{\frac{1}{2}}$, for the Fluxion of the Surface generated by the Curve Line A C, about its Axis A B, whose Fluent may be found after the manner taught in the fifth preceding Example.

EXAMPLE IX.

Let it be required to find the Surface generated by the Rotation of an Equilateral Hyperbola about the Asymptote A B *(See the following Figure.)*

PUT AD $=$ DH $= a$, AB $= x$, BC $= y$, and because, from the Nature of the Curve, $aa = xy$, whence $y = \frac{aa}{x}$, and $\dot{y} = \frac{-aa\dot{x}}{xx}$, therefore $\dot{y}\dot{y} = \frac{a^4\dot{x}\dot{x}}{x^4}$. Again, because $x = \frac{aa}{y}$ (from the Equation of the Curve $aa = xy$) there-

fore

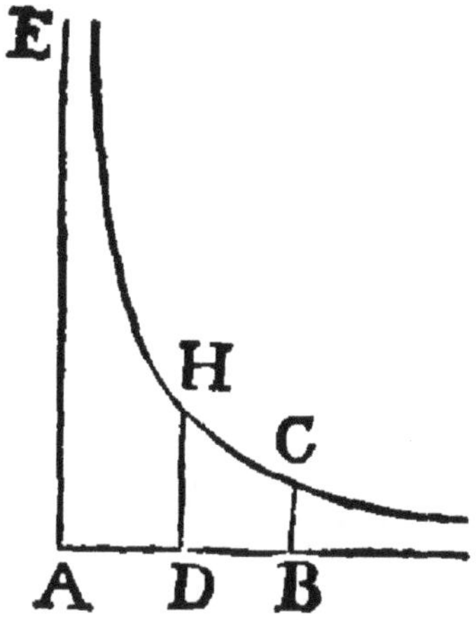

fore $\dot{x} = \frac{-aa\dot{y}}{yy}$, and $\dot{x}\dot{x} = \frac{a^4\dot{y}\dot{y}}{y^4}$, whence $\dot{z} = \overline{\dot{x}\dot{x}+\dot{y}\dot{y}}|^{\frac{1}{2}}$ will be equal to $\overline{\frac{a^4\dot{x}\dot{x}}{x^4} + \frac{a^4\dot{y}\dot{y}}{y^{4\frac{1}{2}}}}|^{\frac{1}{2}}$ $= \overline{\dot{y}\dot{y}+\frac{a^4\dot{y}\dot{y}}{y^4}}|^{\frac{1}{2}}$ (by putting $\dot{y}\dot{y}$ in the room of $\frac{a^4\dot{x}\dot{x}}{x^4}$, to which it is equal) $= \overline{\frac{y^4\dot{y}^2 - a^4\dot{y}^2}{y^4}}|^{\frac{1}{2}}$ $= \frac{\dot{y}}{yy} \times \overline{a^4 + y^4}|^{\frac{1}{2}}$, for the Fluxion of the Curve Line H C, which being multiplied by $\frac{cy}{r}$ (for as $r : c :: y : \frac{cy}{r}$) the Circumference of the Circle generated by the Point C, will give $\frac{cy\dot{y}}{ryy} \times \overline{a^4+y^4}|^{\frac{1}{2}} = \frac{c}{r}\dot{y}y^{-1} \times \overline{a^4+y^4}|^{\frac{1}{2}}$, for the Fluxion of the Surface generated by the Arch H C, revolved about the Asymptote A B as an Axis; but the Square Root of $\overline{a^4 + b^4}$ is $aa + \frac{y^4}{2aa} - \frac{y^8}{8a^6} + \frac{y^{12}}{16a^{10}} - \frac{5y^{16}}{128a^{14}} + \frac{7y^{20}}{256a^{18}}$, &c. This therefore being multiplied by $\dot{y}y^{-1}$, will produce $\frac{aa\dot{y}}{y} + \frac{y^3\dot{y}}{2aa} - \frac{y^7\dot{y}}{8a^6} + \frac{y^{11}\dot{y}}{16a^{10}} - \frac{5y^{15}\dot{y}}{128a^{14}} + \frac{7y^{19}\dot{y}}{256a^{18}}$, &c. whose Fluent being multiplied by $\frac{c}{r}$, will give $\frac{c}{r}aa + \frac{y^4}{8aa}$ $- \frac{y^8}{64a^6} + \frac{y^{12}}{192a^{10}} - \frac{5y^{16}}{2048a^{14}} + \frac{7y^{20}}{5120a^{18}}$, &c $= \frac{c}{r} \times aa$

+

$+\frac{1\times y^4}{2\times4\times a^2}-\frac{1\times1\times y^8}{2\times4\times8\times a^6}-\frac{1\times1\times3\times y^{12}}{2\times4\times6\times12a^{10}}+$

$+\frac{1\times1\times3\times5y^{16}}{2\times4\times6\times8\times16a^{14}}$, &c. for the Surface itself.

EXAMPLE X.

Let it be required to find the Surface generated by the infinite Curve Line A C *of the Logarithmic Curve formed by the Rotation of the same Curve about its Asymptote* E F.

PUT A T, the Subtangent, equal to a, it being an invariable or fixed Quantity, and the Ordinate F C equal to y, then will T C, the Tangent, be equal to $\overline{aa+yy}^{\frac{1}{2}}$, FC being an Ordinate rightly applied, but by *Proposition* II *Sect* I *Part* III as $FC : CT :: \dot{y} : \dot{z}$, that is, as $y : \overline{aa+yy}^{\frac{1}{2}} :: \dot{y} : \dot{z}$, whence $\dot{z}=\frac{\dot{y}}{y}\times\overline{aa+yy}^{\frac{1}{2}}$,

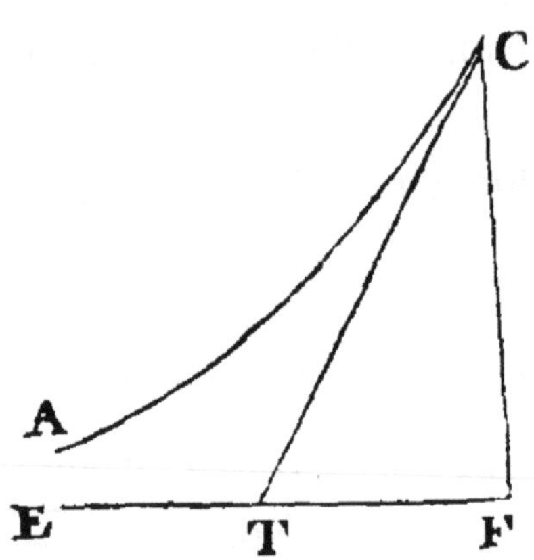

will be the Fluxion of the Curve Line A C. This therefore being multiplied by $\frac{cy}{r}$ (for as $r : c :: y : \frac{cy}{r}$) the Circumference generated by the Point C, will give $\frac{c\dot{y}}{r}\times\overline{aa+yy}^{\frac{1}{2}}$ for the Fluxion of the Surface generated by the Rotation of the Arch A C about its Asymptote E F, or if the Fluxion of the Curve Line A C $=\frac{\dot{y}}{y}\times\overline{aa+yy}^{\frac{1}{2}}$ be multiplied by $2y$,

the

the Product $2y \times \overline{aa+yy}^{\frac{1}{2}}$, will be the Fluxion of a Square, whose Side is equal to the Diameter of a Circle, equal in Area to the Surface of the generated Solid, but the Square Root of $\overline{aa+yy}^{\frac{1}{2}}$ is $a + \frac{yy}{2a} - \frac{y^4}{8a^3} + \frac{y^6}{16a^5} - \frac{5y^8}{128a^7} + \frac{7y^{10}}{256a^9}$, &c This therefore being multiplied by $2y$, will produce $2ay + \frac{y^2 y}{a} - \frac{y^4 y}{4a^3} + \frac{y^6 y}{8a^5} - \frac{5y^8 y}{64a^7} + \frac{7y^{10} y}{128a^9}$, &c whose Fluent $2ay + \frac{y^3}{3a} - \frac{y^5}{20a^3} + \frac{y^7}{56a^5} - \frac{5y^9}{576a^7} + \frac{7y^{11}}{1408a^9}$, &c will give the Side of the same Square, or the Diameter of a Circle, equal in Area to the generated Surface

EXAMPLE XI

Let it be required to find the Surface generated by the Rotation of the infinite Curve Line A C H, *of the Cissoid of* Diocles, *about the Asymptote* D B K.

HAVING drawn B C perpendicular, and E C parallel to the Asymptote D B K, put A D, the Diameter of the generating Circle, equal to d, A E $= x$, then will B C $=$ D E $= d - x$, and (from the Property of the Circle) F F $= \overline{dx - xx}^{\frac{1}{2}}$, and because from the Property of the Curve, as $\overline{DE}^{\frac{1}{2}}$: $\overline{AE}^{\frac{1}{2}}$ :: A E : C E, that is, as $\overline{d-x}^{\frac{1}{2}} : x^{\frac{1}{2}} :: x : x \times \frac{x^{\frac{1}{2}}}{\overline{d-x}^{\frac{1}{2}}} = \frac{x^{\frac{3}{2}}}{\overline{d-x}^{\frac{1}{2}}}$, we shall

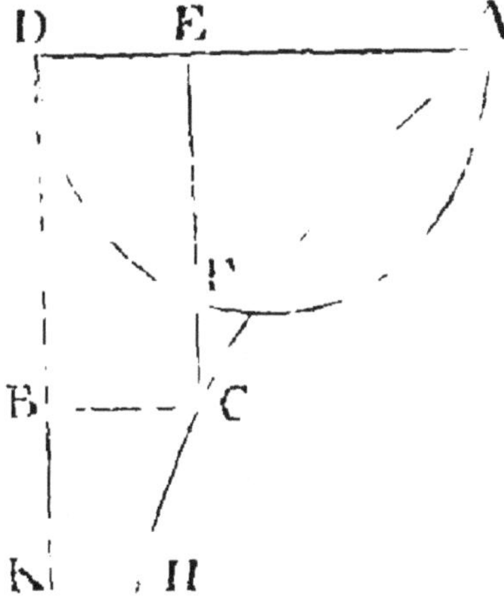

have $\frac{d\dot{x} \times \overline{4d - 3x}^{\frac{1}{2}}}{2 \times \overline{d - x} \times \overline{d - x}^{\frac{1}{2}}}$ for the Fluxion of the Curve Line A C H. This therefore being multiplied by $\frac{c}{r} \times \overline{a - x}^{\frac{1}{2}}$ (for as $r : c :: a - x : \frac{c}{r} \times \overline{a - x}^{\frac{1}{2}}$) the Circumference of the Circle generated by the Point C, will give $\frac{cd\dot{x}}{2r} \times \frac{\overline{d - x} \times \overline{4d - 3x}^{\frac{1}{2}}}{\overline{d - x} \times \overline{d - x}^{\frac{1}{2}}}$ $= \frac{cd\dot{x}}{2r} \times \frac{\overline{4d - 3x}^{\frac{1}{2}}}{\overline{d - x}^{\frac{1}{2}}}$, for the Fluxion of the Surface generated by the Curve Line A C H, equal (by putting d, the Diameter of the generating Circle, $= 1$) to $\frac{c\dot{x}}{2r} \times \frac{\overline{4 - 3x}^{\frac{1}{2}}}{\overline{1 - x}^{\frac{1}{2}}} = \frac{c}{r}$ $\times \dot{x} \times \frac{\overline{4 - 3x}^{\frac{1}{2}}}{\overline{1 - x}^{\frac{1}{2}}}$; but the Square Root of $\overline{4 - 3x}$ is $2 - \frac{3}{4}x$ $- \frac{9}{64}x^2 - \frac{27}{512}x^3 - \frac{405}{16384}x^4$, *&c.* This therefore being divided by $1 - \frac{1}{2}x - \frac{1}{8}xx - \frac{1}{16}x^3 - \frac{5}{128}x^4$, &c the Square Root of $\overline{1 - x}$, will give $2 + \frac{1}{4}x + \frac{15}{64}x^2$ $+ \frac{113}{512}x^3 + \frac{1808}{16384}x^4$, *&c.* which being multiplied by $\dot{x}$, will produce $2\dot{x} + \frac{1}{4}x\dot{x} + \frac{15}{64}x^2\dot{x} + \frac{113}{512}x^3\dot{x} + \frac{1808}{16384}$ $x^4\dot{x}$, *&c.* whose Fluent $2x + \frac{1}{8}x^2 + \frac{15}{192}x^3 + \frac{113}{2048}x^4$

+

$+ \frac{1808}{81920}x^{4}$, *&c.* being multiplied by $\frac{c}{r}$, will give the Value of the Surface generated by the Arch A C H of the Cissoid revolved about the Asymptote D B K.

SECT. IV.

Containing the Use of Fluxions *in the Cubature of* Solids, *or in investigating Methods to find their Contents.*

PROPOSITION VI.

IF the plain Surface G A C *c d* D be revolved about the Line A B *b* as an Axis, I say, that the Fluxion of the Solid generated by the Rotation of the Curvilinear Surface A B C is to the Fluxion of the Solid generated by the Rotation of the Rectangular Space A B D G, as the Square of the Ordinate B C is to the Square of the Ordinate B D.

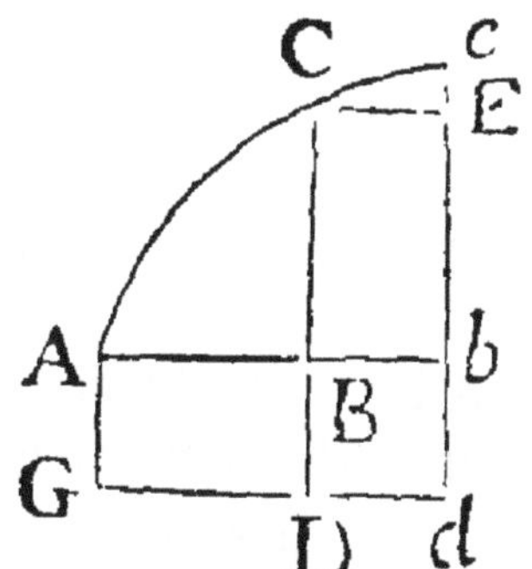

Imagine the Ordinates B C and B D in a flowing State, and let B C *c b*, and B *b d* D represent the nascent Augments of the Surfaces A C B, and A G D B, generated in the same very small Particle of Time, then will the Solids, generated by the Rotation of these nascent Augments, be the nascent Augments of the respective Solids generated in the same very small Particle of Time. Now the Solid generated by the nascent Space B C *c b*, may be conceived as consisting of two Solids, one generated by the rectangular Surface C E *b* B, and the other by the trilinear Space C *c* E, and consequently the nascent Augment of the Solid generated by the Trapezium B C *c* *b*, is to the nascent Augment of the Solid generated by the rectangular Space B *b* *d* D, as the Cylinder generated by the Space B C E *b* *plus*, the *Annulus* generated by the Space C *c* E to the Cylinder generated by the Space B *b* *d* D, but the Cylindric Solids generated by the Spaces C E *b* B, and B *b* *d* D, are as the Squares of their respective Bases, that is, as the Squares of the Ordinates B C and B D

LET us now conceive the nascent Ordinates *b* *c* and *b* *d* in a flowing State, and to move in the Direction *b* A, 'till they arrive at, or coincide with the Ordinates B C and B D, then will the Circles generated by the nascent Ordinates *bc* and *b* *d*, arrive at, or coincide with the Circles generated by the Ordinates B C and B D, the *Annulus* generated by the trilinear Space C *c* E, will vanish, and the Fluxion of the Solid, generated by the Rotation of the Curvilinear Space A B C, will be to the Fluxion of the Solid generated by the Rotation of the rectangular Space A B D G, in the evanescent State, as the Square of the Ordinate B C to the Square of the Ordinate B D

AND since the Cylindric Solid generated by the rectangular Space A B D G, is a constant Quantity, and every where the same, therefore the Solid generated by the Curvilinear Space A B C, will be every where as the Square of the Ordinate B C, or as the generating Circle, Wherefore

TO find the Cubature of any Solid, we must multiply the Area of the Base deduced from the Equation expressing the Nature of the Curve, by the Fluxion of the Axis, and the Fluent thence resulting will give the Solidity.

PUT therefore $AB = x$, $BC = y$, $S =$ Solidity, and r for the Radius of a Circle, whose Circumference is c, and it will be as $r \quad c \quad y \quad \frac{cy}{r}$, for the Circumference of the Circle genera-

generated by the Point C, whence $\frac{cyy}{2r}$, will be the Area, consequently $\frac{cyy\dot{x}}{2r}$ will be the Fluxion of the Solidity. Now if in the room of yy we substitute its Value arising from the Equation expressing the Nature of the generating Curve, the Fluent of this last Expression will give the Cubature of the Solid, as will more evidently appear from the following Examples.

EXAMPLE I.

Let it be required to find the Solidity of a Prism.

LET us suppose the Prism to have a square Base, and put AB $= a$, and r for one Side of the square Base, then will rr be the Area of the Base, and rra $= \dot{S} =$ Fluxion of the Solidity, but inasmuch as the Prism is generated by the uniform Motion of the Square A, according to the Direction of the Line A B, and that the generating Square is a constant or permanent Quantity, therefore $rra = S$, will give the Fluent or Solidity, and if, in the room of rr, we substitute the Area of the Base of any kind of Prism whatsoever, we shall have an Expression, whereby its solid Content may be found. For Example, suppose the Base of the Prism to be a Circle, as in the adjacent Figure, then is the Solid called a Cylinder, and let r stand for the Radius of its Base, c for its Circumference, and a for its Altitude, as before, then will $\frac{rc}{2}$ be the Area of Base, consequently $\frac{arc}{2}$ will be the Solidity Whence it follows,

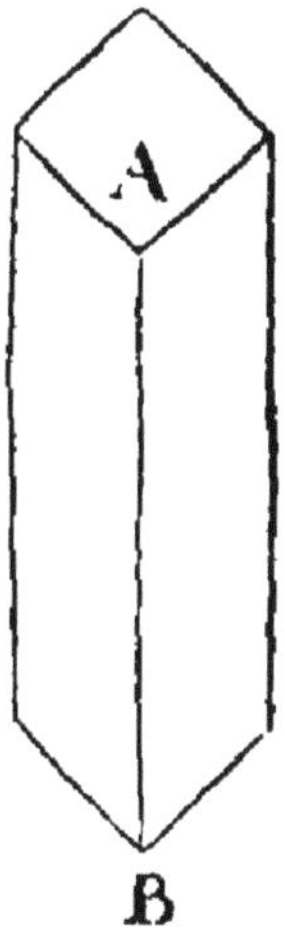

A

B

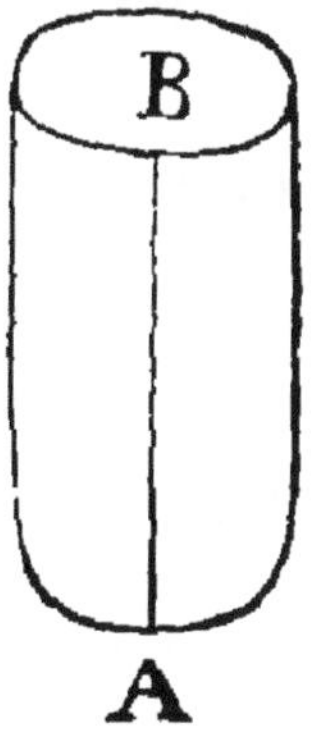

B

A

THAT

THAT the Solidity of the Cylinder is to the Solidity of its circumscribed Prism as $\frac{arc}{2}$ to arr, or as $\frac{rc}{2}$ to rr; that is, as the Circle is to its circumscribed Square.

As in Plain Geometry all Surfaces are compared with the circumscribing Parallelograms, so in Solid Geometry all Solids are compar'd with their circumscribing Prisms, and when the Ratio of the circumscribed Solid to the inscribed Solid is known, the Solidity of the inscribed Solid is known also.

EXAMPLE II.

Let it be required to find the Solid Content of a Pyramid

LET the Pyramid be supposed to stand upon a square Base, and let r stand for one of its Sides Put AD $= a$, AB $= x$, and CC $= y$, then will $yy\dot{x}$ be the Fluxion of the Solid CAC, but because the Triangles CA and EA are similar, it will be as x y a r, wherefore $ya = xr$, and consequently $x = \frac{ya}{r}$, and $\dot{x} = \frac{a\dot{y}}{r}$.

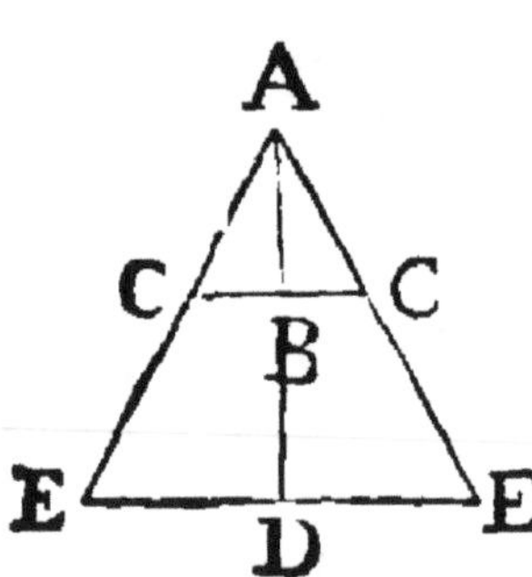

Putting this therefore in the room of $\dot{x}$, in the former Expression $yy\dot{x}$, we shall have $\frac{ayy\dot{y}}{r}$, for the Fluxion of the Solid CAC, the Fluent of which will be $\frac{ayyy}{3r}$. Now when AB, by flowing, becomes equal to AD, y becomes equal to r, and consequently $\frac{ayyy}{3r} = \frac{arrr}{3r} = \frac{arr}{3} = \frac{1}{3}$ $a \times \overline{rr}$, will be the Value of the Pyramid EAE. Whence it it follows, that the Solidity of the Pyramid is to the Solidity of the circumscribing Prism as $\frac{1}{3}$ arr to arr, or as arr to $3\,arr$, or as 1 to 3. So that the Pyramid is $\frac{1}{3}$ of the Prism, having the same Base and Altitude.

AGAIN, if in the room of rr we substitute the Area of the Base of any kind of Pyramid, we shall have an Expression to find the Solidity. For Example, if the Base be a Circle, then the Solid becomes a Cone, and if r stand for the Radius of the Circular Base D E, and C for its Circumference, then $\frac{cr}{2}$ will be the Area of the Base, and consequently the Solidity will be $\frac{acr}{6}$, but the Solidity of the circumscribed Cylinder has been shewn to be $\frac{acr}{2}$; wherefore the Solidity of the circumscribed Cylinder is to the Solidity of the inscribed Cone as $\frac{acr}{2}$ to $\frac{acr}{6}$, or as $6\,acr$ to $2\,acr$, that is, as 6 to 2, or as 3 to 1. Whence it appears, that the Cone is $\frac{1}{3}$ of its circumscribing Cylinder.

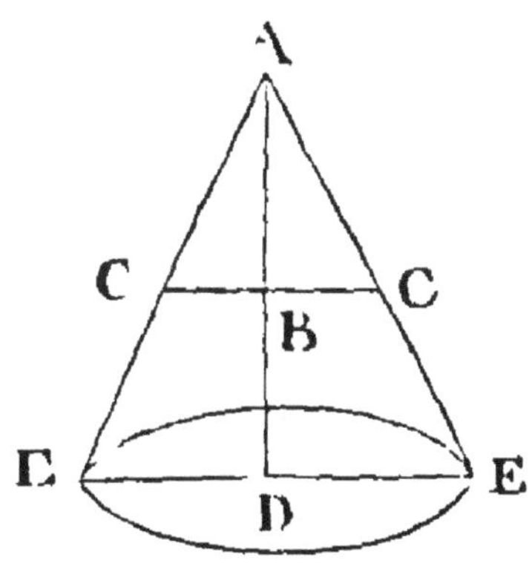

AGAIN let the right Line F H be drawn through A, the Apex of the Triangle A D E, parallel to the Base D E, and imagine the same Triangle A D E to revolve about the Line F H as an Axis; and let it be required to find the Value of the Solid generated by this Rotation.

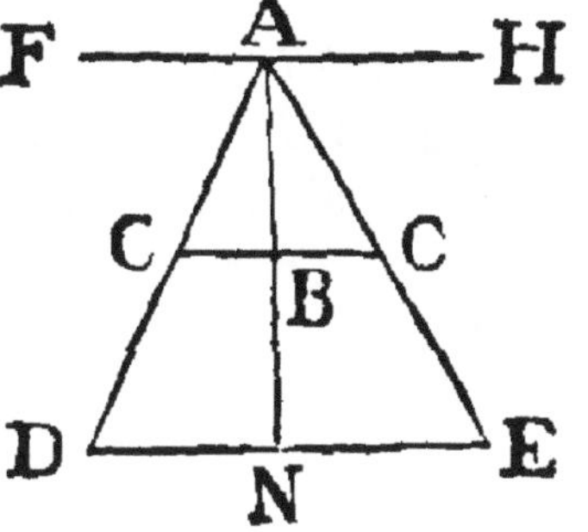

FROM A draw the Line A N, perpendicular to the Base D E, and it will represent the Height. Now if through any Point, as B, in the Line A N, a Line, as C B C, be be drawn parallel to the Base Line D E, this Line CBC, by the Rotation of the Triangle A D E about its Axis F H, will describe a Cylindrical Superficies, which shall be to the Cylindrical Superficies generated by the Line D E, as the Rectangles compounded of their Radii A B, A N, and their Altitudes C C, D E. Put therefore D E $= a$, A N $= r$, C C $= y$, and A B $= x$, and let the Circumference of the Circle generated by the Point D, be equal to c, then will ac be the Cylindric Surface generated by the Line D E. Whence to find the Surface generated by the Line C c, it will be as D E × A N $= ra : ac$, or as $r : C :: CC \times AP = xy : \frac{cxy}{r}$; whence $\frac{cyx\dot{x}}{r}$ will be the Fluxion of the Solidity; but, from the Property of the Triangle, it will be as $a : r :: y : x$, whence $y = \frac{ax}{r}$. Putting this therefore, in the former Equation, in the room of y, we shall have $\frac{acxx\dot{x}}{rr}$, the Fluent of which will be $\frac{acx^3}{3rr}$, but when the Point B, by flowing, arrives at N, x will become equal to r, consequently $\frac{acxxx}{3rr} = \frac{acrrr}{3rr} = \frac{acr}{3} = \frac{1}{3}acr$. Whence it follows,

THAT if the Altitude A N of the Triangle A D E, be equal to D N, half its Base, D E, the Solid thus generated, will be equal to a Sphere formed by the Rotation of a Semi-circle, whose Diameter shall be equal to the Base D E of the Triangle A D E, as will be evident from the following Example.

EXAMPLE III.

To find the Solid Content of a Sphere.

LET A F D E A represent a Semi-circle, B C an Ordinate rightly applied, and imagine the Semi circle to be turned about its Diameter A D as an Axis, 'till it return to the Place from whence it began to move, then will the Semi-circle, by this Motion, generate a Sphere, as will its Ordinate B C generate a Circle, whose Radius is B C

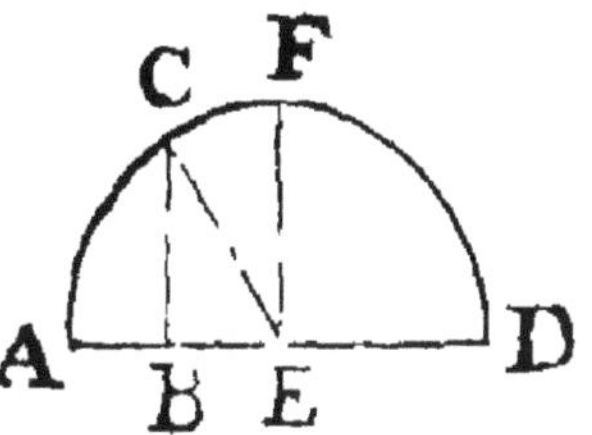

Put A B $= x$, BC $= y$, E F $= r$, and the Circumference generated by the Point F $= c$, then as $r : c :: y : \frac{cy}{r}$, the Circumference of the Circle generated by the Point C, whose Area will be $\frac{cyy}{2r}$, for $\frac{cy}{2r}$ multiplied by y, will be equal to $\frac{cyy}{2r}$, consequently $\frac{cyy\dot{x}}{2r}$ will be the Fluxion of the Solidity; but from the Nature of the Circle $yy = 2rx - xx$; whence $\frac{cyy\dot{x}}{2r}$ will be equal to $\frac{2crx\dot{x} - cxx\dot{x}}{2r}$ (by substituting $2rx - xx$ in the room of yy) $= cx\dot{x} - \frac{cxx\dot{x}}{2r}$, and consequently its Fluent $\frac{cxx}{2} - \frac{cxxx}{6r}$ will be the Solidity of the Portion of the Sphere generated by the Semi Segment A B C, but when A B flows into, or becomes $=$ A D, x becomes equal to $2r$, and consequently we shall have $\frac{4crr}{2} - \frac{8crr}{6}$ by ſubſtituting $2r$ in the room of x, in the Expreſſion $\left.\frac{cxx}{2} - \frac{cxxx}{6r}\right) = \frac{12crr - 8crr}{6} = \frac{4crr}{6}$ $= \frac{2crr}{3} = \frac{2}{3}crr$, for the Value of the whole Sphere.

AND the ſame Value of the Solid may be inveſtigated after the manner following

IMAGINE the Semi circle A F D to revolve about its Diameter A D as an Axis, then will the Semi circle A F D generate a Sphere, while the little Semi-circle C B C will generate a Spherical Surface

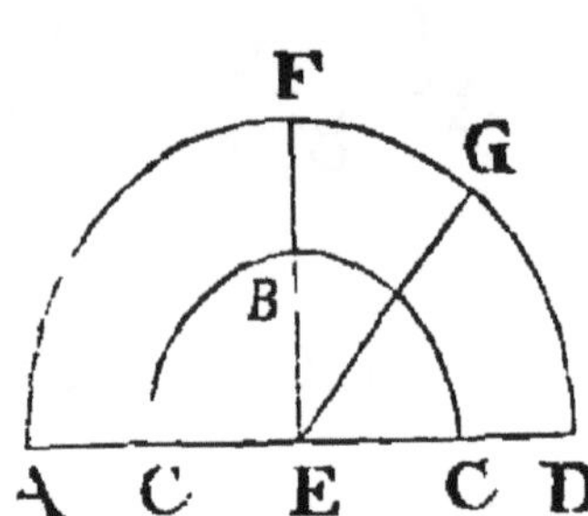

PUT E F $= r$, the Semi-circumference A F D $= \frac{1}{2}c$, E B $= x$, then will the Spherical Surface generated by the Semi-circle A F D $= 2cr$, and to find the Spherical Surface generated by the Semi-circle C B C (becauſe the Surfaces of Spheres are to each other as the Squares of their Radii) it will be as $rr \quad xx$

$2cr . \frac{2cxx}{r}$, whence $\frac{2cxx\dot{x}}{r}$ will be the Fluxion of the Solidity, and $\frac{2cxxx}{3r}$, the Fluent thence reſulting, will be the Value of the Sphere generated by the Semi-circle C B C Imagine the Semi circle C B C in a flowing State, and to move 'till it arrives at, or coincides with the Semi-circle A F D, then will the Point B coincide with the Point F, the Radius E B will become equal to the Radius E F, and x will become equal to r, whence we ſhall have $\frac{2crrr}{3r} = \frac{2}{3}crr$, for the Value of the

the whole Sphere, by substituting r in the room of x, in the Expression $\frac{2cxxx}{3r}$.

AGAIN, from E, the Center of the Semi-circle A F D, draw the Radius E G, then while the whole Semi circle A F D E A generates a Sphere, the Sector G E D will generate a Cone, whose Altitude E D will be the same with the Radius of the Sphere, and its Base the Space described by the little Arch of the Circle G D, let this be put equal to z, then will the Solidity of this Cone be $z \times \frac{r}{3}$, but when the Ray E G, revolving about the Point E, coincides with the Line E A, that is, when the Point G arrives at A, the Surface of the Base of the little Cone z, generated by the Arch G D, will become equal to the entire Surface of the Sphere generated by the Semi-circumference A F D, equal to $2cr$, and consequently the whole Solidity will be $\frac{2cr}{3} \times \frac{r}{3} = \frac{2crr}{3}$, the same as was before investigated. Whence it follows,

First, THAT the Sphere is to the Cube of its Diameter as $\frac{2}{3}$ of its Circumference is to four times its Diameter, for as $\frac{4}{3}crr : 8rrr :: \frac{2}{3}c : 8r = 4d$, and consequently, that the Sphere is to two Thirds of the Cube of its Diameter as the Circumference is to four times its Diameter

Secondly, THAT the Sphere is to its circumscribing Cylinder as 2 to 3, since, in this Case, the Cylinder is $\frac{1}{2}cr \times 2r = crr$

Thirdly, THAT the Sphere is to the Cone (which hath for its Base the great Circle of the Sphere, and for its Altitude the Diameter of the same Sphere) as 2 to 1, for the Solidity of the Cone, in this Case, is $\frac{1}{2}cr \times \frac{2}{3}r = \frac{1}{3}crr$.

Fourthly, THAT the Cone, the Sphere, and the Cylinder having the same Height, and the same Diameter, are as the Numbers 1, 2, 3

Fifthly, THAT the Cone is equal to the Excess of the Cylinder above the Sphere

EXAMPLE IV.

Let it be required to find the Value of a Parabolic Conoid, generated by the Revolution of the Semi-Parabola A C E D *about its Axis* A D.

FROM any Point, as B, in the Axis A D, let the Ordinate B C be drawn parallel to the Base D E, then put A B $= x$, B C $= y$, and D E $= r$, also A D $= a$, and the Circumference described by the Point E $= c$, whence to find the Circumference generated by the Ordinate B C, it will be as $r : c :: y : \frac{cy}{r} =$ to the Circumference described by the Point E, whence $\frac{cy}{2r} \times y = \frac{cyy}{2r}$, will be the Area of the same Circle. This therefore being multiplied by $\dot{x}$, the Fluxion of the Absciffe, will give $\frac{cyy\dot{x}}{2r} = \frac{cx\dot{x}}{2r}$ (by putting x in the room of yy, because, from the Nature of the Parabola, $1x = yy$) for the Fluxion of the Solid generated by the Space A B C, whose Fluent $\frac{cxx}{4r} = \frac{cyyx}{4r}$ (by putting yy in the room of x) equal to $\frac{carr}{4r} = \frac{1}{4}acr$ (by putting a in the room of x, and r in the room of y) will be the

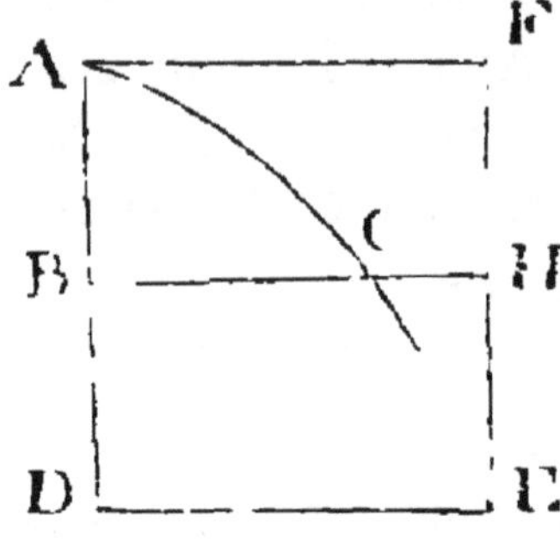

 Value

Value of the Solid generated by the whole Parabolic Space A D E, for if we imagine the Ordinate B C in a flowing State, and to move 'till it arrives at, or coincides with the Ordinate D E, then A B will become equal to A D, x will become equal to a, and y will become equal to r. Whence it follows,

First, THAT the Parabolic Conoid is to the circumscribed Cylinder as 1 to 2, for the Cylinder is equal to $\frac{acr}{2}$.

Secondly, THAT the inscribed Cone is to the Cylinder as 1 to 3.

Thirdly, THAT the Cylinder, the Parobolic Conoid, and the Cone, are to each other as the Numbers 3, $\frac{3}{2}$, 1.

IN the Equation expressing the Nature of the Curve, if instead of $x = yy$, we assume $x = y^m$, which is a general Equation for all Kinds of Parabolas whatsoever, we shall have $y = x^{\frac{1}{m}}$, and $yy = x^{\frac{2}{m}}$. Putting therefore $x^{\frac{2}{m}}$ in the former Equation $\frac{cyy}{2r}$ in the room of yy (to which it is equal) we shall have $\frac{cx^{\frac{2}{m}}}{2r}$ for the Area of the Circle described by the Ordinate B C, whence $\frac{cx^{\frac{2}{m}}\dot{x}}{2r}$, will be the Fluxion of the Solid generated by the Rotation of the Space A B C, whose Fluent $\frac{mcx^{\frac{2}{m}+1}}{2mr+4r} = \frac{mcxyy}{2mr+4r}$ (by putting yy in the room of $x^{\frac{2}{m}}$) will give the Value of the same Solid.

BUT when A B flows into, and becomes equal to A D, then B C flows into, and becomes equal to D E, consequently y will become $= r$, and x will become $= a$, and we shall have $\frac{mcarr}{2mr+4r} = \frac{m}{2m+4}acr$, for the Value of the Solid

lid generated by the Space A D E, by putting r in the room of y, and a in the room of x, in the Expression $\frac{m c x y y}{2 m r + 4 r}$

If $m = 3$, the Equation will be $y^3 = x$, and we shall have $\frac{3}{10} a r c$ for the Value of the Solid, which is to the Cylinder circumscribed as 3 is to 5, for as $\frac{3 a c r}{10}$ $\frac{a c r}{2}$ 3 5.

EXAMPLE V

Let it be required to find the Value of the Solid formed by the Rotation of the Parabolic Space A D E, *about the Line* F E, *parallel and equal to the Axis* A D (*See the preceding Figure*)

Let A C E represent a Semi-Parabola, A D its Axis, B C an Ordinate rightly applied, which being produced to cut F E in the Point H, imagine the Semi-Parabola to revolve about the Line F E, as an Axis, then will the Line B H generate a Circle. Putting therefore F E $=$ A D $= a$, A B $= x$, B C $= y$, A F or D E $= r$, c for the Circumference of the Circle described by the Point D, we shall have C H $= r - y$, and $\frac{c r - c y}{r}$ for the Circumference of the Circle generated by the Point C, for as r c $r - y$ $\frac{c r - c y}{r}$; whence $\frac{r - y}{2} \times \frac{c r - c y}{r} = \frac{c r r - 2 c r y + c y y}{2 r}$, will be the Area of the Circle described by the Line C H. This therefore being taken from $\frac{c r}{2}$, the Area of the Circle described by the Line B H, will give $\frac{2 c r y - c y y}{2 r}$ for the Area of the *Annulus* described

described by the Ordinate B C, and this being multiplied by x, will give $\frac{2cryx - cyyx}{2r}$ for the Fluxion of the Solid generated by the Space A B C equal to $\frac{2rcx^{\frac{1}{2}}x - cxx}{2r}$ by putting $x^{\frac{1}{2}}$ in the room of y, and x in the room of yy, to which they are respectively equal, from the Nature of the Parabola, whose Fluent $\frac{2crx^{\frac{1}{2}}x}{3r} - \frac{cxx}{4r} = \frac{2cryx}{3r} - \frac{cxyy}{4r}$ (by substituting y in the room of $x^{\frac{1}{2}}$, and yy in the room of x) $= \frac{8cryx - 3cxyy}{12r}$, will give the Value of the Solid generated by the same Space A B C. Now if we consider the Ordinate B C in a flowing State, and to move 'till it arrive at, or coincide with the Ordinate D E, then A B will become equal to A D, x will become equal to a, y will become equal to r, and $\frac{8crxy - 3cxyy}{12r}$ will become $\frac{8crar - 3carr}{12r} = \frac{8acr - 3acr}{12} = \frac{5acr}{12}$ the Value of the Solid generated by the whole Space A D E. Whence it is evident, that the Solid thus formed is to its circumscribed Cylinder as 5 to 6, for the Value of the Cylinder is $\frac{acr}{2}$, and $\frac{5}{12}acr$ is to $\frac{acr}{2}$ as $\frac{5}{12}$ to $\frac{1}{2}$, or as $\frac{5}{12}$ to $\frac{6}{12}$, or as 5 to 6.

EXAM-

EXAMPLE VI.

Let it be required to find the Value of the Solid formed by the Rotation of the Parobolic Space ACED, *about the Line* AF, *as an Axis, touching the Parabola in the Vertical Point* A.

FROM any Point H, in the Axis AD, draw the Ordinate HC, parallel to the Base DE, it is evident, that while the Curvilinear Space AED is revolved about the Line AF as an Axis, that this Line HC will describe a Cylindrical Surface. Put therefore $AD = r$, $DE = AF = a$, $AB = HC = x$, $BC = AH = y$, then $\dot{y}$ will be the Fluxion of the Ordinate $BC = AH$, and let the Circumference of the Circle formed by the Point C be put equal to c, whence ac will be the Cylindric Surface formed by the Line DE, whence to find the Cylindric Surface formed by the Line HC, it will be as $DE \times DA = ar$ ac, or as r to c

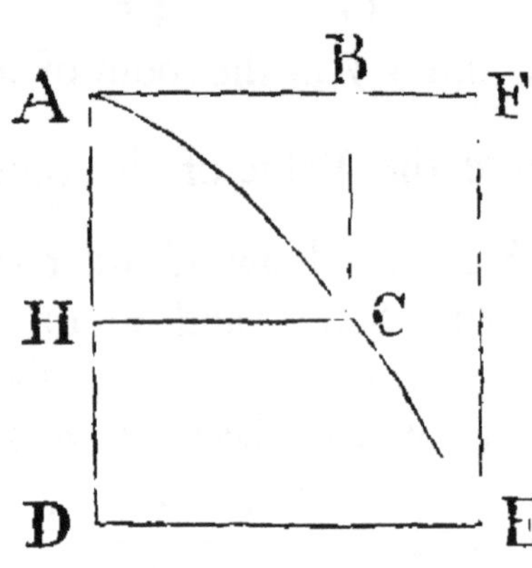

$HC \times HA = xy$ $\frac{cxy}{r}$; whence $\frac{cxy\dot{y}}{r}$, will be the Fluxion of the Solid generated by the Space AHC, and because, from the Nature of the Parabola, $xx = y$, whence $x = y^{\frac{1}{2}}$, if we substitute $y^{\frac{1}{2}}$, in the former Equation, in the room of x, to which it is equal, we shall have $\frac{cyy^{\frac{1}{2}}\dot{y}}{r} = \frac{cy^{\frac{3}{2}}\dot{y}}{r}$ for the Fluxion of the same Solid, whose Fluent $\frac{2cy^{\frac{1}{2}}y^{2}}{5r}$

=

$= \frac{2cxyy}{5r}$, by putting x in the room of $y^{\frac{1}{2}}$, will give the Value of the Solid itself.

Now if we conceive the Ordinate H C in a flowing State, and to move according to the Direction A D, 'till it arrives at, or coincides with the Ordinate D E, then A H will become equal to A D, y will become equal to r, x will become equal to a, consequently $\frac{2}{5}\frac{cxyy}{r}$ will become $\frac{2}{5}\frac{carr}{r} = \frac{2}{5}acr$, for the Value of the Solid generated by the whole Parabolic Space A D E

Again, if the Value of the Solid be required in the Terms of x, because $y^2 = a\,x$, therefore $y = 2\,x\,x$. Now if we substitute these Values of y and y^2 in the general Equation $\frac{cxyy}{r}$ in the room of y and y, we shall have $\frac{2cxxxxx}{r} = \frac{2cx^4x}{r}$, for the Fluxion of the Solid generated by the Space AHC, whose Fluent $\frac{2cx^4x}{5r}$, will give the Value of the Solid itself, but because, from the Nature of the Curve $yy = x^4$, if we substitute yy, in the former Equation, in the room of x^4, we shall have $\frac{2cxyy}{5r}$ for the Value of the same Solid, equal to $\frac{2acr}{5}$ for the Value of the Solid generated by the whole Space A D E, the same as was before investigated, for when x, by flowing, becomes equal to a, y becomes equal to r. Whence it follows.

First, That the Solid is to the circumscribed Cylinder as 4 to 5

Secondly, THAT the Solid generated by the Concave, or Supplemental Part of the Parabola ACEF is equal to $\frac{1}{10}acr$, and that this may more evidently appear, put FE $= r$, the Circumference of the Circle generated by the Point E $= c$, then to find the Circumference generated by the Point C, it will be as $r : c :: y \; \frac{cy}{r}$, whence $\frac{cyy}{2r}$ will be the Area of the same Circle, consequently $\frac{cyy\dot{x}}{2r}$, will be the Fluxion of the Solid generated by the Space ABC equal to $\frac{cx^4\dot{x}}{2r}$, by putting x^4 in the room of yy, to which it is equal, whence $\frac{cx^4x}{10r}$, will be the Value of the same Solid equal to $\frac{cyyx}{10r}$, by putting yy in the room of x^4, whence we shall have $\frac{crra}{10r} = \frac{1}{10}acr$, for the Value of the Solid generated by the whole Space ACEF, the same as was before found, for when x becomes equal to a, y becomes equal to r

EXAMPLE VII.

Let it required to find the Value of the Solid generated by the Rotation of the Parabolic Space ADE, *about the Base* DE, *as an Axis.*

PUT AD $= r$, DE $= a$, BC $= y$, AB $= x$, and c for the Circumference of the Circle generated by the Point A, then will BD $= r - x$, and $\frac{cr - cx}{r}$ the Circumference of the

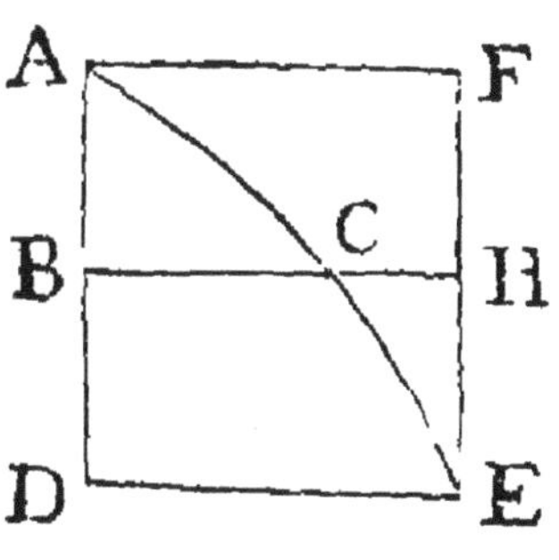

the Circle generated by the Point C (for as $r : c :: r - x : \frac{cr - cx}{r}$), whence $\frac{cry - cxy}{r}$ will be the Cylindrical Surface generated by the Ordinate B C, and $\frac{cry\dot{x} - cyx\dot{x}}{r}$, the Fluxion of the Solid. But because, from the Nature of the Parabola, $1x = yy$, therefore $\dot{x} = 2y\dot{y}$. Substituting therefore $2y\dot{y}$, in the former Equation, in the room of $\dot{x}$, and yy in the room of x, and we shall have $\frac{2cryy\dot{y} - 2cy^4\dot{y}}{r}$, whose Fluent $\frac{2cry^3}{3r} - \frac{2cy^5}{5r}$ will be the Value of the Solid generated by the Space A B C. Now if we imagine the Ordinate B C in a flowing State, and to move 'till it arrives at, or coincides with the Ordinate D E, then AB will become equal to AD, x will become equal to r, and y become equal to a, consequently $\frac{2cry^3}{3r} - \frac{2cy^5}{5r} = \frac{2cryx}{3r} - \frac{2cxxy}{5r}$ (by substituting x in the room of yy) will become equal to $\frac{2arc}{3} - \frac{2arc}{5} = \frac{10arc - 6arc}{15} = \frac{4arc}{15} = \frac{4}{15}acr$, the Value of the Solid generated by the whole Space A D E. Whence it follows,

THAT the Solid thus generated is to the circumscribed Cylinder as 8 to 15, for the Solidity of the Cylinder is ½ of acr.

EXAMPLE VIII

Let it be required to find the Value of the Solid formed by the Rotation of the Parabolic Space A E D *about* A D, *when the Ordinates* B C *and* D E *are not perpendicular to* A D, *in which Caſe* A D *is a Diameter of the Section.*

PUT A D $= b$, A B $= x$, D E $= r$, and c for the Circumference of the Circle deſcribed by the Point E.

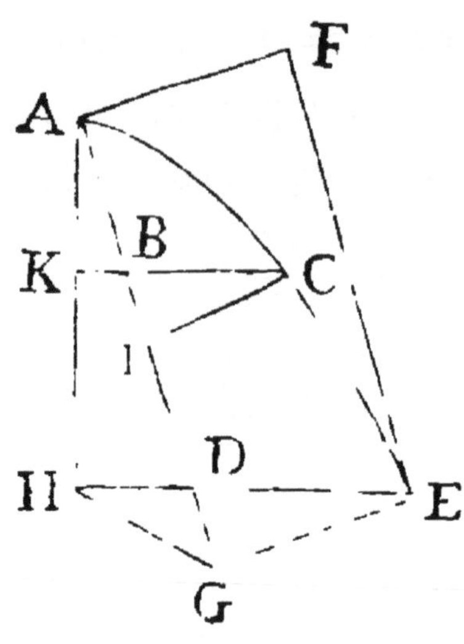

NOW foraſmuch as the Ordinates B C and D E, by their Rotation about A D, as an Axis, will deſcribe Conical Superficies parallel amongſt themſelves, and inaſmuch as theſe Surfaces are to each other as the Squares of their Sides B C and D E, and theſe being to each other as the reſpective Portions A B and A D of the Diameter A D, and ſince $\frac{1}{2}cr$ will be the Conic Surface deſcribed by the Ordinate D E, to find that deſcribed by the Ordinate B C, we muſt ſay as b : x :: $\frac{cr}{2}$: $\frac{crx}{2b}$.

FROM A let fall the Perpendicular A H upon the Ordinate E D produced, and continue the Ordinate C B till it meet the Perpendicular A H in K. Now putting A H $= a$, and A K $= z$, we ſhall have $\frac{crxz}{2b}$ for the Fluxion of the Solid, but by reaſon of the Similitude of the Triangles A B K, A D H, it will be as $x : z :: b . a$. Wherefore $z = \frac{ax}{b}$, and $\dot{z} = \frac{a\dot{x}}{b}$. Putting therefore $\frac{a\dot{x}}{b}$, in the former Expression $\frac{crx\dot{z}}{2b}$, in the room of $\dot{z}$, we shall have $\frac{acrx\dot{x}}{2bb}$, the Fluent of which $\frac{acrxx}{4bb}$ will be Value of the Solid described by the Space ABC; but when the Ordinate BC, by flowing, arrives at or coincides with the Ordinate DE, then AB will be equal to AD, consequently x will become equal to b, and $\frac{acrxx}{4bb}$, will become $\frac{acrbb}{4bb} = \frac{1}{4}acr$, the Value of the Solid generated by the whole Parabolic Space ADE. Whence it is evident, that this Solid is to that formed by the Rotation of the Parallelogram AFED as 1 to 2; for this Solid is equal to the Conic Surface formed by DE, multiplied into the Height AH $= \frac{1}{2}acr$.

EXAMPLE IX.

The same Things being supposed, as in the former Example, let it be required to find the Value of the Solid formed by the Rotation of the Parabolic Space ADE, about the Line AF, a Tangent to the Curve in the Vertex A. (See the preceding Figure.)

It is evident, that the Ordinates BC and DE, by their Rotation about the Line AF, as an Axis, will describe Cylindrical Surfaces, which will be to each other in a Ratio compounded of their Radii, and of their Altitudes. So that the Cylindric Surface described by the Ordinate DE, is to the Cylindric Surface described by the Ordinate BC, as DE × AH is to BC × AK, or as DL × AD is to CB × AB. Putting therefore

therefore D E $= a$, A D $= b$, A H $= r$, the Circumference described by the Point H $= c$, A B $= x$, B C $= y$, A K $= z$ it will be as A D × D E $= ab$ ac (= the Cylindric Surface described by D E) (A B × B C =) xy $\frac{cxy}{b}$ equal to the Cylindric Surface describ'd by B C, and multiplying this Quantity by z, we shall have $\frac{cxyz}{b}$ for the Fluxion of the Solid But because, from the Property of the Parabola, $x = y^{\frac{1}{2}}$, and $z = \frac{ry}{b}$. Putting then these Values in the former Equation in the room of z and x, we shall have $\frac{cry^{\frac{1}{2}}y}{bb}$, the Fluent of which will be $\frac{2cry^{\frac{5}{2}}}{5bb} = \frac{2crxyy}{5bb}$, in putting for $y^{\frac{1}{2}}$ its Value, x, equal to $\frac{2}{5}acr$, for the Value of the whole Solid For when x flows into, or becomes equal to a, then y becomes equal to b Whence it follows,

THAT this Solid is to the Cylindric Superficies, described by D E, and multiplied by A H, as 2 to 5, for the Cylindric Superficies, described by D E, and multiplied by A H $= acr$.

EXAMPLE X.

Let it be required to find the Value of the Solid formed by the Rotation of the Hyperbolic Space E G H A B F, *about the Asymptote* G E

DRAW the Asymptote H G $= r$, (*See the following Figure*) the Ordinate Q B $= y$, put H A $= a$, G Q = C B $= x$, and the Circumference described by the Point H $= c$, then will

† the

the Cylindrical Surface, described by the Ordinate HA, be equal to ac. Whence to find the Value of the Cylindric Surface, described by the Ordinate QB, it will be as GH $\times$ HA $= ar : ac ::$ GQ$\times$QB $= xy : \frac{cxy}{r}$. Whence

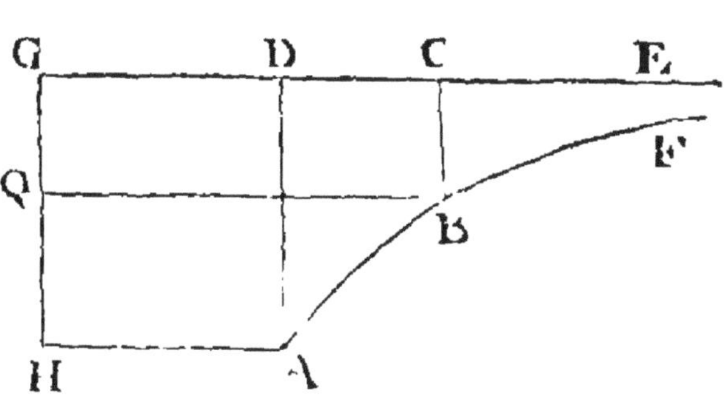

$\frac{cxy\dot{x}}{r}$ will be the Fluxion of the Solid, but because, from the Nature of the Hyperbola, $xy = ar$, therefore $x = \frac{ar}{y}$, consequently $\frac{cxy\dot{x}}{r} = ac\dot{x}$ (by substituting $\frac{ar}{y}$ in the room of x) and acx, the Fluent thence resulting will be the Value of the Solid described by the Space EGHABF, but when the Ordinate QB, by flowing, becomes equal to HA, GQ will become equal to GH, and x will become equal to r, and consequently the whole Solid will be equal to acr.

WHENCE it is evident, that the Solid thus formed is double of the Cylinder formed by the Rectangle GDAH, notwithstanding the Hyperbolic Solid is formed by an infinite Space, and universally if $x = y^m$, which expresses the Nature of all Kinds of Hyperbola's whatsoever, then $y = x^{\frac{1}{m}}$, and consequently if we put $x^{\frac{1}{m}}$ in the room of y, in the Expression $\frac{cxy\dot{x}}{r}$, the Fluxion of the Solid, we

shall

shall have $\frac{c x^{\frac{1}{m}+1} \dot{x}}{r}$, whose Fluent will be $\frac{m c x^{\frac{1}{m}+2}}{\overline{2m+1} \times r}$ $= \frac{m c x x y}{\overline{2m+1} \times r}$ (by substituting y in the room of $x^{\frac{1}{m}}$, to which it is equal Whence $\frac{m}{2m+1} a c r$, will be the Value of the whole Solid.

EXAMPLE XI.

The same Things being supposed, as in the former Example, let it be required to find the Value of the Solid formed by the Rotation of the Hyperbolic Space EGHABF, *about the other Asymptote* GH (*See the preceding Figure.*)

PUT AH $= r$, and the Circumference described by the Point A $= c$, and it will be as r c y $\frac{c y}{r}$ equal to the Circumference of the Circle described by the Point B, whence $\frac{c y y}{2r}$ will be the Area of the Circle described by the Ordinate QB, consequently $\frac{c y y \dot{x}}{2r}$ will be the Fluxion of the Solid But because, from the Nature of the Curve, $x y = a r$, therefore $y = \frac{a r}{x}$, and $y y = \frac{a a r r}{x x}$ Substituting therefore $\frac{a a r r}{x x}$ in the room of $y y$ in the former Equation, we shall have $\frac{a a c r \dot{x}}{2 x x} = \frac{a a c r x^{-2} \dot{x}}{2}$, the Fluent of which will be

$a a c r$

$\frac{aacr}{-2x}$ for the Value of the Solid described by the Space H A B Q, which will give $\frac{acr}{-2}$ for the Value of the whole Solid, for when the Point Q arrives at H, x becomes equal to a, and universally, if $y^m = x$, then $\dot{x} = my^{m-1}\dot{y}$, and substituting this Quantity $my^{m-1}\dot{y}$, in the Expression $\frac{cyy\dot{x}}{2r}$, the Fluxion of the Solid, in the room of $\dot{x}$, we shall have $\frac{mcy^{m+1}\dot{y}}{2r}$, whose Fluent will be $\frac{mcy^{m+2}}{2m+4\times r} = \frac{mcxyy}{2m+4\times r}$ (by putting x in the room of y^m), whence the Value of the whole Solid will be $\frac{m}{2m+4}acr$, because when x, by flowing, becomes equal to a, y, by flowing, will become equal to r

EXAMPLE XII.

Let it be required to find the Value of the Hyperbolic Conoid formed by the Rotation of the Hyperbola A C F D, *about its Axis* A D

HAVING drawn an Ordinate, as B C, put D F = r, B C = y, A B = x, A D = a, and A E = $2b$ then will E D = $a + 2b$, and E B = $x + 2b$, and the Area of the Circle generated by the Ordinate B C = $\frac{cyy}{2r}$, whence $\frac{cyy\dot{x}}{2r}$ will be the Fluxion of the Solid and because, from the Nature of the Hyperbola, as ED × AD : DF² :: EB × AB : BC², therefore

fore $aa + 2ab \quad rr \quad xx + 2bx \quad yy$, whence $yy = \frac{rrxx + 2brrx}{aa + 2ab}$. Putting thefore this last Expression in the room of yy, in the Fluxion of the Solid $\frac{cyy\dot{x}}{2r}$, we shall have $\frac{crxx\dot{x} + 2bcrx\dot{x}}{2aa + 4ab}$, whose Fluent $\frac{crx^3}{6aa + 12ab} + \frac{bcrxx}{2aa + 4ab} = \frac{crx^3 + 3bcrx^2}{6aa + 12ab}$, for the Value of the Solid formed by the Space A B C, whence $\frac{aacr + 3abcr}{6a + 12b}$ will be the Value of the whole Solid, for when A B flows into, or becomes equal to A D, x will become equal to a Whence it follows,

THAT the circumscribed Cylinder is to the inscribed Hyperbolic Conoid, as $3a + 6b$ is to $a + 3b$, for the Cylinder is $\frac{1}{2}acr$.

EXAMPLE XIII

Let it be required to find the Value of the Solid formed by the Rotation of the Hyperbolic Space A C D F E, *about the Line* E F, *the half of the Conjugate Axis of the Hyperbola* A C D.

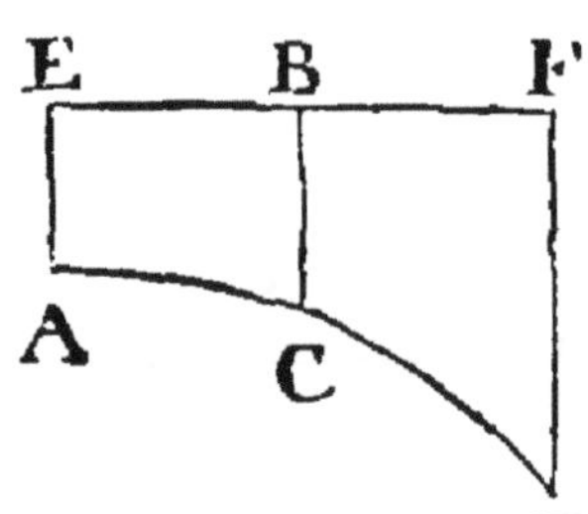

FROM any Point, as C, let the Ordinate C B be drawn, it is manifest that this Ordinate will, by the Rotation of the Hyperbolic Space about the Line E F, describe a Circle, put therefore c for the Circumference of the Circle described by the Point D, also E A $= a$, E F $= b$, E B $= x$, B C $= y$, and D F $= r$, then will the Area of the Circle, described by the Ordinate B C, be be $\frac{cyy}{2r}$; whence $\frac{cyy\dot{x}}{2r}$, will be the Fluxion of the Solid; because, from the Nature of the Hyperbola, as $xx : yy - aa :: bb : aa$, therefore $aaxx = bbyy - bbaa$, and $bbyy = aaxx + aabb$, and $yy = \frac{aaxx + aabb}{bb}$. Putting therefore this Value in $\frac{cyy\dot{x}}{2r}$, the Fluxion of the Solid, we shall have $\frac{aacxx\dot{x} + aabbc\dot{x}}{2bbr}$, whose Fluent will be $\frac{aacx^3}{6bbr} + \frac{aacx}{2r}$, and putting $\frac{bbyy}{xx+bb}$ in the room of aa, we shall have $\frac{cx^3yy}{6rxx+6bbr} + \frac{bbcyyx}{2rxx+2bbr}$ for the Value of the Solid formed by the Rotation of the Space ACBE.

Now if we consider the Ordinate BC in a flowing State, and to move 'till it arrive at, or coincide with the Ordinate DF, then EB will become equal to EF, x will become equal to b, y will become equal to r, and we shall have $\frac{1}{3}bcr$ for the Value of the Solid formed by the Rotation of the whole Space AEFD.

Whence it is evident, that the circumscribed Cylinder is to the inscribed Solid, as 3 to 2, for $\frac{1}{2}bcr : \frac{1}{3}bcr$, as 3 to 2.

EXAMPLE XIV.

Let it be required to find the Value of a Spheroid formed by the Rotation of the Semi Ellipsis ACD, *about its longer Axis, or transverse Diameter* AD.

Having drawn the Semi conjugate Diameter $FE = r$, and the Ordinate $CB = y$, put $AD = 2a$, $EB = x$, then

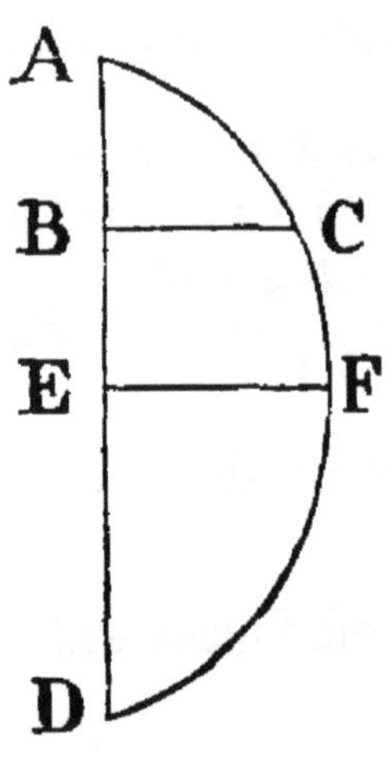

$AB = a - x$, and $BD = a + x$ whence we shall have $\frac{cy}{2r} \times y = \frac{cyy}{2r}$ for the Area of the Circle described by the Ordinate BC. This therefore being multiplied by $\dot{x}$, the Fluxion of the Diameter AD, will give $\frac{cyy\dot{x}}{2r}$, for the Fluxion of the Solid, but because, from the Nature of the Ellipsis, as $\overline{CB}^2 : \overline{AB} \times \overline{BD} :: \overline{FE}^2 : \overline{AE}^2$; therefore as $yy : aa - xx :: rr : aa$, whence $yy = rr - \frac{rrxx}{aa}$, and putting this Value of yy, in the Fluxion of the Solid, instead of yy, we shall have $\frac{cr\dot{x}}{2} - \frac{crxx\dot{x}}{2aa}$, for the Fluxion of the Solid formed by the Rotation of the Space CBEF, whose Fluent $\frac{crx}{2} - \frac{crx^3}{6aa}$, will give the Value of the same Solid. Now if we imagine the Ordinate BC in a flowing State, and to move 'till the Point B arrives at, or coincides with the Point A, then EB will become equal to EA, and x will become equal to a, and we shall have $\frac{cra}{2} - \frac{cra^3}{6aa} = \frac{1}{3}cra$ for the Value of the Solid formed by the Rotation of the Quadrantal Space AEF; whence $\frac{2}{3}cra$ will be the Value of the whole Spheroid. Whence it follows,

First, THAT the Spheroid described about the longest Axis, is to its circumscribing Cylinder as 2 to 3, and since the Cylinder is to the Cone as 3 to 1, it follows, that the Spheroid is to the Cone as 2 to 1.

Secondly, THAT the Spheroid is to the circumscribing Sphere, as the Square of the lesser Axis of the Ellipsis is to the Square of the greater Axis.

Thirdly, THAT the Spheroid is to its inscribed Sphere, as the longest Axis is to the shortest; and so is any Segment of the Spheroid to the correspondent Segment of the inscribed Sphere; whence the Value of any Segment of a Spheroid, or any Portion of it cut off by two parallel Planes, may be easily found.

Fourthly, THAT the Sphere has the same Ratio to its circumscribing Cylinder as the Spheroid has to its circumscribing Cylinder; also that the Sphere and Spheroid are in the same Ratio as their inscribed Cones and circumscribed Cylinders, which have for their Base the great Circle of the Sphere, and the same common Height.

AFTER the same manner it may be proved, that the Spheroid formed by the Rotation of an Ellipsis, about its shortest Diameter, is to its circumscribed Cylinder as 2 to 3, and that the Spheroid formed by the Rotation of an Ellipsis about its longest Axis, is to the Spheroid formed by the Rotation of an Ellipsis about its shortest Axis, as the longest Axis to the shortest.

EXAMPLE XV.

To find the Value of the Solid formed by the Rotation of the Logarithmic Space A C D F E, *about its Asymptote* F E.

HAVING drawn the Ordinate BC $= y$, (*See the following Figure*) put EB $= x$, FD $= r$, and c for the Circumference described by the Point D, then will $\frac{cyy}{2r}$ be the Area of the Circle described by the Ordinate BC. This therefore being multiplied by $\dot{x}$, the Fluxion of the Asymptote FE, will give $\frac{cyy\dot{x}}{2r}$ for the Fluxion of the Solid; but because, from the

Pro-

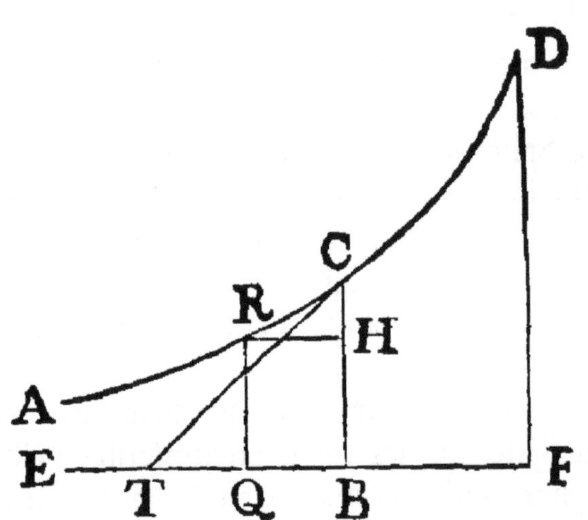

Property of the Logarithmic Curve $x = \frac{ay}{\dot{y}}$, if we substitute this Value of x in the Expression $\frac{cyyx}{2r}$, in the room of x, we shall have $\frac{acy\dot{y}}{2r}$, for the Fluxion of the Solid generated by the Rotation of the infinite Space E B C A, whose Fluent $\frac{acyy}{4r}$, will give the Value of the same Solid

Now if we imagine the Ordinate B C to move in the Direction B F, 'till it arrive at, and coincide with the Ordinate F D, then y will become equal to r, and we shall have $\frac{1}{4}acr$ for the Value of the Solid formed by the Rotation of the whole Logarithmic Space A C D F E Whence it follows,

That the Solid formed by the Rotation of the infinite Space E F D A, is to the Cone, which hath for its Altitude the Subtangent of the Curve, and for its Base the same as the Solid, as 3 to 2, for the Value of the Cone is $\frac{acr}{6}$, and as

$\frac{1}{4}$ $\frac{1}{6}$ 3 2

EXAMPLE XVI

On O, as a Center, (*See the following Figure*) with the Radius O D, describe the Semi-circle A D G, and produce D O 'till O E be equal to D O; then on E, as a Center, with the Radius E A, describe the Quadrant A F G, and compleat the Parallelogram A H I G A.

Let

Let now the whole Space H A F G I be turned about the Line H I, as an Axis, and let it be required to find the Value of the Solid thus described.

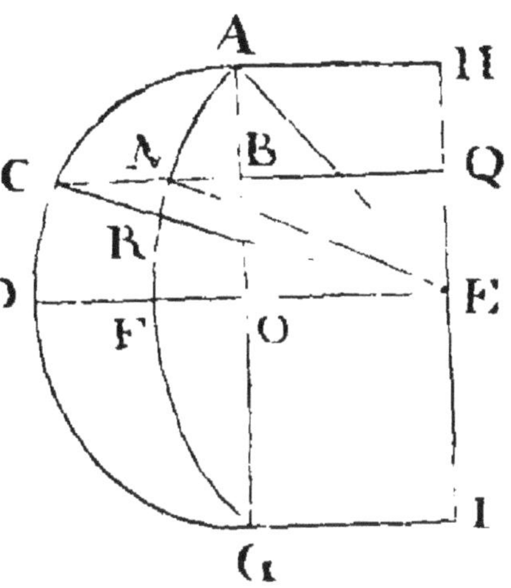

From any Point N of the Arch A F G, let an Ordinate, as N B, be drawn, and let it be produced 'till it cut the Line H I in Q, then put c for the Circumference of the Circle described by the Point F, N B $=z$, B Q $=r$, A B $=x$, N Q $=r+z$, and because the Circumference of the Circle described by the Point F, is to the Circumference of the Circle described by the Point N, as F E to N Q, it will be as $r\sqrt{2}$

c $r+z$ $\frac{cr+cz}{r\sqrt{2}}$ equal to the Circumference described by the Point N, and multiplying this Quantity by $\frac{r\dot{x}+z\dot{x}}{2}$, we shall have $\frac{crr\dot{x}+2crz\dot{x}+czz\dot{x}}{2r\sqrt{2}}$, for the Fluxion of the Solid. But from the Nature of the Space $\overline{NQ}^2-\overline{BQ}^2$ $=AB\times BG$, therefore $2rz+zz=2rx-xx$. Putting then $2rx-xx$, in the room of $2rz+zz$, we shall have $\frac{crr\dot{x}+2crx\dot{x}-cxx\dot{x}}{2r\sqrt{2}}$, whose Fluent $\frac{crx}{2\sqrt{2}}+\frac{cxx}{2\sqrt{2}}$ $-\frac{cx^3}{6r\sqrt{2}}$, will give the Value of the Solid formed by the Rotation of the Space H A N Q. Now if we imagine the Ordinate N B to move according to the Direction B G, 'till the Point B arrives at, and coincides with the Point G, then x will

will become equal to $2r$, and we ſhall have $\frac{crr}{\sqrt{2}} + \frac{2crr}{\sqrt{2}} - \frac{4crr}{3 \times \sqrt{2}}$ for the Value of the Solid formed by the Rotation of the whole Space A H F G I

It is evident, that the firſt Member $\frac{crr}{\sqrt{2}} =$ to the Cylinder deſcribed by the Rotation of the Rectangle A H I G about the Line H I, and that the two other Members $\frac{2crr}{\sqrt{2}} - \frac{4crr}{3\sqrt{2}} = \frac{2crr}{3\sqrt{2}}$ are equal to the Sphere deſcribed by the Rotation of the Semi-circle A D G about the Diameter A G; for in this Caſe the Circumference is equal to $\frac{c}{\sqrt{2}}$. Whence the Solid formed by the Segment A F G A, is equal to the Sphere formed by the Semi-circle A D G.

EXAMPLE XVII

The ſame Things being ſuppoſed, as in the former Example, let it be required to find the Value of the Solid formed by the Rotation of the Lunula A D G F A *about the Line* H I, *as an Axis (See the Figure belonging to the former Example)*

Produce the Ordinate Q B to meet the Semi circumference in C, and let the whole Surface H A C D G I be turned round the Line H I, as an Axis, then will the Line Q C generate a Circle, and putting D E $= 2r$, C B $= y$, A B $= x$, then will C Q $= r + y$, alſo let c ſtand for the Circumference

ci

of the Circle described by the Point D; and to find the Circumference of the Circle generated by the Point C, it will be as $2r$ $c \cdot r+y$ $\frac{cr+cy}{2r}$, whence $\frac{crr+2cry+cyy}{4r}$ will be the Area of the same Circle; and because $yy=2rx-xx$, and $y=\overline{2rx-xx}^{\frac{1}{2}}$ Putting then $\overline{2rx-xx}^{\frac{1}{2}}$ in the room of y, and multiplying by $\dot{x}$, we shall have $\frac{crr\dot{x}+2crx\dot{x}-cx x\dot{x}+2cr\dot{x}\times\overline{2rx-xx}^{\frac{1}{2}}}{4r}$ for the Fluxion of the Solid, whose Fluent $\frac{crx}{4}+\frac{cxx}{4}-\frac{cx^3}{12r}$ +, the Fluent of $\frac{c\dot{x}\times\overline{2rx-xx}^{\frac{1}{2}}}{2}=\frac{crx}{4}+\frac{cxx}{4}-\frac{cx^3}{12r}$ $+\frac{c}{2}\times$ ABCA, will give the Value of the indeterminate Portion of the Solid described by the Space HACQ, which gives $\frac{crr}{2}+crr-\frac{2}{3}crr+\frac{c}{2}\times$ ADGA $=\frac{crr}{2}+\frac{1}{3}$ $crr+\frac{ccr}{16}$ (for the Space ADGA $=\frac{cr}{8}$) for the whole Solid; because when the Point B, by flowing, arrives at G, x becomes equal to $2r$

Now the first Member $\frac{crr}{2}$ is equal to the Cylinder described by the Rectangle AHIG, for its Circumference is equal to $\frac{c}{2}$, then the two other Members are equal in Value to the Solid formed by the Rotation of the Semi circle ADG about the Line HI. Taking away then from this Value the Solid formed by the Rotation of the Segment AFGA equal to $\frac{1}{3}crr$ (by the preceding Example) equal to the Value of the Sphere formed

formed by the Rotation of the Semi circle A D B, the Remainder $\frac{1}{16} c r r$, will be the Value of the Solid formed by the Rotation of the *Lunula* A D G F A about the Line H I.

WHENCE it is evident, that if the Value of this Solid could be exactly determined, the Quadrature of the Circle would be determined also.

EXAMPLE XVIII.

Let it be required to find the Value of the Solid formed by the Rotation of the Cissoidal Space G A D F, *about its Asymptote* D F

PUT B C $= y$, A B $= x$, A D $= 2r$, then will B D $= 2r - x$, and, from the Nature of the Circle, B C $= \overline{2rx - xx}^{\frac{1}{2}}$, but because, from the Property of the Cissoid, as D B : B C :: A B : B N, it will be as $r - x$: $\overline{2rx - xx}^{\frac{1}{2}} :: x : \frac{x \times \overline{2rx - xx}^{\frac{1}{2}}}{r - x}$ = B N, but as $r : c :: $ (D B =) $r - x . \frac{c \times \overline{r - x}}{r}$, the Circumference generated by the Point B. This therefore being multiplied by $\frac{x \times \overline{2rx - xx}^{\frac{1}{2}}}{r - x}$, the Value of B N, will give $\frac{cx \times \overline{2rx - xx}^{\frac{1}{2}}}{r}$, for the Surface generated by the Rotation of the Ordinate B N. This again being multiplied by $\dot{x}$, will give $\frac{cx\dot{x} \times \overline{2rx - xx}^{\frac{1}{2}}}{r}$, for the Fluxion of the Solid

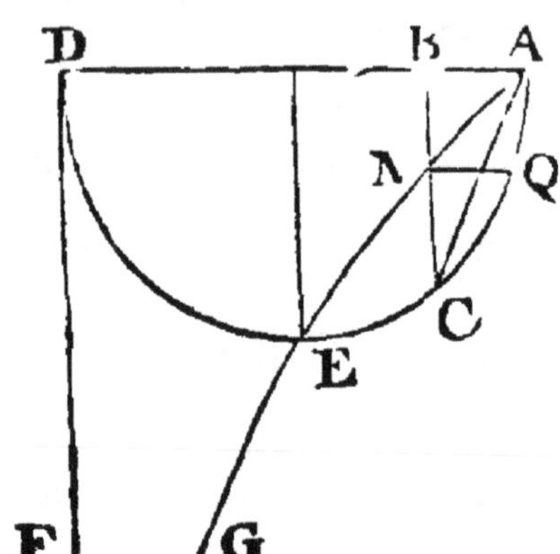

genera-

generated by the Rotation of the Space G A D F about the Asymptote D F.

AND to find its Fluent, imagine the generating Semi-circle A E D, to revolve about an Axis parallel to the Asymptote D F, and to pass by the Point A, then will the Ordinate BC describe a Cylindrical Surface, whence we shall have $\frac{c\,x\,x \times \overline{2rx - xx}^{\frac{1}{2}}}{r}$, for the Fluxion of this Solid, which being the same with the Fluxion of the former Solid, it is manifest, that the Solid formed by the Rotation of the Cissoidal Space, infinitely extended about one of its Asymptotes, is equal to a Solid formed by the Rotation of its generating Semi circle about a right Line parallel to its Asymptote passing through the Point A.

AGAIN, because $\frac{c\,x\,x \times \overline{2rx - xx}^{\frac{1}{2}}}{r} = \frac{c}{r} \times x^{\frac{1}{2}}\,x \times \overline{2r - x}^{\frac{1}{2}}$ $= \frac{c}{r} \times x^{\frac{1}{2}}\,x \times \overline{1 - x}^{\frac{1}{2}}$ (by putting $2r$, the Diameter of the generating Circle, equal to 1) if we multiply $1 - \frac{1}{2}x - \frac{1}{8}x^2 - \frac{1}{16}x^3 - \frac{5}{128}x^4 - \frac{7}{256}x^5$, &c. the Square Root of $\overline{1 - x}$ by $x^{\frac{1}{2}}\,x$, we shall have $\frac{c}{r}$ $x^{\frac{1}{2}}x - \frac{1}{2}x^{\frac{3}{2}}x - \frac{1}{8}x^{\frac{5}{2}}x - \frac{1}{16}x^{\frac{7}{2}}x - \frac{5}{128}x^{\frac{9}{2}}x - \frac{7}{256}x^{\frac{11}{2}}x$, &c. for the Fluxion of the Solid generated by the Rotation of the Space G A D F about the Asymptote D F, whose Fluent $\frac{c}{r} \times \frac{2}{5}x^{\frac{5}{2}} - \frac{1}{7}x^{\frac{7}{2}} - \frac{1}{36}x^{\frac{9}{2}} - \frac{1}{88}x^{\frac{11}{2}} - \frac{5}{832}x^{\frac{13}{2}} - \frac{7}{1920}x^{\frac{15}{2}}$, &c. $= \frac{c}{r}x^{\frac{3}{2}} \times \frac{2}{5}x - \frac{1}{7}xx - \frac{1}{36}x^3$

$$x^3 - \frac{1}{88}x^4 - \frac{5}{832}x^5 - \frac{7}{1920}x^6, \text{\&c.} = \frac{c}{r}x^{\frac{1}{2}} \times \frac{1\times2}{1\times5}x -$$

$$-\frac{1\times2}{1\times7}xx - \frac{1\times1\times2}{2\times4\times9}x^3 - \frac{1\times1\times3\times2}{2\times4\times6\times11}x^4 -$$

$$-\frac{1\times1\times3\times5\times2}{2\times4\times6\times8\times13}x^5 - \frac{1\times1\times3\times5\times7\times2}{2\times4\times6\times8\times10\times15}x^6, \text{\&c.}$$

will give the Value of the Solid generated by the Rotation of the same Space.

EXAMPLE XIX.

Let it be required to find the Value of the Solid formed by the Rotation of the Conchoidal Space F B A D N E, *about its Asymptote* D E.

LET the Conchoid be such, that having drawn from some Point in the Curve, as B, to its Pole C, a Line, as B C cutting the Asymptote in the Point N, the Rectangle under C N and N B, that is, C N × N B may be equal to the Rectangle C D × D A, and let it be required to find the Value of the Solid generated by the Conchoidal Space

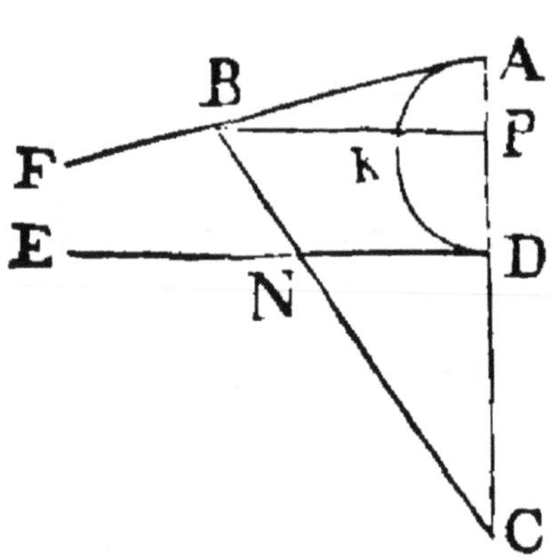

HAVING described upon the Diameter A D a Semi-circle A K D, from some Point, as P, in the Diameter draw an Ordinate, as P B, it is manifest that this Ordinate P B will, by the Rotation of the Conchoidal Space about the Line E D, describe a Cylindric Surface

PUT A C $= a$, A D $= 2r$, A P $= x$; then C P $= a - x$, and P D $= 2r - x$. Put also P B $= z$, and P K $= y$, and because, from the Nature of the Conchoid, as A P . P D

1 PB²

$\overline{PB}^2$ $\overline{CP}^2$, therefore as x $\overline{2r-x}$ zz $\overline{aa-2ax+xx}$, whence $zz\times\overline{2r-x}=aax-2ax^2+x^3$, whence you will have $z=\overline{a-x}\times\sqrt{\frac{x}{2r-x}}$, and to find the Cylindric Surface described by P B, we must say, as r c P D $\times$ P B $=\overline{2r-x}\times\overline{a-x}\sqrt{\frac{x}{2r-x}}$. $\frac{2acr-acx}{r}$

$\frac{-2crx+cxx}{r}\times\sqrt{\frac{x}{2r-x}}$, which being multiplied by x we shall have the Fluxion of the Solid.

Now in order to find the Fluent, imagine the Semi-circle AKD to revolve about a Line parallel to the Asymptote D E, and to pass through the Point C, the Pole of the Conchoid, it is then manifest, that the Line PK will describe a Cylindrical Surface. Wherefore as r c PK$\times$PC $=\overline{a-x}\sqrt{2rx-xx}$ $\frac{\overline{ac-cx}\times\overline{2rx-xx}^{\frac{1}{2}}}{r}$ equal to the Cylindric Surface described by the Line PK, but KP$\times$PC $=\overline{a-x}\times\overline{2rx-xx}^{\frac{1}{2}}$ $=$ PD$\times$PB $=\overline{2r-x}\times\overline{a-x}\sqrt{\frac{x}{2r-x}}$; for as AP PD $\overline{PK}^2$ $\overline{PD}^2$, whence as PK PD PB CP, whence the Fluxion of these two Solids are equal, consequently their Fluents will be the same. Wherefore the Solid formed by the Rotation of the Conchoidal Space, infinitely extended about its Asymptote, is equal to a Solid formed by the Revolution of a Semi-circle A K D, about a Line parallel to its Asymptote passing through its Pole.

EXAM-

EXAMPLE XX.

Let it be required to find the Value of the Solid formed by the Rotation of the Curvilinear Space A C D *about the Axis* A D, *the general Equation, expressing the Nature of the Curve, being* $y = \frac{\overline{a-x} \times x^{\frac{m}{n}}}{a^{\frac{m}{n}}}$.

Having drawn the Ordinate B C $= y$, and putting r for the greater Ordinate, and c for the Circumference of the Circle generated by it, we shall have $\frac{cyy}{2r}$ for the Circumference described by the Ordinate B C, and $\frac{cyy\dot{x}}{2r}$ for the Fluxion of the Solidity, but because y

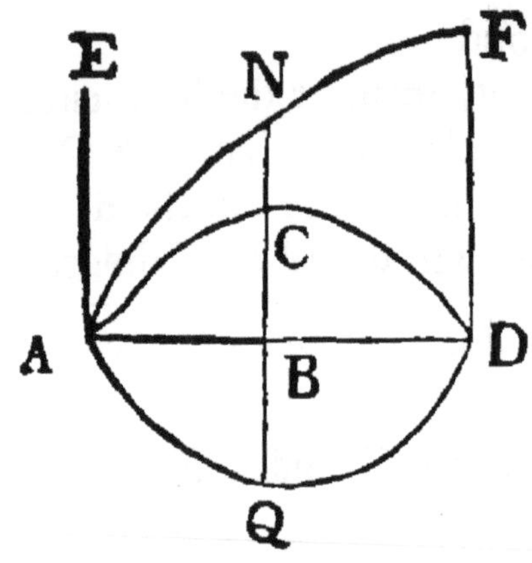

$= \frac{\overline{a-x} \times x^{\frac{m}{n}}}{a^{\frac{m}{n}}}$ then $yy = \frac{aax^{\frac{2m}{n}} - 2ax^{\frac{2m}{n}+1} + x^{\frac{2m}{n}+2}}{a^{\frac{2m}{n}}}$; and putting this Value in the room of yy, in the Fluxion of the Solid $\frac{cyy\dot{x}}{2r}$, we shall have $\frac{aacx^{\frac{2m}{n}}\dot{x} - 2acx^{\frac{2m}{n}+1}\dot{x} + cxc^{\frac{1m}{n}+1}\dot{x}}{2ra^{\frac{2m}{n}}}$

the Fluent of which $\frac{naacx^{\frac{2m}{n}+1}}{\overline{4m+2n}r \times a^{\frac{1m}{n}}} - \frac{nacx^{\frac{2m}{n}+2}}{\overline{2m+2n}r \times a^{\frac{2m}{n}}} +$

+

$+ \frac{n c x^{\frac{2m}{n}+3}}{4m+6nr \times a^{\frac{2m}{n}}}$, will be the Value of the Solid formed by the Revolution of the Space A C B, whence the whole Solid, described by the Revolution of the Space A C D, will be $\frac{n a^3 c}{4m+2nr} - \frac{n a^3 c}{2m+2nr} + \frac{n a^3 c}{4m+6nr} =$

$\frac{n^3 a^3 c}{8m^3 + 24mmn + 22mnn}$; for when B, by flowing, arrives at D, x becomes equal to a

IF $m = 2$, and $n = 1$, the Value of the Solid found by the Rotation of the Space A B C, will be found to be equal to $\frac{c x^5}{10 a a r} - \frac{c x^6}{6 a^3 r} + \frac{c x^7}{14 a^4 r}$, and the entire Solid will be equal to $\frac{a^3 c}{210 r}$. Now by the Method *de Maximis & Minimis*, x being equal to $\frac{2}{3} a$, we shall have, by putting this Value in the Equation of the Curve $a a y = a x x - x^3$ for the greatest Ordinate $y = r$, $\frac{4}{27} a$. Whence $\frac{a^3 c}{210 r} = \frac{9 a a c}{280}$. Now the circumscribing Cylinder having for the Radius of its Base the greatest Ordinate, and for its Height the Axis A D, its Value will be $\frac{2}{27} a a c$ Whence the Solid formed by the Rotation of the Curve A C D, is to its circumscribed Cylinder as 243 to 560.

THE Value of the Solids formed by the Rotation of the Curves A N F, A Q D, and their Ratio to each other, may be found with the same Ease.

SECT. V.

Containing the Uſe of FLUXIONS *in finding the Centers of* Gravity *of Lines and Surfaces.*

DEFINITION

THE Center of Gravity of a Body, is a Point within that Body ſo placed, that the Particles of the Body, at equal Diſtances from that Point, conſiſt of equal *Momenta*, or have equal Propenſities, or Tendencies to Motion; ſo that by the mutual and contrary Endeavours of all the Particles of which the Body is compoſed, if the Body be ſuſpended or ſuſtained by this Point, in whatſoever Situation it is placed, it will retain it, and remain at Reſt.

NOW ſince by the *Momentum* of any Body, we are to underſtand a Reſult ariſing from the Multiplication of the Quantity of Matter it contains, into the Velocity it is moved with, and as the ſame Body may be impelled with different Degrees of Force

HENCE it is, that the *Momenta* of the ſame Body are of different Values, according to the different Velocities with which it may be moved, or according to its different Propenſities, or Tendencies to Motion.

FOR Example, If two Bodies, A and B, of equal Denſity, and containing equal Quantities of Matter, be made to move with different Velocities, that is, if the Velocity with which the Body A is made to move, be double to the Velocity with which the Body B is made to move, then the *Momentum* of the Body A is, in this Caſe, double to the *Momentum* of the Body B, and ſince the Bodies A and B are equally denſe, and contain equal Quantities of Matter, one may be taken indifferently for the other, and either of them may be conſidered as one and the ſame Body impelled at different Times with different Degrees of Force, and conſequently the *Momentum* of the ſame Body, in one Caſe, is to its *Momentum* in the other Caſe as 2 to 1,

AND hence it is, that the different *Momenta* of the ſame Body, are in a direct Ratio of the different Velocities with which the Body may be made to move, or according to its different Propenſities, or Tendencies to Motion.

AND hence it is that the *Momentum* of one and the ſame Body may become equal to the *Momentum* of any other Body, how great or ſmall ſoever it be, for if the Velocities with which they move, or would move with, were they at liberty to move, be in a reciprocal Ratio to their Maſſes of Matter, the *Momentum* of one will be equal to the *Momentum* of the other, and conſequently if placed on contrary Sides of their common Center of Gravity, will counterpoiſe one another. For Example, if the Quantity of Matter in the Body A be to the Quantity of Matter in the Body B as 6 to 4, and the Velocity that the Body A moves with, or would move with, were it at liberty to move, be to the Velocity that the Body B moves with, or would move, were it at liberty to move, as 2 to 3, the *Momentum* of the Body A, in this Caſe, will be equal to the *Momentum* of the Body B, ſince $2 \times 6 = 3 \times 4 = 12$

NOW if the Bodies A and B be fixed at the Ends A and B of an inflexible right Line AB, void of Gravity, and that right Line be ſo divided in the Point C, that the Segment CA be to the Segment BC as the Velocity the Body B moves with, or would move with, were it at liberty, to the Velocity the Body A moves with or

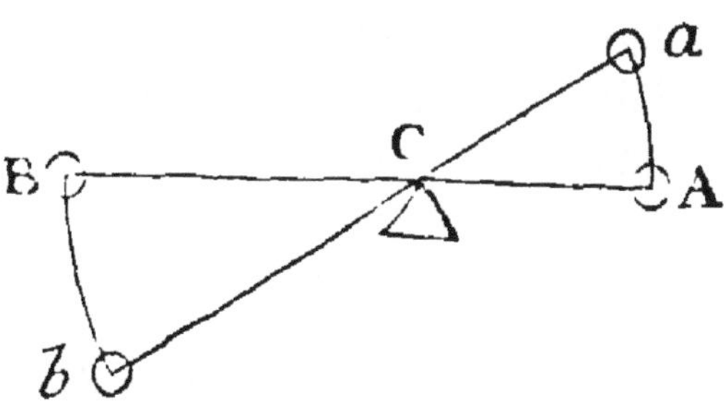

would move with, were it at liberty to move, then their *Momenta* will be equal, and if the inflexible right Line AB be

 ſuſpended

ſuſpended, or ſuſtained by the Point C, inaſmuch as their Propenſities or Tendencies to Motion are equal, and contrary, both will remain at Reſt, and this Point C is called the common Center of Gravity of the two Bodies A and B

FOR let us ſuppoſe the Line B C A to revolve about the Point C as a Center, and to remove from its Situation B C A, into the Situation *b* C *a*, in which time the Body A will move over the Arch A *a*, as will the Body B move over the Arch B *b*, and ſince the Velocities are proportional to the Spaces that the Bodies run over in the ſame Time, and ſince theſe Arches are as their reſpective Radii C A and C B; and moreover, ſince theſe Radii C A and C B are in a reciprocal Ratio to the Quantities of Matter contained in the Bodies C and A, it follows, that the *Momentum* of the Body A is equal to the *Momentum* of the Body B, that their Propenſities, or Tendencies to Motion, are contrary and equal, and both muſt remain at Reſt

AND the ſame Conſequences will follow, if ſeveral Bodies, or Weights, as D, E, F, G, *&c* are fixed to the ſame inflexible Line A B, void of Gravity, ſuſpended, or ſuſtained by the Point C, provided that the Sum of the Products of the Bodies, or Weights on one Side of the Point C, multiplied by their reſpective Diſtances from the ſame Point, be equal to the Products ariſing from the Multiplication of the Bodies on the other Side of the Point C, into their reſpective Diſtances from the ſame Point, for if we ſuppoſe the Body A be divided into two Bodies F and G, and the Bodies F and G, ſuſpended at ſuch Diſtances C K and C B, from the Center C, that $CK \times F + CB \times G = CA \times A$ And again, if we ſuppoſe the Body B, divided in like manner into two Bodies D and E, and each of theſe ſuſpended at ſuch Diſtances C H and C A, from the ſame Point C, ſo that $CH \times E + CA \times D = CB \times B$ Now inaſmuch as $CA \times A = CB \times B$, therefore $CK \times F + CB \times G = CH \times E$

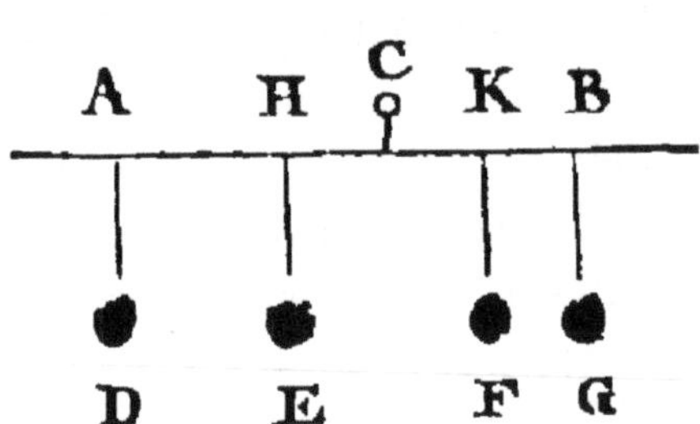

$\times$ E + C A $\times$ D, and the same will hold good, into how great soever a Number of Parts the Bodies A and B be divided, provided the Law of Suspension be observed.

LET us therefore imagine the Matter contained in the Bodies A and B (*See Fig in Pag* 369) which we will suppose to consist of ten Parts, to be equally diffused through the whole Line A B, then will the Quantity contained in the Segment C B, be to the Quantity contained in the Segment C A, as the Line B C is to the Line A B, that is, as 6 to 4, but the Velocity of every conceivable Point of the Segment C B is to the Velocity of every conceivable Point in the Segment C A, at proportional Distances from the Point C, as 3 to 2, consequently the Velocity of the whole Line B C is to the Velocity of the whole Line C A as 3 to 2, whence the *Momentum* of the Segment B C is to the *Momentum* of the Segment A C as 3 $\times$ 6 is to 2 $\times$ 4, or as 18 to 8, or as 9 to 4, and consequently the Segment B C will preponderate. And in order to find the Center of Gravity arising from this new Disposition of the Matter, let us suppose the Line B A to be suspended at one End, as A, then will the Line B A represent the whole Quantity of Matter, as well as the whole Velocity. Putting therefore A B $= x$, $\dot{x}$ will represent the Fluxion of the Line A B; that is, of the Weight or Matter represented by it Now if we consider the Line A B in a flowing State, and beginning to revolve about the Point A, as a Center, it is manifest, that $x\dot{x}$ will be the Fluxion of the *Momentum* of the whole Mass into the whole Velocity, whence $\frac{1}{2}xx$, its Fluent, will give the whole *Momentum*, this therefore being divided by x, the whole Weight or Mass, will give $\frac{1}{2}x$ for the Distance of the Center of Gravity from the Point of Suspension A, equal to half the Line A B, for as the *Momentum* is a Result of the Multiplication of the Velocity into the Quantity of Matter, so the Velocity (which is in every conceivable Point of the Line A B, as the Distance of the Center of Gravity from the Point of

B A

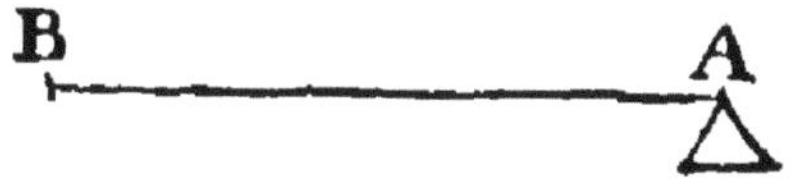

Suspension, and is therefore analogous to it, and may be represented by it) is a Result of the Division of the *Momentum* by the Quantity of Matter contained in the Mass, and as the *Momentum* of each Particle of which a Surface or Solid consists, arises from the Multiplication of the Quantity of Matter it contains, into its respective Distance from the Axis of Suspension, so if the whole *Momentum* be divided by the total Gravity, the Quotient will give the Distance of a Point from the Point of Suspension, by which if the Body be sustained, or suspended, it will remain at Rest; from whence we may draw this general Rule for finding the Center of Gravity.

DIVIDE the *Momentum* of the whole Weight, or Mass, by the whole Weight, or Mass, and the Quotient thence resulting will give the Distance of the Center of Gravity from the Point or Axis of Suspension, which will always be found in that right Line that divides the Surface into two equal Parts, which, for Distinction sake, I call the Axis of *Equilibrium*, as I do the Point, where this Axis cuts the Perimeter of the Surface, the Point of Suspension

WHEREFORE let C A C B C represent a Curvilinear Space, A B its Axis, and A the Point of Suspension Put A B $= x$, B C $= y$, and let the Nature of the Curve be such, that $x = yy$, then will $x^{\frac{1}{2}} = y$, and $\dot{x}y = x^{\frac{1}{2}}\dot{x}$, be the Fluxion of the Mass, or whole Weight, whence $\frac{2}{3}x^{\frac{3}{2}}$ will be the Mass, and $x^{\frac{3}{2}}\dot{x}$ will be the Fluxion of the *Momentum*, consequently its Fluent $\frac{2}{5}x^{\frac{5}{2}}$ will be the *Momentum* itself. This therefore being divided by $\frac{2}{3}x^{\frac{3}{2}}$ the Mass, will give $\frac{3}{5}x$ for the Distance of the Center of Gravity D from the Point of Suspension A, and by the same Method of Investigation may the Center of Gravity of any other Surface be found, as will appear from the following Examples.

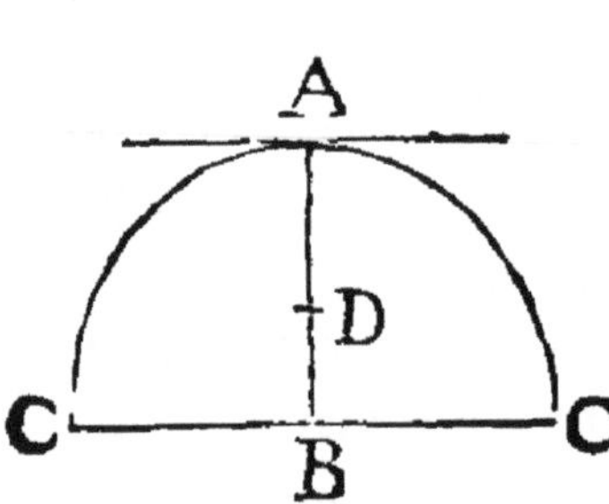

EXAM-

EXAMPLE I

Let it be required to find the Center of Gravity of a Parallelogram A H I D

LET S E repreſent the Axis, and S the Point of Suſpenſion. Put $A D = S E = a$, $A H = C C = b$, and $S B = x$, then will $b \dot{x}$ be the Fluxion of the Maſs, and $b x$ the Fluent thence reſulting will be the Maſs itſelf Now if we multiply $b \dot{x}$ by x the Velocity, we ſhall have $b \dot{x} x$ for the Fluxion of the *Momentum*, whoſe Fluent $\frac{b x x}{2}$ will be the *Momentum* This therefore being divided by $b x$, the whole Maſs, will give $\frac{x}{2}$ for the Diſtance of the Center of Gravity from the Point of Suſpenſion S, but when S B, by flowing, becomes equal to S E, x becomes equal to a, and conſequently $\frac{1}{2} a$ will be the Diſtance of the Center of Gravity of the Parallelogram A H I D, from the Point of Suſpenſion S, equal to $\frac{1}{2}$ the Axis S E

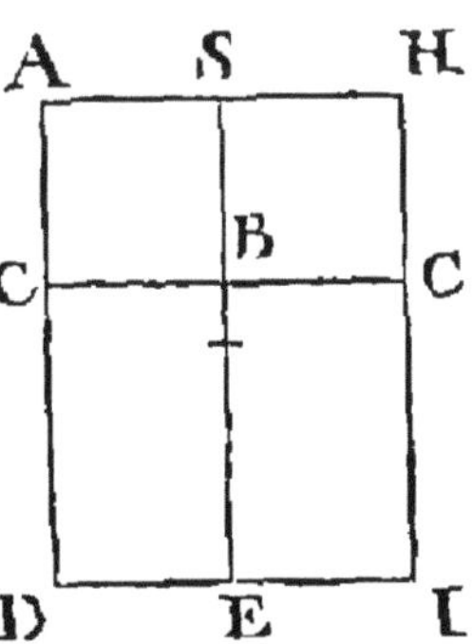

EXAMPLE II.

Let it be required to find the Center of Gravity of a Triangle D A E

DRAW the Line A H, cutting the Baſe D E in equal Parts in the Point H, then will the Triangles D A H and E A H be equal, and conſequently the Center of Gravity will be found ſomewhere in the Line A H Alſo from A draw the Line A F perpendicular to the Baſe D E, and put $A F = h$, $A H = a$, $D E = b$, $A N = z$, $A B = x$, and $C C = y$, then will $y \dot{z}$ be the

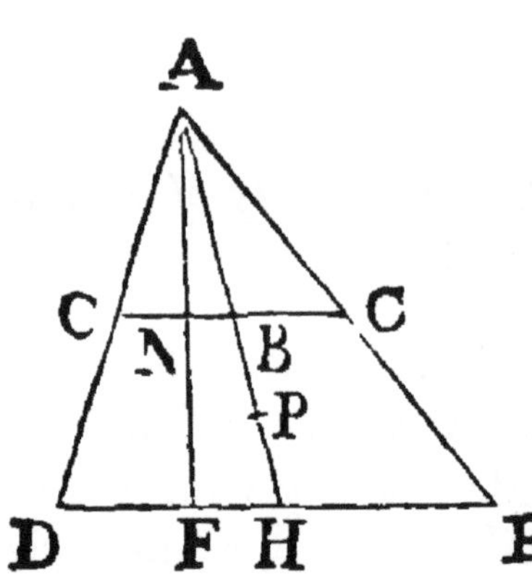

the Fluxion of the Mass; but because the Triangles N A B and F A H are similar, as $z . x \therefore h . a$; therefore $z = \frac{xh}{a}$, and $\dot{z} = \frac{h\dot{x}}{a}$; consequntly $y\dot{z} = \frac{hy\dot{x}}{a}$. Again, because of the Similitude of the Triangles A C C and A D E, it will be as $y \cdot x \therefore b . a$. Wherefore $y = \frac{bx}{a}$, and substituting $\frac{bx}{a}$ in $\frac{hy\dot{x}}{a}$ in the room of y, we shall have $\frac{bhx\dot{x}}{aa}$ for the Fluxion of the Mass, or whole Weight, whose Fluent $\frac{bhxx}{2aa}$ will be the Mass. Again, if $\frac{bhx\dot{x}}{aa}$ be multiplied by the Velocity x, we shall have $\frac{bhxx\dot{x}}{aa}$ for the Fluxion of the *Momentum*, the Fluent of which is $\frac{bhxxx}{3aa}$. This therefore being divided by $\frac{bhxx}{2aa}$, the whole Mass, will give $\frac{2}{3}x$ for the Center of Gravity of the Triangle C A C, but when C C flows into the Place of D E, then A B will become equal to A H, x will become equal to a, and we shall have $\frac{2}{3}a$ for the Distance of the Center of Gravity of the Triangle D A E, from the Point of Suspension A.

Wherefore if the Line A H, which divides the Triangle D A E into two equal Parts, be divided in the Point P, so that A P be to P H as 2 to 1, the Point P will be the Center of Gravity of the Triangle.

CO-

COROLLARY

If the Triangle A D E be an Isosceles Triangle, then the Lines A H, A F will coincide, and the Distance of the Center of Gravity from A, the Point of Suspension, will be $\frac{2}{3}$ of A F, the Perpendicular let fall from the Vertex of the Triangle on the Base D E

EXAMPLE III.

Let it be required to find the Center of Gravity of the Parabolic Space E A E

Put AD $= a$, EE $= b$, AB $= x$, BC $= y$, then will $2 y \dot{x}$ be the Fluxion of the Mass, or whole Weight; but because, from the Nature of the Parabola, $1 x = y y$, whence $x^{\frac{1}{2}} = y$, and $2 x^{\frac{1}{2}} = 2 y$ Substituting therefore $2 x^{\frac{1}{2}}$ instead of $2 y$ in the Expression $2 y \dot{x}$, we shall have $2 x^{\frac{1}{2}} \dot{x}$ for the Fluxion of the Mass, whose Fluent $\frac{4 x^{\frac{3}{2}}}{3}$ will be the Mass, or whole Weight.

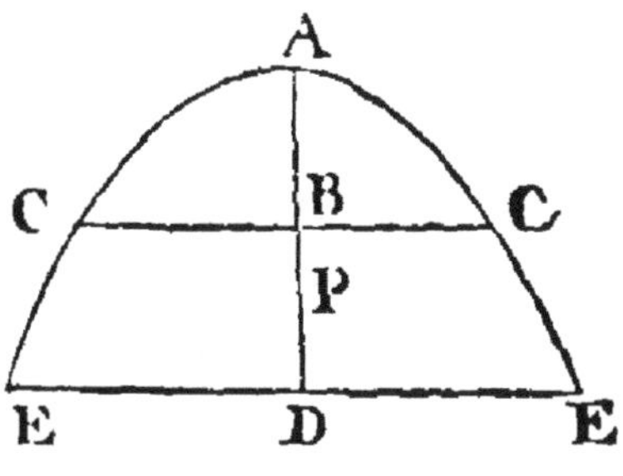

Now if we multiply $2 x^{\frac{1}{2}} \dot{x}$ by x, the Velocity, we shall have $2 x^{\frac{1}{2}} x \dot{x}$, for the Fluxion of the *Momentum*, whose Fluent $\frac{4 x^{\frac{5}{2}}}{5}$ will be the *Momentum* itself. This therefore being divided $\frac{4 x^{\frac{3}{2}}}{3}$, the whole Weight, will give $\frac{12}{20} x^{\frac{5}{2}-\frac{3}{2}} = \frac{3}{5} x$ for the Distance of the Center of Gravity of the Space C A C B, from the Point of Suspension A; but when the Line C B C flows into the Place of E D E, A B becomes equal to A D, the Points B and D will coincide, and x will become equal to a; whence

whence $\frac{1}{5}a$ will be the Diſtance of the Center of Gravity from the Point of Suſpenſion A, of the whole Parabolic Space EAEDE.

Now if we ſuppoſe $y^m = 1\,x$, which is a general Equation for all kinds of Parabolas, we ſhall have $y = x^{\frac{1}{m}}$, conſequently $x^{\frac{1}{m}}\dot{x}$ will be the Fluxion of the whole Maſs, as will $x^{\frac{1}{m}+1}\dot{x}$ be the Fluxion of the *Momentum*. Now if the Fluent of this laſt Fluxion, which is $\frac{m}{2m+1}x^{\frac{1}{m}+2}$, be divided by the Fluent of $x^{\frac{1}{m}}\dot{x}$, which is $\frac{m}{m+1}x^{\frac{1}{m}+1}$, we ſhall have $\frac{m+1}{2m+1}x$, for the Diſtance of the Center of Gravity of the Space CBC from the Point of Suſpenſion A, whence $\frac{m+1}{2m+1}a$, will be the Diſtance of the Center of Gravity of the whole Parabolic Space EAE, from A, the Point of Suſpenſion, along the Axis of the Parabola AD, for when AB, by flowing, becomes equal to AD, x, by flowing, becomes equal to a

If $m = 2$, as in the common Parabola, then $\frac{m+1}{2m+1} = \frac{2+1}{4+1} = \frac{3}{5}a$ will be the Diſtance of the Center of Gravity from the Point of Suſpenſion.

If $m = 3$, as in the Cubic Parabola, then $\frac{m+1}{2m+1}a = \frac{3+1}{6+1}a = \frac{4}{7}a$ will be the Diſtance of the Center of Gravity, but if $m = 4$, we ſhall have $\frac{5}{9}$ of the Axis for the Diſtance.

If $m = \frac{1}{2}$, which is the Property of the Concave, or Supplemental Space, then the Axis will become a Tangent to the Vertical Point, and we ſhall have $\frac{3}{4}$ of a for the Diſtance required.

EXAM-

EXAMPLE IV

Let it be required to find the Center of Gravity of the Semi-Parabolic Space ACEDA

PUT AD $= a$, DE $= b$, AB $= x$, BC $= y$, and let the Parabolical Space ACEDA be suspended by the Axis ABD. Conceive the Line ANH to divide the Space AED into two equal Parts, then will the Center of Gravity be found some where in this Line, and CN will be equal to $\frac{1}{2} y$, and let this represent the Velocity. Wherefore if $y x$, the Fluxion of the Mass (equal to $x^{\frac{1}{2}} x$, from the Nature of the Curve, whose Fluent is $\frac{2}{3} x^{\frac{3}{2}}$) be multiplied by this Velocity, we shall have $\frac{y y x}{2}$ for the Fluxion of the *Momentum* equal to $\frac{x x}{2}$ (by substituting x in the room of $y y$, to which it is equal) whose Fluent $\frac{1}{4} x x$ will be the *Momentum*. Wherefore if this Quantity be divided by $\frac{2}{3} x^{\frac{3}{2}}$, the Quotient $\frac{3}{8} x^{\frac{1}{2}}$, equal to $\frac{3}{8} y$ (because $x^{\frac{1}{2}}$ is equal to y) will be the Distance of the Center of Gravity from the Axis of Suspension ABD of the Space ABC.

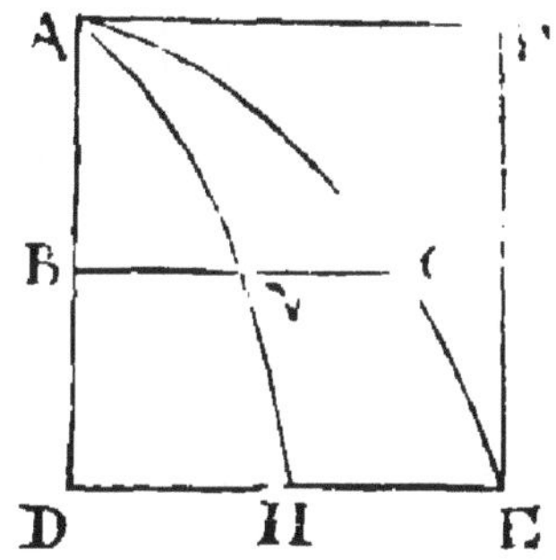

BUT when AB, by flowing, becomes equal to AD, then BC becomes equal to DE, and consequently y becomes equal to b, and $\frac{3}{8} b = \frac{3}{8}$ DE, will be the Distance of the Center of Gravity from the Axis ABD.

IT was shewn in the last Example, that when the Parabolic Space was suspended by the Tangent Line AF, that the Distance of the Center of Gravity from the Point of Suspension A, was equal to $\frac{3}{5} a$, or the Axis of the Curve. Wherefore if through the Point P, distant from the Vertex A, $\frac{1}{5}$ of A D, be drawn a Line, as P C, parallel to D E, and through the Point Q, distant from D $\frac{3}{8}$ of D E, a Line, as Q C, be be drawn parallel to A D, where these two Lines intersect each other, as in the Point C, will be the Center of Gravity of the Space A F D.

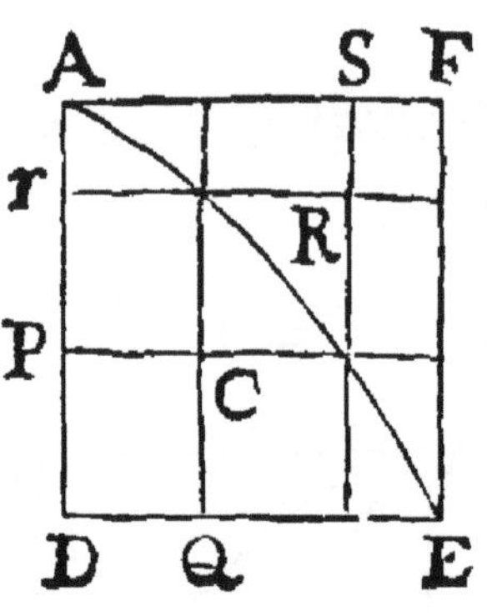

AND universally if $x = y^m$, then $x^{\frac{1}{m}} = y$, and $\frac{y y \dot{x}}{2} = \frac{x^{\frac{2}{m}} \dot{x}}{2}$ (by substituting x^{m} in the room of y)) will be the Fluxion of the *Momentum*, whose Fluent $\frac{m}{2m+4} x^{\frac{2}{m}+1}$, will be the *Momentum*. This Quantity therefore divided by $\frac{m}{m+1} x^{\frac{1}{m}+1}$, the Fluent of $x^{\frac{1}{m}} \dot{x}$, the Fluxion of the Mass, or whole Weight, will give $\frac{m+1}{2m+4} x^{\frac{1}{m}}$, for the Distance of the Center of Gravity of the Space A B C from the Axis of Suspension A B (*See the Figure in Page* 377), but when A B flows into, or becomes A D, B C becomes equal to D E, and y becomes equal to b, whence we shall have $\frac{m+1}{2m+4} b$, or D E, for the Distance of the Center of Gravity of the whole Space A D E from the Axis of Suspension A B D. Wherefore

IF $m = 2$, as in the common Parabola $\frac{m+1}{2m+4} b$, will give $\frac{3}{8} b$ for the Distance of the Center of Gravity from the Axis of Suspension A B D, the same as was before determined.

IF

If $m = 3$, as in the Cubic Parabola, then A P will be $\frac{4}{7}$ of A D, and D Q $= \frac{2}{5} b$

If $m = 4$, as in the Biquadrat Parabola, then A P $= \frac{5}{9}$ of A D, and D Q $= \frac{5}{12}$ D E

If $m = 5$, as in the Sur-Solid Parabola, then A P $= \frac{6}{11}$ of A D, and D Q $= \frac{3}{7}$ D E

If $m = \frac{1}{2}$, as in the Supplemental or Concave Parabola, then A S $= \frac{3}{4}$ A F, and A $r = \frac{3}{10}$ A D

If $m = \frac{1}{3}$, as in the Complement of the Cubic Parabola, then A S $= \frac{4}{5}$ A F, and A $r = \frac{2}{7}$ A D.

If $m = \frac{1}{4}$, as in the Complement of the Biquadrat Parabola, then A S $= \frac{5}{6}$ A F, and A $r = \frac{5}{18}$ A D

If $m = \frac{1}{5}$, as in the Complement of the Sur-Solid Parabola, then A S $= \frac{6}{7}$ A F, and A $r = \frac{3}{11}$ A D.

EXAMPLE V.

Let it be required to find the Center of Gravity of the Space A D F, *inclosed between two equal Parabolas* A C D, A C F, *touching one another in the Point* A, *and the right Line* D F *parallel to the common Axis* E K.

Put A B $= y$, B C $= x$, A H $= a$, D H $= b$, and the Parameter $= 1$, then because, from the Nature of the Curve, $x = yy$, therefore $xy = yyy$, will be the Fluxion of the Mass, whose Fluent $\frac{1}{3} y^3$ will be the Mass itself, but $y^3 y$ is the Fluxion of the *Momentum*, wherefore $\frac{1}{4} y^4$ will give the *Momentum*. This therefore being divided by $\frac{1}{3} y^3$, the

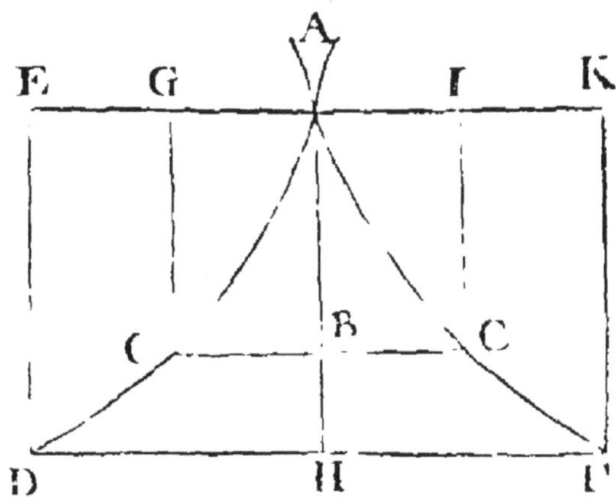

 the

the Mass will give $\frac{1}{4}y$ for the Distance of the Center of Gravity of the Space A C B C from the Point of Suspension A. Now if we suppose the Line C B C in a flowing State, and to move 'till it arrives at, or coincides with the Line D H F, then A B will become equal to A H, y will become equal to a, and we shall have $\frac{3}{4}a$ for the Distance of the Center of Gravity of the whole Space A D F from the Point of Suspension A

Now if we suppose $1x^n = y^m$, which is a general Equation for all Kinds of Parabolas whatsoever, then $x = y^{\frac{m}{n}}$, and $x\dot{y} = y^{\frac{m}{n}}\dot{y}$, will be the Fluxion of the Mass, whose Fluent $\frac{n}{m+n}y^{\frac{m+n}{n}}$ will be the Mass itself, but $y^{\frac{m}{n}+1}\dot{y} = y^{\frac{m+n}{n}}\dot{y}$ will be the Fluxion of the *Momentum*, wherefore $\frac{n}{m+2n}$ $y^{\frac{m+n}{n}+1}$, its Fluent, will give the *Momentum* This therefore being divided by $\frac{n}{m+2n}y^{\frac{m+n}{n}}$, the whole Mass, will give

$$\frac{\frac{n}{m+2n}y^{\frac{m+n}{n}+1}}{\frac{m}{m+n}y^{\frac{m+n}{n}}} = \frac{m+n}{m+2n}y,$$ for the Distance of the Center of Gravity of the Space A C B C from the Point of Suspension A, but when A B, by flowing, becomes equal to A H, y will become equal to a, and consequently we shall have $\frac{m+n}{m+2n}a$, for the Distance of the Center of Gravity of the whole Space A D F from the Point of Suspension A

If $n = 1$, and $m = 2$, as in the common Parabola, then $\frac{m+n}{m+2n}$

$\frac{m+n}{m+2n}a = \frac{2+1}{2+2}a = \frac{3}{4}a$, will be the Distance of the Center of Gravity from the Point of Suspension, the same as was deduced from the former Investigation.

If $n = 2$, and $m = 3$, as in the Cubic Parabola, then the Distance of the Center of Gravity from the Point of Suspension will be $\frac{3+2}{3+4}a = \frac{5}{7}a$.

EXAMPLE VI.

Let it be required to find the Center of Gravity of the Arch of a Circle.

LET the Arch of the Circle, whose Center of Gravity is to be found, be E H F, less than the Semi-circle D H I. It is evident that the Center of Gravity of this Arch will be found somewhere in the Ray A H, which divides the Arch E H F into two equal Parts in the Point H.

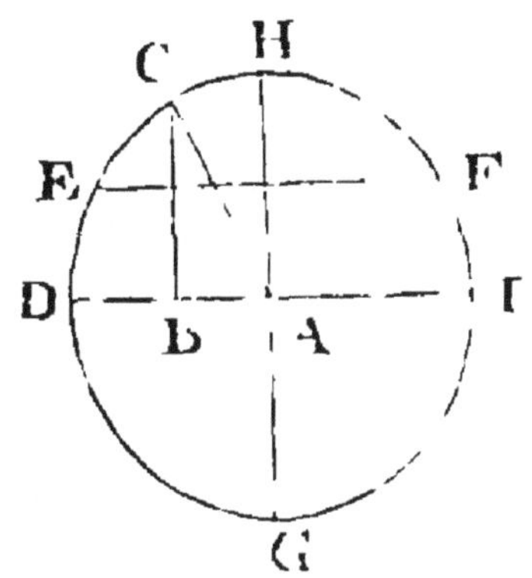

DRAW D I, a Diameter, parallel to E F, the Chord of the given Arch E H F, and C B an Ordinate rightly applied. Put D I = 2 r (which we consider as the Axis of Suspension) E F = 2 a, the Arch E H F = 2 c, the Arch C H = z, A B = x, and B C = y, then will $y\dot{z}$ be the Fluxion of the *Momentum*, but as $y : r :: \dot{x} : \dot{z}$ (for when the Point C arrives at H, y becomes equal to r, and $\dot{z}$ and $\dot{x}$, in their evanescent State, become equal to each other), wherefore $y\dot{z} = r\dot{x}$, consequently $r\dot{x}$ will be the Fluxion of the *Momentum*, whose Fluent xr will be the *Momentum*

after

itself. This therefore being divided by the whole Mass z, will give $\frac{rx}{z}$ for the Distance of the Center of Gravity of the Arch CH from the Point of Suspension A, but when the Point C arrives at E, x becomes equal to a, and z becomes equal to c, and consequently the Distance of the Center of Gravity of the Arch E H I, from the Point of Suspension A, will be $\frac{ar}{c}$. Put this equal to d, then will $dc = ar$, and consequently as $d : r :: a : c :: 2a : 2c$. Whence it follows

First, THAT the Distance d of the Center of Gravity of an Arch from the Point of Suspension, is to the Radius r as the Chord of the Arch a to the Arch itself c, whence in the Semicircumference it will be as the Diameter to half the Circumference.

Secondly, BECAUSE $\frac{a}{c} = \frac{d}{r}$, and r being a known and constant Quantity, it follows, that if the Ratio of the Chord of an Arch to the Arch itself be known, the Center of Gravity of the Arch is given, and on the contrary, if the Center of Gravity of an Arch of any Circle be known, or given, the Ratio of this Arch to its Chord, is likewise given, and consequently the Ratio of the Diameter of a Circle to its Circumference will be known also, which gives the Quadrature of the Circle.

Thirdly, THAT the Distances of the Centers of Gravity of similar Arches of different Circles from the Center of the Circle, or Point of Suspension, are in the same Ratio to their respective Semi-diameters.

HENCE it will be easy to find the Center of Gravity of any Portion of the Surface of a right Cylinder, intercepted between two right Lines drawn from the Extremities of the generating Arch, perpendicular to the Base of the Cylinder, for the middle of that right Line, which passes through the Centers of

Gravity of the Line cut off at Top and Bottom, will be the Center of Gravity required

EXAMPLE VII.

Let it be required to find the Center of Gravity of the Sector of a Circle.

LET CFCAC be the Sector of a Circle, draw the Line FBA bisecting the same, then will the Center of Gravity be found somewhere in this Line.

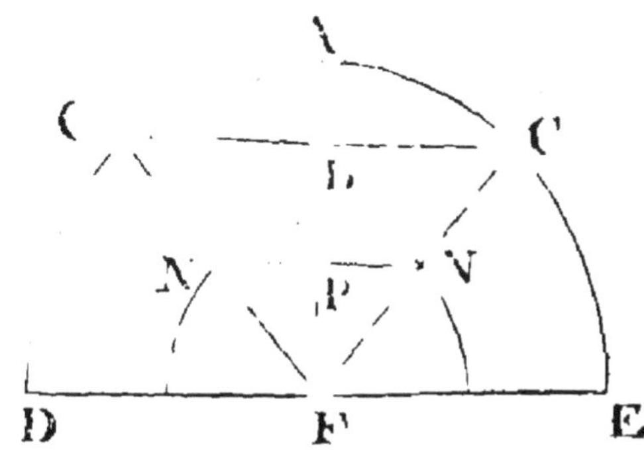

ON F, as a Center, with the Distance FN, describe the Arch NPN, and draw the Chords, CC, NN, then put FC $= r$, the Chord CC $= 2a$, the Arch CAC $= 2c$, and FN $= x$

NOW the *Momentum* of any Arch CAC, in respect to the Axis of Suspension, is equal to the Chord of that Arch multiplied into the Radius, therefore the *Momentum* of one Arch is to the *Momentum* of another Arch in a Ratio compounded of the Ratios of their Semi-diameters and Chords, that is, because the Chords are as the Radii or Semi diameters in a duplicate Ratio of their Semi diameters, whence to find the *Momentum* of the Arch NPN, it will be as rr to xx, so is the *Momentum* of the Arch CAC $= 2ar$, to the *Momentum* of the Arch NPN $= \frac{2axx}{r}$, and multiplying this by x, we shall have $\frac{2axxx}{r}$ equal to the Fluxion of the Sector NFNP, whose Fluent $\frac{2axxx}{3r}$, will be the

Mo-

Momentum of the Sector N F N P This therefore being divided by cr, the Value of the Mass, will give $\frac{2ax^3}{3crr}$ for the Distance of the Center of Gravity of the Sector N F N, but when the Arch N P N flows into, and becomes C A C, then x becomes equal to r, and $\frac{2axxx}{3crr}$ will become $\frac{2ar}{3c}$ for the Distance of the Center of Gravity of the Sector C F A C, from the Point of Suspension F.

WHENCE it follows, that the Distance of the Center of Gravity of any Sector of a Circle from the Center of Suspension, is to $\frac{2}{3}$ of the Radius, as the Chord of the Arch is to the Arch itself, for if d be put for the Distance of the Center of Gravity, then $d = \frac{2ar}{3c} = \frac{2}{3}\,\frac{ar}{c}$. Wherefore as $d \quad \frac{2}{3}r \quad a \quad c \quad 2a \quad 2c$. Whence to find the Distance of the Center of Gravity of a Semi circle, from the Center or Point of Suspension, we must say, as half of the Circumference is to the Diameter, so is $\frac{2}{3}$ of the Radius, or $\frac{1}{3}$ of the Diameter to the Distance required

Secondly, BY knowing the Distance of the Center of Gravity of the Sector C F C A, and of the Triangle C F C B C, from the Point of Suspension, we may find the Distance of the Center of Gravity of the Sector C A C from the Center F

Thirdly, IT is evident, that the Distances of the Centers of Gravity of similar Sectors of different Circles, from the Center or Point of Suspension, are as the Radii themselves, forasmuch as like Parts are in the same Proportion as their Wholes

EXAM-

EXAMPLE VIII

Let it be required to find the Center of Gravity of the Space inclosed by an Hyperbola, and its Asymptote.

LET ABF represent a Semi-Hyperbola, GE, GH its Asymptotes, BC an Ordinate, and put $GC = x$, $BC = y$, $GH = GD = a$, and because, from the Nature of the Hyperbola, $y = x^{-1}$, therefore $x^{-1}\dot{x}$ will be the Fluxion of the Mass, or whole Weight, and multiplying this by $x = GC$, we shall have $x^{-1+1}\dot{x}$, for the Fluxion of the *Momentum*, whose Fluent is $\frac{x}{1}$, which being divided by the whole Weight, $= \frac{xy}{0}$, an infinite Quantity, shews that the Distance of the Center of Gravity from the Axis of Suspension, is infinitely small.

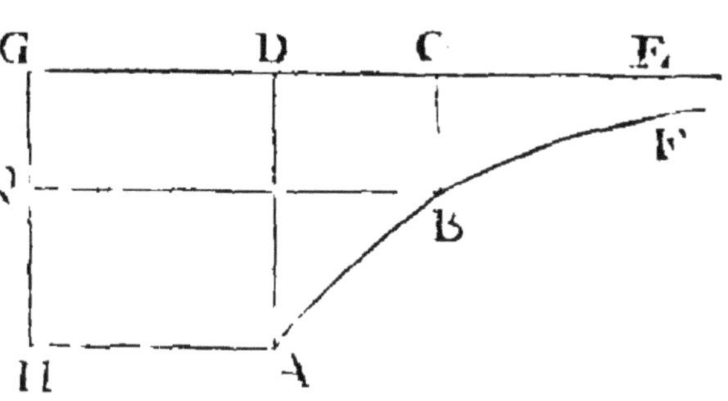

AND universally if $y^m = x$ which expresses the Nature of all Hyperbola's to Infinity with regard to their Asymptotes, m representing a Negative or Positive, whole Number or Fraction, we shall have $y = x^{\frac{1}{m}}$, and $x^{\frac{1}{m}}\dot{x}$, equal to the Fluxion of the whole Mass, or Weight, and $x^{\frac{1}{m}+1}\dot{x}$, equal to the Fluxion of the *Momentum*, whence the Fluent $\frac{m}{2m+1} x^{\frac{1}{m}+2}$, will be the *Momentum*, which being divided by $\frac{m}{m+1} x^{\frac{1}{m}+1}$, the Fluent of $x^{\frac{1}{m}}\dot{x}$, the Fluxion of the Mass, will give $\frac{m+1}{2m+1}x$, for

 the

the Distance of the Center of Gravity of the Hyperbolical Space ECHABF, from the Axis of Suspension GE, but when CB flows into the Place of DA, then GC becomes equal to GD, and x becomes equal to a, whence we shall have $\frac{m+1}{2m+1}a$, for the Distance of the Center of Gravity of the whole Space EGHABF, from the Axis of Suspension GE.

AND because in such Cases the Value of m is negative, the Distance of the Center of Gravity from the Axis of Suspension is equal to $\frac{-m+1}{-2m+1}a = \frac{m-1}{2m-1}a$. Wherefore if m be negative, as in the common Hyperbola, then the Distance of the Center of Gravity from GE, the Axis of Suspension, is equal to $\frac{0}{1}$, which shews, that the Distance is infinitely small, as was determined in the former Investigation.

IF m be equal to -2, as in the Cubical Hyperbola, we shall have $\frac{1}{3}a$ for the Distance required.

IF $m = -3$, we shall have $\frac{2}{5}a$ for the Distance sought.

LET it now be required to find the Center of Gravity of one half of the Hyperbolic Space EGHABF, and let the Asymptote GH be the Axis of Suspension. Put, as before, GC $= x$, CB $= y$, then will $y\dot{x}$ be the Fluxion of the whole Mass, which being multiplied by $\frac{1}{2}y$, the Velocity, will give $\frac{yy\dot{x}}{2}$ for the Fluxion of the *Momentum*, equal to $\frac{x^{\frac{2}{m}}\dot{x}}{2}$ (because in the Hyperbola $y^m = x$), whence the *Momentum* itself will be equal to $\frac{m}{2m+4}x^{\frac{2}{m}+1}$, which being divided by $\frac{m}{m+1}x^{\frac{1}{m}+1}$, the Fluent of $x^{\frac{1}{m}}\dot{x}$ equal to $y\dot{x}$ (because $y = x^{\frac{1}{m}}$, the Fluxion of the whole Mass, will give $\frac{m+1}{2m+4}x^{\frac{1}{m}}$ equal

equal to $\frac{m+1}{2m+4}y$ (by substituting y in the room of $x^{\frac{1}{m}}$) for the Distance of the Center of Gravity of the indeterminate Space E G H A B F, from the Axis of Suspension G H, and putting H A $=b$, we shall have $\frac{m+1}{2m+4}b$, for the Distance of the Center of Gravity of the entire Space, for when G C, by flowing, becomes equal to G D, C B becomes equal to D A, and y becomes equal to b.

BUT it has been shewn in the former Part of this Example, that the Distance of the Center of Gravity from the Axis of Suspension G E, is $\frac{m+1}{2m+1}a$, where a is put equal to G H. Wherefore if a Line be drawn parallel to the Asymptote G E, at the Distance $\frac{m+1}{2m+1}a$, and another Line parallel to the Asymptote G H, at the Distance of $\frac{m+1}{2m+4}b$, where these two Lines intersect each other, will be the Place of the Center of Gravity.

IF $m=-3$, the Distance of the Center of Gravity from the Asymptote G F considered as the Axis of Suspension, will be $\frac{2}{5}a$, and from the Asymptote G H, the Distance will be equal to b, or G H itself. $\frac{m+1}{2m+1}a=\frac{-3+1}{-6+1}a=\frac{2}{5}a$, and $\frac{m+1}{2m+4}b=\frac{-3+1}{-6+4}a=\frac{2}{2}b=b$.

IF $m=-4$, then $\frac{m+1}{2m+1}a$ will be $\frac{3}{7}a$, for the Distance from the Asymptote G F, and $\frac{m+1}{2m+4}b=\frac{3}{4}b$, for the Distance from the Asymptote G H.

SECT. VI.

Containing the Use of FLUXIONS *in finding the Centers of* Gravity *of Solids.*

AS the Center of Gravity of a Plane Surface is found in that Line that divides the Surface into two equal Parts, so the Center of Gravity of a Solid will be found in the Axis of *Equilibrium* of that Plane, which passing through the Point of Suspension of the Solid, will divide the Solid into two equal Parts, or, which is the same thing, in that Line about which the Generating Surface is revolved; or if the Solid be generated by the uniform Motion of a Plane Surface moving constantly parallel to itself, which is the Case of all Prisms, then the Center of Gravity will be found in that Line which is described by the Center of Gravity of the Generating Surface. Wherefore in

EXAMPLE I.

Let it be required to find the Center of Gravity of a Prism.

LET the Prism ABDC (*See the following Figure*) be a square Prism, then it is evident that the Center of Gravity will be found somewhere in the Line ABD, described by the Point A, the Center of Gravity of the describing Plane. Put the Side of the generating Square $= y$, $AD = a$, $AB = x$, and $BC = y$, then will $yy\dot{x}$, be the Fluxion of the whole Mass, and $\frac{yyx}{1}$, the Mass itself. Also $yy\dot{x}x$ will be the Fluxion of the *Momentum*, and $\frac{yy\dot{x}x}{2}$, the *Momentum*. Now if this

Quantity

Quantity $\frac{yy\dot{x}x}{2}$ be divided by $\frac{yy\dot{x}}{1}$, the whole Mass, the Quotient will be $\frac{x}{2}$, the Distance of the Center of Gravity of the Part A B C from the Point of Suspension A, but when A B, by flowing, becomes equal to A D, then x becomes equal to a, and consequently the Distance of the Center of Gravity from the Point of Suspension A, of the whole Prism, will be equal to $\frac{1}{2}a$; and the same will hold good of any other Prism, let the Base be of what Form soever.

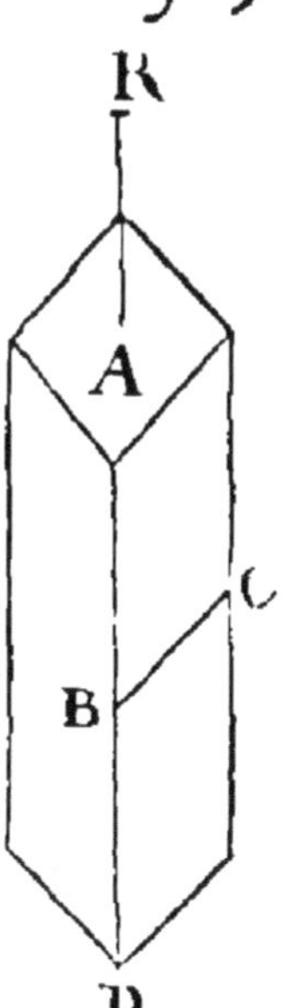

EXAMPLE II.

Let it be required to find the Center of Gravity of a Cylinder.

IT is manifest, that the Center of Gravity will be found somewhere in the Axis A B H. Put therefore A H = a, H E = r, and the Circumference of the Circle D H E = c, then will the Circle itself be equal to $\frac{cr}{2}$, equal to the Circle generated by the Line B C, because, from the Nature of the Solid, B C = H E. Put A B = x, then will $\frac{cr\dot{x}}{2}$ be the Fluxion of the whole Mass, and $\frac{cr\dot{x}x}{2}$ the Fluxion of the *Momentum*, whose Fluent is $\frac{crxx}{4}$, which being divided by $\frac{cr\dot{x}}{2}$, the Fluent of $\frac{crx}{2}$, the Fluxion

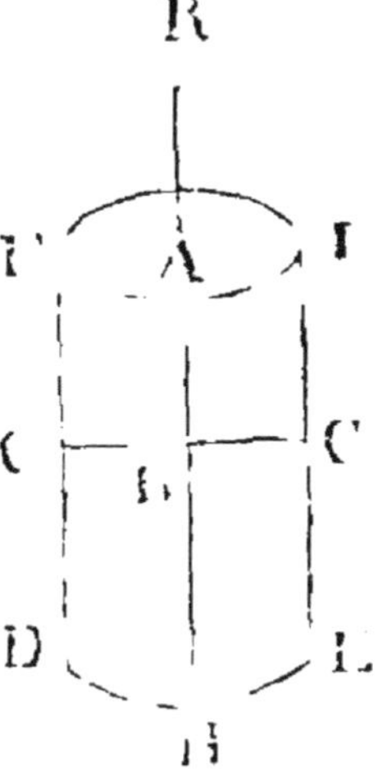

Fluxion of the Mass, will give $\frac{x}{2}$ for the Distance of the Center of Gravity of the Segment of the Cylinder C F I C from the Axis of Suspension C, equal to $\frac{1}{2}a$, for the whole Cylinder, for when C B C flows into the Place of D H E, A B becomes equal to A H, and x becomes equal to a.

EXAMPLE III.

Let it be required to find the Center of Gravity of a Pyramid.

LET the Pyramid be supposed to stand upon a square Base, and let r represent one of the Sides. Put A D $= a$, A B $= x$, and C C $= y$, then will $yy\dot{x}$ be the Fluxion of the Solidity, but as $y : x :: r : a$, because the Triangles A C C and A E E are similar, therefore $y = \frac{rx}{a}$ and $yy = \frac{rrxx}{aa}$. Putting then $\frac{rrxx}{aa}$ in the room of yy, in the Fluxion $yy\dot{x}$, we shall have $\frac{rrxx\dot{x}}{aa}$, which being multiplied by x, the Velocity, we shall have $\frac{rrxxx\dot{x}}{aa}$, for the Fluxion of the *Momentum*, whose Fluent is $\frac{rrx^4}{4aa}$. This therefore being divided by $\frac{rrxxx}{3aa}$, the Fluent of $\frac{rrxx\dot{x}}{aa}$, the Fluxion of the Mass, will give $\frac{3}{4}x$ for the Distance of the Center of Gravity from the Point of Suspension A, of that Part of the Pyramid whose Altitude is A B, but when A B, by flowing, becomes equal to A D, x

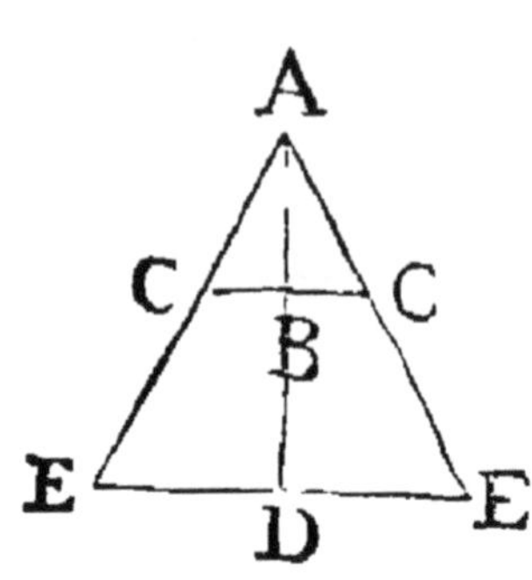

becomes equal to a, and consequently we shall have $\frac{1}{4}a$, or AD the Altitude, for the Distance of the Center of Gravity of the whole Pyramid E A E, from the Point of Suspension A, and the same Law will hold good, let the Base be of what Form soever, as will more evidently appear in the following Example.

EXAMPLE IV.

Let it be required to find the Center of Gravity of a Cone.

PUT A D $= a$, D E $= r$, the Circumference of the Base E D E $= c$, also A B $= x$, and B C $= y$, then as $r : c :: y : \frac{cy}{r}$, the Circumference of the Circle C B C, which being multiplied by $\frac{y}{2}$, will give $\frac{cyy}{2r}$ for the Circle described by the Radius B C; but as $y : x :: r : a$, therefore $y = \frac{rx}{a}$, and $yy = \frac{rrxx}{aa}$,

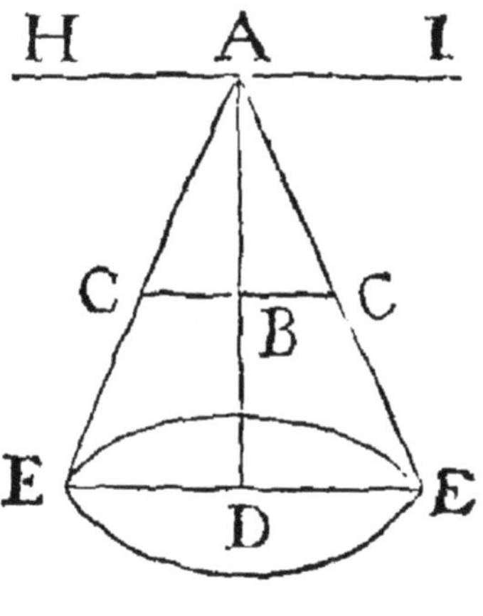

consequently $\frac{crxx\dot{x}}{2aa}$ will be the Fluxion of the Mass, and $\frac{rcxxx\dot{x}}{2aa}$ the Fluxion of the *Momentum*, whose Fluent is $\frac{crx^4}{8aa}$, which being divided by $\frac{crxxx}{6aa}$, the Fluent of $\frac{crxx\dot{x}}{2aa}$, the Fluxion of the Mass, will give $\frac{1}{4}x$ for the Distance of the Center of Gravity of the Portion of the Cone described

described by the Triangle CAC from the Point of Suspension A, which will give $\frac{3}{4}a$ for the Distance of the Center of Gravity of the whole Cone from the same Point A, for when AB, by flowing, becomes equal to AD, x becomes equal to a.

EXAMPLE V

Let it be required to find the Center of Gravity of a Sphere.

LET PAM be the Axis of Suspension, touching the Sphere in the Point A, whence it is evident, that the Center of Gravity will be found somewhere in the Diameter AD.

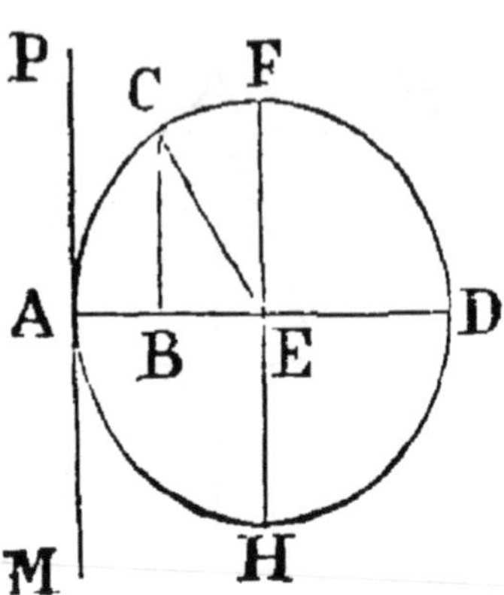

PUT $AB = x$, $BC = y$, $EF = r$, and the Circumference of the Circle generated by the Point $F = c$, then will $\frac{cyy}{2r}$ be the Area of the Circle generated by the Point C, and because, from the Nature of the Circle, $yy = 2rx - xx$, therefore $\frac{cyy}{2r} = \frac{2crx - cxx}{2r}$, whence $\frac{2crx\dot{x} - cxx\dot{x}}{2r} = cx\dot{x} - \frac{cxx\dot{x}}{2r}$ will be the Fluxion of the whole Weight. This therefore multiplied by x, will give $cxx\dot{x} - \frac{cx^3\dot{x}}{2r}$, for the Fluxion of the *Momentum*, whose Fluent $\frac{cx^3}{3} - \frac{cx^4}{8r}$, being divided

ded by $\frac{cxx}{2} - \frac{cxxx}{6r}$, the whole Weight, will give $\frac{8crxxx - 3cxxxx}{12crxx - 4cxxx} = \frac{8rx - 3xx}{12r + 4x}$ for the Distance of the Center of Gravity of the Segment of the Sphere formed by the Rotation of the Semi-Segment of the Circle ABC about the Axis AD, but when the Point B, by flowing, arrives at D, x becomes equal to $2r$, and $\frac{8rx - 3xx}{12r - 4x}$ becomes $\frac{16rr - 12rr}{12r - 8r} = \frac{4rr}{4r} = r$, for the Distance of the Center of Gravity of the whole Sphere from the Point of Suspension A, from whence it is evident, that the Center of Gravity is the same with the Center of the Sphere.

If x be put equal to r, then $\frac{8rx - 3xx}{12r - 4x}$ will become $\frac{8rr - 3rr}{12r - 4r} = \frac{5rr}{8r} = \frac{5}{8}r$ for the Distance of the Center of Gravity of the Hemisphere generated by the Quadrant AFE from the Point of Suspension A

Hence we are taught how to find the Center of Gravity of any Segment of a Sphere, or of any Portion cut off by two parallel Planes.

EXAMPLE VI

Let it be required to find the Center of Gravity of a Solid formed by the Rotation of the Semi Parabolic Space ACED, *about its Axis* AD

It is manifest, that the Center of Gravity will be found somewhere in the Axis AD (*See the following Figure*), put therefore $AD = a$, $DE = r$, $AB = x$, $BC = y$, and the Cir-

Circumference generated by the Point E, equal to c, then will

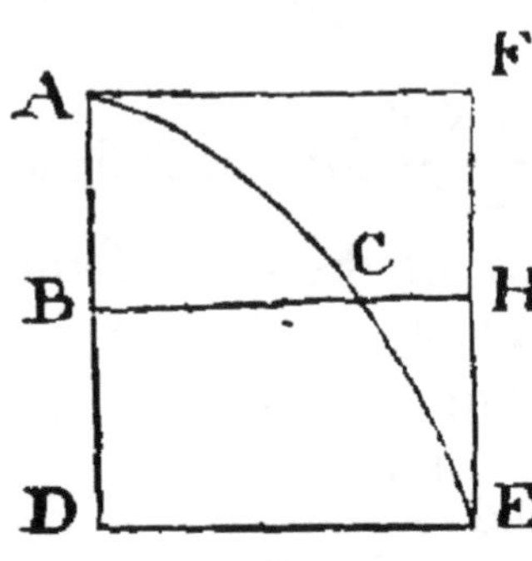

$\frac{cy}{r}$ be the Circumference of the Circle generated by the Ordinate BC, and $\frac{cyy}{2r}$ its Area; but because, from the Nature of the Curve, $1x = yy$, if we substitute x in the room of yy, in the Expression $\frac{cyy}{2r}$, we shall have $\frac{cx}{2r}$ for the Area of the same Circle, whence $\frac{cx\dot{x}}{2r}$ will be the Fluxion of the whole Mass, and $\frac{cxx\dot{x}}{2r}$, the Fluxion of the *Momentum*, whose Fluent will be $\frac{cxxx}{6r}$. This therefore being divided by $\frac{cxx}{4r}$, the Fluent of $\frac{cx\dot{x}}{2r}$, the Fluxion of the whole Mass, or Weight, will give $\frac{2}{3}x$ for the Distance of the Center of Gravity of the Solid generated by the Space A B C, from A the Point of Suspension; but when B C, by flowing, arrives at, or coincides with D E, x becomes equal to a, and consequently the Distance of the Center of Gravity from the Point of Suspension A of the whole Solid, will be $\frac{2}{3}a$, or $\frac{2}{3}$ A D.

AND universally if $1x = y^m$, which is the general Equation for all Kinds of Parabolas whatsoever, then $y = x^m$, and $yy = x^{\frac{2}{m}}$, whence we shall have $\frac{cx^{\frac{2}{m}}\dot{x}}{2r}$ for the Fluxion of the Mass, and $\frac{cx^{\frac{2}{m}+1}\dot{x}}{2r}$ for the Fluxion of the *Momentum*,

whose

whose Fluent is $\frac{mcx^{\frac{2}{m}+2}}{4m+4\times r}$, which being divided by $\frac{mcx^{\frac{2}{m}+1}}{2m+4\times r}$, the Fluent of $\frac{cx^{\frac{2}{m}}\dot{x}}{2r}$, the Fluxion of the Mass, will give $\frac{m+2}{2m+2}x$, for the Distance of the Center of Gravity of the Solid generated by the Space A B C from the Point of Suspension A, and when B C flows into the Place of D E, then x becomes equal to a, whence we shall have $\frac{m+2}{2m+2}a$, for the Distance of the Center of Gravity of the whole Solid from the same Point A.

If $m=2$, as in the common Parabola, then $\frac{m+2}{2m+2}a = \frac{2+2}{4+2}a = \frac{4}{6}a = \frac{2}{3}a$, for the Distance, &c.

If $m=3$, as in the Cubic Parabola, then $\frac{m+2}{2m+2}a = \frac{3+2}{6+2}a = \frac{5}{8}a$, for the Distance, &c.

If $m=4$, as in the Biquadrate Parabola, then $\frac{m+2}{2m+2}a = \frac{4+2}{8+2}a = \frac{6}{10}a = \frac{3}{5}a$, for the Distance, &c.

EXAMPLE VII

Let it be required to find the Center of Gravity of a Solid formed by the Rotation of a Semi-Parabola A C E D, *about the Line* F E *parallel to the Axis* A D. (See the preceding Figure.)

IT is manifest, that the Center of Gravity will be found somewhere in the Line F E, the Axis of Rotation.

PUT $FE = a$, $AB = FH = x$, $BC = y$, $AF = DE = r$, then will $CH = r - y$, and put c for the Circumference of the Circle generated by the Point D; then will $\frac{cr - cy}{r}$ be the Circumference of the Circle generated by the Point C, and $\frac{crr - 2cry + cyy}{2r}$ the Area of the same Circle, which taken from $\frac{cr}{2}$, the Area of the Circle, whose Radius is H B, will give $\frac{2cry - cyy}{2r} = \frac{2crx^{\frac{1}{2}} - cx}{2r}$ (by putting $x^{\frac{1}{2}}$ in the room of y, and x in the room of yy) for the Area of the Circle described by the Ordinate B C; whence $\frac{2crx^{\frac{1}{2}}x - cxx}{2r}$ will be the Fluxion of the Mass, and $\frac{2crx^{\frac{1}{2}+1}x - cxxx}{2r}$, the Fluxion of the *Momentum*, whose Fluent will be $\frac{2crx^{\frac{1}{2}+2}}{5r} - \frac{cxxx}{6r} = \frac{12crx^{\frac{1}{2}+2} - 5cx^3}{30r}$, which being divided by $\frac{8crx^{\frac{1}{2}+1} - 3cxx}{12r}$, the Fluent of of $\frac{2crx^{\frac{1}{2}}\dot{x} - cx\dot{x}}{2r}$, the Fluxion of the Mass, will give for the Quotient $\frac{24rx^{\frac{1}{2}+1} - 10xx}{40rx^{\frac{1}{2}} - 15x} = \frac{24rx - 10yx}{40r - 15y}$ (by dividing by $x^{\frac{1}{2}}$, and substituting y in the room of $x^{\frac{1}{2}}$), but when BC flows into or becomes equal to DE, AB becomes equal to AD, at which time x becomes equal to a, and y becomes equal to r; whence we shall have $\frac{24ra - 10ra}{40r - 15r} = \frac{14}{25}a$, for the Distance of the Center of Gravity of the whole Solid from the Point of Suspension F.

EXAMPLE VIII.

Let it be required to find the Center of Gravity of a Solid formed by the Rotation of the Semi Parabolic Space about the Line A F *(as an Axis) touching the Parabola in the Vertical Point* A.

It is manifest, that the Center of Gravity will be found somewhere in the Line A F Put D E = A F = a, A D = F E = r, c for the Circumference of the Circle described by the Point D, also A B = H C = x, A H = B C = y, whence ac will be the Cylindric Surface formed by D E, and $\frac{cxy}{r}$ for the Cylindric Surface formed by H C,

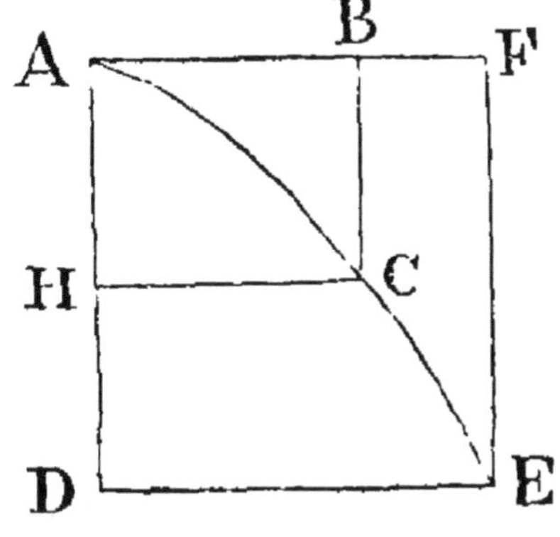

whence $\frac{cxy\dot{y}}{r} = \frac{cy^{\frac{1}{2}}\dot{y}}{r}$ (by putting $y^{\frac{1}{2}}$ in the room of x) will

be

be the Fluxion of the Mass, and multiplying this by $y^{\frac{1}{2}}$, we shall have $\frac{c y^{\frac{1}{2}} y^{\frac{1}{2}} \dot{y}}{r}$ for the Fluxion of the *Momentum*, whose Fluent will be $\frac{c y y y}{3r}$, which being divided by $\frac{2cy^{\frac{5}{2}}}{5r}$, the Fluent of $\frac{c y^{\frac{3}{2}} \dot{y}}{r}$, will give $\frac{5}{6} y^{\frac{1}{2}}$, equal to $\frac{5}{6} x$; but when H C flows into or becomes equal to D E, then x becomes equal to a, which gives $\frac{5}{6} a$ of A F for the Distance of the Center of Gravity of the whole Solid from the Point of Suspension F.

EXAMPLE IX.

Let it be required to find the Center of Gravity of the Solid formed by the Rotation of the Semi-Parabola A C E D *about the Base* D E

It is evident that the Center of Gravity will be found somewhere in the Line D E.

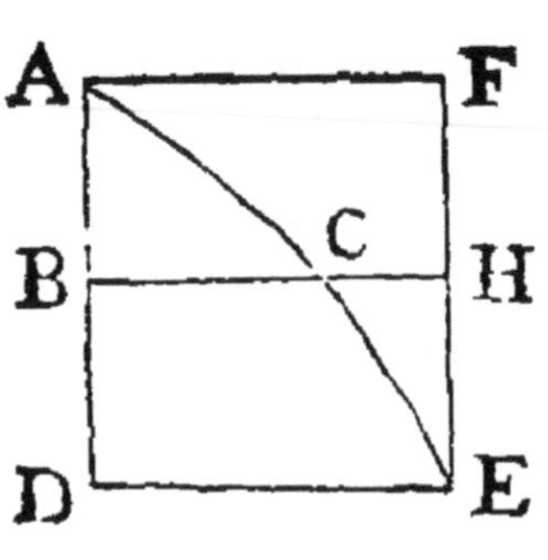

Put D E $= a$, A B $= x$, B C $= y$, A D $= r$, and c for the Circumference of the Circle described by the Point A, then will B D $= r - x$, consequently $\frac{cr - cx}{r}$ will be the Circumference of the Circle described by the Point C (for as $r : c :: r - x : \frac{cr - cx}{r}$); whence $\frac{cr - cx}{r} \times \dot{y} = \frac{cr\dot{y} - cx\dot{y}}{r}$, will be the Area of the Circle described by the Ordinate B C, but because, from the Nature of the Curve, $x = yy$, whence $\dot{x} = 2y\dot{y}$ Substituting therefore these Values of x, and $\dot{x}$ in the

Expreſſion $\frac{cry - cxy}{r}$, and we ſhall have $\frac{2cryyy - 2cy^4\dot{y}}{r}$ for the Fluxion of the Maſs, which being multiplied by $\frac{1}{2}y$, will give $\frac{cry^3y - cy^5y}{r}$ for the Fluxion of the *Momentum*, whoſe Fluent $\frac{cry^4}{4r} - \frac{cy^6}{6r} = \frac{3cry^4 - 2cy^6}{12r}$, being divided by $\frac{10cry^3 - 6cy^5}{15r}$, the Fluent of $\frac{2cryyy - 2cy^4y}{r}$ the Fluxion of the Maſs, will give $\frac{15ry - 10y^3}{40r - 24yy}$, equal to $\frac{15xy - 10yx}{40x - 24x} = \frac{5xy}{16x} = \frac{5}{16}y = \frac{5}{16}a$ for the Diſtance of the Center of Gravity of the whole Solid from the Point of Suſpenſion F, for when B C, by flowing, becomes equal to D E, the Point B will coincide with the Point D, then x will become equal to r, and y become equal to a.

EXAMPLE X.

Let it be required to find the Center of Gravity of any Portion of a Solid, generated by the Rotation of a Semi Parabola about its Axis, cut by one or more Planes paſſing through the ſame Axis

As the whole Solid is formed by the uniform Motion of the Space A E D about its Axis A D, (*See the Figure in the preceding Page*) ſo any Portion of it, generated in any Part of Time, will be to the entire Solid, as the Baſe of the Portion is to the Baſe of the entire Solid, and conſequently the Portions ariſing from the Section of the Solid by Planes paſſing through the Axis, will be ſimilar to each other, and conſequently the Diſtance of their Centers of Gravity from the

the Axis of Suſpenſion A F will be $\frac{m+2}{2m+2}a$, the ſame with that of the whole Solid found in the laſt Example. It remains therefore to determine the Diſtance of the Center of Gravity of any one of theſe Portions from the Axis A D, conſidered as the Axis of Suſpenſion.

Put $AB = x$, $BC = y$, $DE = r$, $AD = a$, and the Circumference deſcribed by the Point E equal to c; whence $\frac{cy}{r}$ will be the Circumference, and $\frac{cyy}{2r}$ will be the Area, whence $\frac{cyy\dot{x}}{2r}$ will be the Fluxion of the Maſs. But it has been ſhewn in *Example* VII, *Section* V, that the Diſtance of the Center of Gravity from the Center of the Circle, is to $\frac{2}{3}$ of the Radius, as the Chord of the Sector is to the Arch, whence putting c for the Arch of the Sector of the Baſe, and a for the Chord, we ſhall have $\frac{2ay}{3c}$, for the Diſtance of the Center of Gravity from the Axis of Suſpenſion A D, and $\frac{ay^3\dot{x}}{3r} = \frac{ax^{\frac{3}{m}}\dot{x}}{3r}$ (becauſe $x^{\frac{1}{m}} = y$) for the Fluxion of the *Momentum*, whoſe Fluent $\frac{max^{\frac{3}{m}+1}}{\overline{3m+9}\,r}$ being divided by $\frac{mcx^{\frac{2}{m}+1}}{\overline{2m+4}\,r}$, the Fluent of $\frac{cx^{\frac{2}{m}}\dot{x}}{2r}$, the Fluxion of the Maſs, will give $\frac{\overline{2m+4}\,ax^{\frac{1}{m}}}{\overline{3m+9}\,c} = \frac{\overline{2m+4}}{3m+4c} \times \frac{ay}{c}$, for the Diſtance of the Center of Gravity from the Axis of Suſpenſion A D of the Portion of the Solid formed by the Rotation A B, but when B C flows into the Place of D E, y becomes equal to r, and

and consequently we shall have $\frac{2m+4}{3m+9}\ \frac{ar}{c}$, for the Distance of the Center of Gravity of the whole Solid.

If $m = 2$, as in the common Parabola, we shall have $\frac{2}{3}a$ for the Distance of the Center of Gravity from the Axis of Suspension A F, and $\frac{8ar}{15c}$ for the Distance from the Axis of Suspension A D.

If $m = 3$, as in the Cubic Parabola, the Distance of the Center of Gravity from A F, will be $\frac{5}{8}a$, and from A D $\frac{5ar}{9c}$.

If $m = \frac{1}{2}$, we shall have $\frac{7}{10}a$ for the Distance from A F, and $\frac{14ar}{27c}$ for the Distance from A D

EXAMPLE XI.

Let it be required to find the Center of Gravity of a Solid formed by the Rotation of a Parabola, about one of its Diameters A D

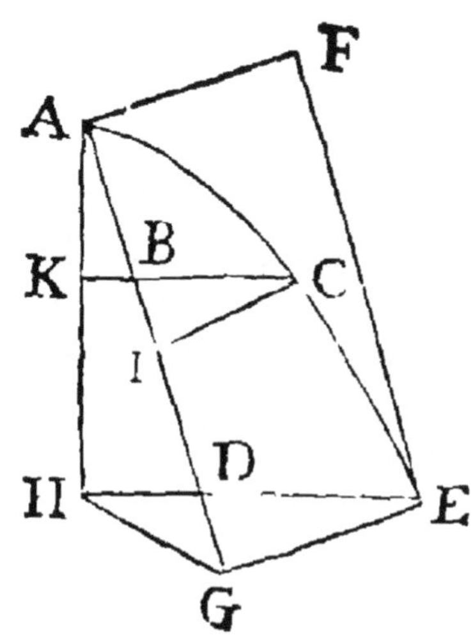

Put A D $= b$, A B $= x$, D E $= r$, and c for the Circumference of the Circle described by the Point E

Because the Ordinates B C and D E describe Conical Surfaces parallel to each other, and that the Conic Surface described by the Ordinate D E is $\frac{cr}{2}$, the Conic Surface described by the Ordinate B C, will be $\frac{crx}{2b}$

Fcc FROM

FROM the Points C and E draw the Perpendiculars C I and E G, it is manifest, that D G and B I, will be Axes of right Cones described by the right-angled Triangles E G D and C I B, by the Rotation of the Space about its Axis, but it has been already shewn, that the Center of Gravity of a Conic Surface is distant from the Point of Suspension $\frac{2}{3}$ of the Length of the Axis

PUT therefore D G $= a$, whence we shall have $a \times \sqrt{\frac{x}{b}}$ equal to B I; consequently $\frac{2}{3} a \sqrt{\frac{x}{b}}$ is the Distance of the Center of Gravity of the Conic Surface described by B C from the Point B, whence $\frac{2}{3} a \sqrt{\frac{x}{b}} + x$, will be the Distance from the Vertex A Multiplying therefore $\frac{acrxx}{2bb}$ by $\frac{2}{3} a \sqrt{\frac{x}{b}} + x$, we shall have $\frac{aacrx^{\frac{1}{2}}x}{3b^{\frac{1}{2}+1}} + \frac{acrxxx}{2bb}$ equal to the Fluxion of the *Momentum*, whose Fluent $\frac{2aacrx^{\frac{5}{2}}}{15b^{\frac{1}{2}+1}} + \frac{acrx^3}{6bb}$ being divided by the Mass, or whole Weight $\frac{acrxx}{4bb}$ will give $\frac{8}{15} a \sqrt{\frac{x}{b}} + \frac{2}{3} x$, for the Distance of the Center of Gravity of the Solid form'd by the Space A B C, from the Point of Suspension A, but when B C flows into, or becomes equal to D E, the Points B and D will coincide, and x will become equal to b, whence we shall have $\frac{8}{15} a + \frac{2}{3} b$ for the Distance of the Center of Gravity of the whole Solid, from the Point of Suspension A

EXAMPLE XII

Let it be required to find the Center of Gravity of the Solid formed by the Rotation of the Parabolic Space A D E, *about the Tangent* A F (See the preceding Figure)

IT is evident, that the Ordinates B C and D E will describe Cylindrical Surfaces, which will be to each other in a Ratio compounded of their Radii and their Altitudes. Putting therefore D E $= a$, A D $= b$, A H $= r$, A B $= x$, B C $= y$, and c for the Circumference generated by the Point E, we shall have $\frac{cxy}{b} = \frac{cy^{\frac{1}{2}}}{b}$ (by putting yy in the room of x, to which it is equal, from the Property of the Curve) for the Value of the Cylindric Surface generated by the Ordinate B C But forasmuch as the Center of Gravity of a Cylindrical Surface is placed in the middle of its Axis, putting therefore D H $= d$, we shall have B K $= \frac{dy}{b}$, and $\frac{x}{2} + \frac{dy}{b}$ will be the Distance of the Center of Gravity from the Axis of Suspension A H. Multiplying therefore the Fluxion of the Mass, or whole Weight, equal to $\frac{cry^{\frac{1}{2}}y}{bb}$ by $\frac{x}{2} + \frac{dy}{b}$, and putting for x, its Value, $y^{\frac{1}{2}}$, we shall have $\frac{cryyy}{2bb} + \frac{cdry^{\frac{1}{2}+1}y}{bbb}$, for the Fluxion of the *Momentum*, whose Fluent will be $\frac{cry^{3}}{6bb}$ $+ \frac{2cdry^{\frac{1}{2}+2}}{7bbb}$, which being divided by the Mass, or whole Weight $\frac{2cry^{\frac{1}{2}+1}}{5bb}$, will give $\frac{5}{12}y^{\frac{1}{2}} + \frac{5dy}{7b}$ for the Distance of the Center of Gravity of the Solid described by the Space

 A B C

A B C from the Axis of Suspension, whence we shall have $\frac{5}{12}a + \frac{1}{2}d$ for the Distance of the Center of Gravity of the whole Solid, for when A B, by flowing, becomes equal to A D, then B C, by flowing, will become equal to D E

EXAMPLE XIII.

Let it be required to find the Center of Gravity of the Solid formed by the Rotation of an Hyperbola about one of its Asymptotes G E.

Put $GH = r$, $QB = y$, $HA = a$, $GQ = BC = x$, and the Circumference described by the Point $H = c$, whence the Cylindric Surface generated by $HA = ac$, as will the Cylindric Surface generated by Q B equal

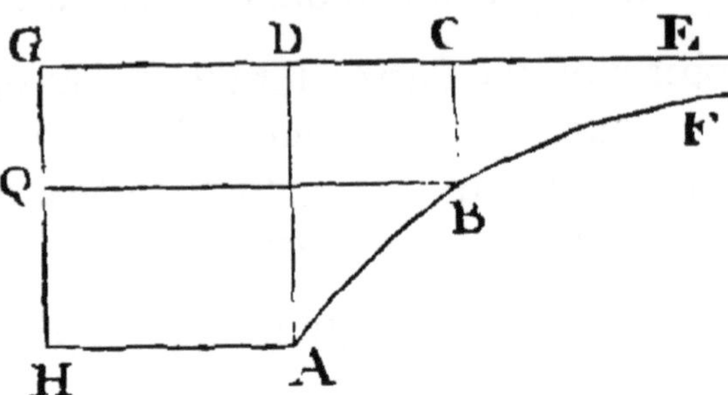

to $\frac{cxy}{r}$, but because from the Nature of the Hyperbola $xy = ar$, therefore $x = \frac{ar}{y}$, whence $\frac{cxy}{r}$ will be equal to ac, and consequently acx will be the Fluxion of the Mass, or whole Weight, and because the Center of Gravity will be found somewhere in the Line that passes through the Middle of the several Ordinates, put it equal to $\frac{1}{2}y$, whence we shall have $\frac{acyx}{2}$ for the Fluxion of the *Momentum*, but because $y = \frac{ar}{x}$, therefore $\frac{acyx}{2} = \frac{aacrx}{2x} = \frac{aacrx^{-1}x}{2}$, whose Fluent

will

will be $\frac{aacr}{2\times o}$, which being divided by the Mass acx, will give $\frac{ar}{2x\times o}$ for the Distance of the Center of Gravity from the Axis of Suspension G H; whence the Distance of the Center of Gravity of the whole Solid will be $\frac{a}{2\times o}$, because when Q B flows into the Place of H A, x becomes equal to r, whence it appears, that the Distance of the Center of Gravity from the Axis of Suspension is infinite

AND universally if $y^m = x$, then $y = x^{\frac{1}{m}}$, whence we shall have $\frac{cx^{\frac{1}{m}+1}\dot{x}}{r}$ for the Fluxion of the Mass, or whole Weight. This therefore being multiplied by $\frac{1}{2}y$, or its Value $\frac{x^{\frac{1}{m}}}{2}$, we shall have $\frac{cx^{\frac{2}{m}+1}\dot{x}}{2r}$ for the Fluxion of the *Momentum*, whose Fluent $\frac{mcx^{\frac{2}{m}+2}}{4m+4\times r}$ being divided by $\frac{mcxxy}{2m+1\times r}$, the Fluent of the Mass, or whole Weight, will give $\frac{2m+1}{4m+4}y$, for the Distance of the Center of Gravity of the Solid formed by the Rotation of the Space E G H A B F about G E, from the Axis of Suspension G H, whence we shall have $\frac{2m+1}{4m+4}a$, for the Distance of the Center of Gravity of the whole Solid, for when the Point Q, by flowing, arrives at H, y becomes equal to a.

EXAM-

EXAMPLE XIV

Let it be required to find the Center of Gravity of the Solid formed by the Rotation of the same Hyperbolic Space about the other Asymptote G H. (See the Figure in the former Example)

PUTTING then A H $= r$, the Circumference described by the Point A $= c$, we shall have $\frac{cy}{r}$ for the Circumference described by the Point B, whence $\frac{cyy}{2r}$ will be the Area, and $\frac{cyy\dot{x}}{2r}$ will be the Fluxion of the whole Mass, equal to $\frac{mcy^{m+1}\dot{y}}{2r}$ (by substituting $my^{m-1}\dot{y}$ in the room of $\dot{x}$, to which it is equal from the Equation of the Curve). Multiplying this therefore by x, or its equal y^m, we shall have $\frac{mcy^{2m+1}\dot{y}}{2r}$ for the Fluxion of the *Momentum*, whose Fluent is $\frac{mcy^{2m+2}}{\overline{4m+4}\times r} = \frac{mcyyxx}{\overline{4m+4}\times r}$, which being divided by the Mass, or whole Weight $\frac{mcxyy}{\overline{2m+4}\times r}$, will give $\frac{m+2}{2m+2}\ x$, for the Distance of the Center of Gravity of the Solid formed by the Rotation of the Space E G H A B F about G H, from the Axis of Suspension G E, whence we shall have $\frac{m+2}{2m+2}\ a$, for the Distance of the Center of Gravity of the whole Solid, for when Q, by flowing, arrives at H, x becomes equal to a.

If m be a negative Quantity, as it really is in the common Hyperbola, then we shall have $\frac{2-m}{2-2m}a$, for the Distance of the Center of Gravity, whence it is easy to see which Solids have Centers of Gravity, and which have none, in supposing m to be greater, equal or less than some positive Number taken at Pleasure

EXAMPLE XV

Let it be required to find the Center of Gravity of a Solid formed by the Rotation of the Semi-Hyperbolic Space ACFD *about the Axis* AD.

Put DF $= r$, AD $= a$, AE $= 2b$, AB $= x$, BC$= y$, then will ED$= a + 2b$, and EB$= x + 2b$. But as $c \quad r \quad y \quad \frac{cy}{r}$, the Circumference of the Circle generated by the Ordinate BC, whence $\frac{cy}{2r} \times y = \frac{cyy}{2r}$, will be the Area. This therefore being multiplied by x, will give $\frac{cyyx}{2r}$ for the Fluxion of the Mass, but because, from the Nature of the Curve, as EB × AB   ED × AD $\overline{BC}^2$ $\overline{DF}^2$, it will be as $(\overline{x+2b} \times x =)\ xx + 2bx\ \ (\overline{a+2b} \times a =)\ aa + 2ab$ $yy \quad rr$, whence $yy = \frac{rrxx + 2brrx}{aa + 2ab}$. Substituting therefore this Value of yy, in the Expression $\frac{cyyx}{rr}$, in the

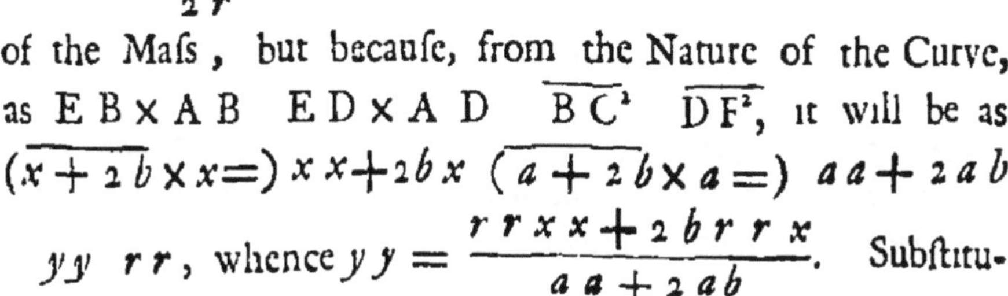

room

room of yy, and we shall have $\frac{crxx\dot{x}+2bcrxx}{2aa+4ab}$ for the Fluxion of the Mass, and consequently $\frac{crx^3\dot{x}+2bcrxxx}{2aa+4ab}$ for the Fluxion of the *Momentum*, whose Fluent $\frac{crx^4}{8aa+16ab}$ $+\frac{bcrx^3}{3aa+6ab}=\frac{3crx^4+8bcrx^3}{24aa+48ab}$, being divided by $\frac{crx^3+3bcrxx}{6aa+12ab}=\frac{4crx^3+12bcrxx}{24aa+48ab}$, the Fluent of the Mass or whole Weight, will give $\frac{3xx+8bx}{4x+12b}$ for the Distance of the Center of Gravity of the Solid formed by the Rotation of the Space A B C about A B, from the Point of Suspension A, whence we shall have $\frac{3aa+8ab}{4a+12b}$, for the Distance of the Center of Gravity of the whole Solid from the Point of Suspension A, for when the Point B, by flowing, arrives at, or coincides with the Point D, x becomes equal to a.

WHENCE it is evident, that the Distance of the Center of Gravity of the Hyperbolic Conoid from the Point of Suspension, or Vertex of the Solid, is to the whole Axis as $3a+8b$ is to $4a+12b$.

EXAMPLE XVI.

Let it be required to find the Center of Gravity of a Solid form'd by the Rotation of the Hyperbolic Space E A D F E, *about the Semi-Conjugate Axis* E F.

PUT C for the Circumference of the Circle generated by the Point D (*See the following Figure*), also E A $=a$, F E $=b$,

$EB = x$, $BC = y$, and $FD = r$, then will the Area of the Circle described by the Ordinate $BC = \frac{cyy}{2r}$ (for as $r : c :: y : \frac{cy}{r}$, but $\frac{cy}{2r} \times y = \frac{cyy}{2r}$), whence $\frac{cyy\dot{x}}{2r}$ will be the Fluxion of the Mass,

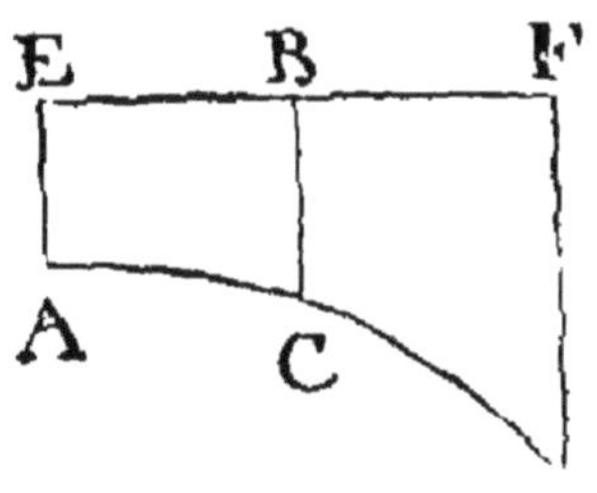

or whole Weight, equal to $\frac{aacxx\dot{x} + aabbc\dot{x}}{2bbr}$ (because, from the Nature of the Curve $yy = \frac{aaxx + aabb}{bb}$, consequently $\frac{aacx^3\dot{x} + aabbcx\dot{x}}{2bbr}$ will be the Fluxion of the *Momentum*, whose Fluent $\frac{aacx^4}{8bbr} + \frac{aabbcxx}{4bbr} =$ $= \frac{cx^4yy + 2bbcxxyy}{8rxx + 8bbr}$ (by substituting in the room of aa, its Value $\frac{bbyy}{xx + bb}$) being divided by the Fluent of the Mass, or whole Weight $\frac{cx^3yy + 3bbcxyy}{6rxx + 6bbr}$, will give $\frac{3x^3 + 6bbx}{4xx + 12bb}$ for the Distance of the Center of Gravity of the Solid formed by the Rotation of the Space AEBC about EB, from the Axis of Suspension AE; whence we shall have $\frac{9}{16}b$, for the Distance of the Center of Gravity of the whole Solid, for when BC flows into and becomes equal to FD, x flows into or becomes equal to b

 Whence

WHENCE it follows, that the Distance of the Center of Gravity of this Solid from the Point of Suspension E, is to the whole Axis E F as 9 to 16

EXAMPLE XVII

Let it be required to find the Center of Gravity of a Solid formed by the Rotation of a Semi Ellipsis A F D *about its Axis* A D, *the Axis of Suspension* A H *being perpendicular to* A D, *and passing through the Vertex* A

IT is evident the Center of Gravity will be fouud somewhere in the Axis A D of the Solid

PUT $FE = r$, $CB = y$, $AD = 2a$, $AB = x$; then will $\frac{cyy}{2r}$ be the Area of the Circle described by the Ordinate B C, and $\frac{cyy\dot{x}}{2r}$, the Fluxion of the Mass, or whole Weight, but because in the Ellipsis as $yy : 2ax - xx :: rr : aa$, therefore $yy = \frac{2arrx - rrxx}{aa}$ Putting this therefore in the room of yy, in the Fluxion of the Mass $\frac{cyy\dot{x}}{2r}$, and we shall have $\frac{2acrx\dot{x} - crxx\dot{x}}{2aa}$ for the Fluxion of the Mass This being again multiplied by x, will give $\frac{2acrxx\dot{x} - crx^3\dot{x}}{2aa}$ for the Fluxion of the *Momentum*, whose Fluent $\frac{crx^3}{3a} - \frac{crx^4}{8aa} = \frac{8acrx^3 - 3crx^4}{24aa}$ being divided by $\frac{12acrxx - 4crx^3}{24aa}$, the Fluent of the Mass, or whole

whole Weight, will give $\frac{8ax - 3xx}{12a - 4x}$ for the Distance of the Center of Gravity of the Solid formed by the Rotation of the Space A B C about A B, as an Axis, from the Point of Suspension A, but when the Point B, by flowing, arrives at, or coincides with the Point D, then x becomes equal to $2a$, and we shall have $\frac{16aa - 12aa}{12a - 8a} = \frac{4a}{4} = a$, for the Distance of the Center of Gravity of the Spheroid from the Point of Suspension A, equal to $\frac{1}{2}$ A D, equal to A E, which shews, that the Center of the Solid is the Center of Gravity.

WHENCE it follows, that the Distance of the Center of Gravity of the Semi Spheroid, formed by the Rotation of the Space A E F, about the Semi-Axis A E, is distant from A, the Point of Suspension $\frac{5}{8}a$, or $\frac{5}{8}$ of the Semi-transverse Diameter A E, for in this Case x becomes equal to a, consequently $\frac{8ax - 3xx}{12a - 4x}$ will become $\frac{8aa - 3aa}{12a - 4a} = \frac{5aa}{8a} = \frac{5}{8}a$

THE Center of Gravity of any Plane or Solid Figure being given, together with that of one of its Parts, the Center of Gravity of the other Part may be readily found.

LET the Parabolic Conoid, formed by the Rotation of the Semi-Parabolic Space A D E about the Axis A D, be the Solid proposed, and let G be its Center of Gravity, and let it be required to find the Center of Gravity of the Frustrum E C C E, cut off by a Plane passing through C B C

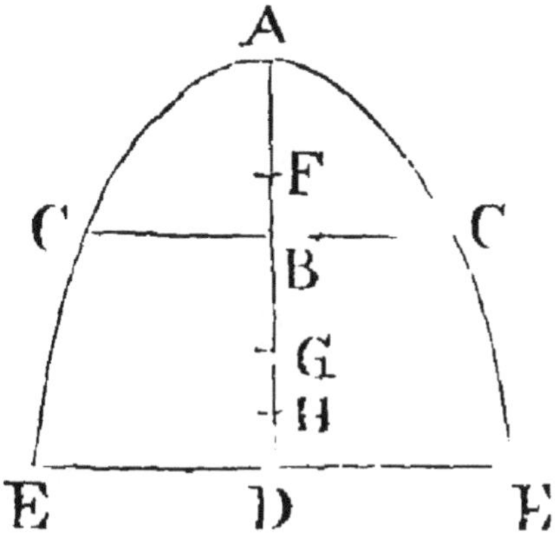

A
F
C
C
B
G
H
E
D
E

LET the Conoid be suspended by the Point A, and suppose F to be the Center of Gravity of the Segment C A C. Put F G $= a$, the Mass

C A C $= n$, alſo the Maſs, or whole Weight, E C C E $= m$, and becauſe the Diſtances of the Centers of Gravity are reciprocally proportional to their Maſſes, it will be as $m \,.\, n \,..\, a \,.\, \frac{an}{m}$ equal to G H, the Diſtance of the Center of Gravity of the Maſs E C C E from G the Center of Gravity of the whole Solid E C A C E

By the Help of the Center of Gravity may the Value of any Surface or Solid be found.

For if we imagine the Line A B, whoſe Center of Gravity is C, to be carried with an uniform Motion along the Line A D, according to the Direction A D, it is manifeſt, that while the deſcribing Line A B generates the parallelogramic Spaces A H Q B, A D E B, the Center of Gravity C, will deſcribe the Lines C P, C K; but the parallelogramic Spaces A H Q B, A D E B are as the Lines C P, C K (*by the 1ſt of* Euclid *the 6th*). Wherefore (*by Example* I. *of Section* II *of Part* III.) the Areas of the Parallelograms A H Q B, A D E B, are as the Rectangles made of the generating Line A B, and the Lines C P, C K, deſcribed by the Center of Gravity C in the ſame Time.

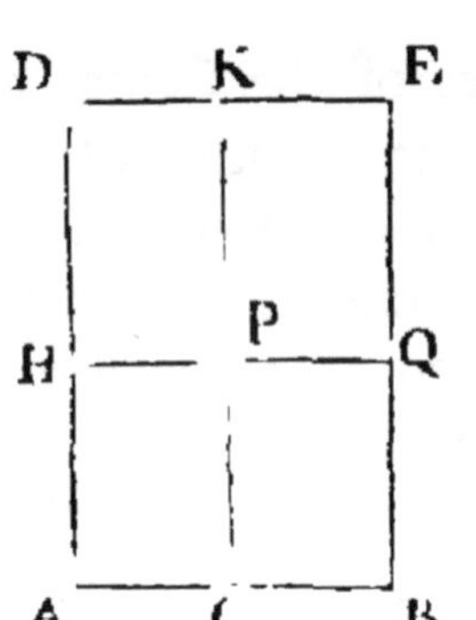

Again, if we imagine the ſame Line A B, whoſe Center of Gravity is C, to revolve about the Point A as a Center, it is manifeſt, that the Line A B will deſcribe the Circular Space A B D E, while the extreme Point B will deſcribe the Circumference B D E, and at the ſame time the Center of Gravity C will deſcribe the Periphery C F G

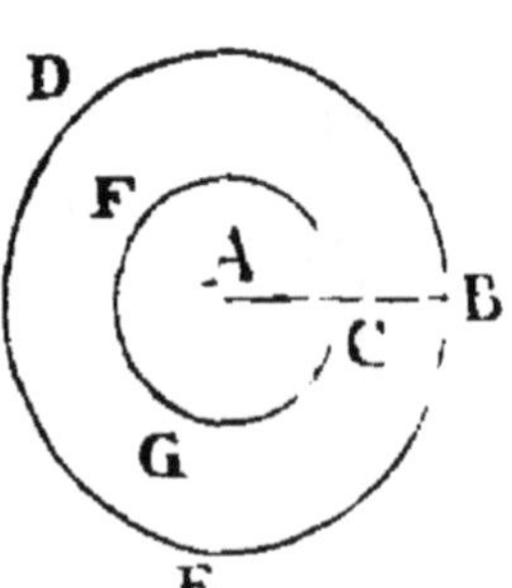

Now if we put the generating Line A B $= r$, and the Circumference B D E generated by the Point B $= c$, becauſe the Center of Gravity C,

C, of the Line A B, is in the middle of the Line A B; therefore the Circumference C F G, generated by the Center of Gravity C, will be equal to $\frac{1}{2}c$, but the Area of the whole Circle A B E D has been shewn to be equal to $\frac{1}{2}cr$, equal to $\frac{1}{2}c$, the Circumference of the Circle generated by the Center of Gravity C, and r the generating or describing Line A B.

AGAIN, inasmuch as in the same time that the describing Line A B, generated the Circular Space A B D E, the Part C B generated the Annular Space C B D E G F, and because the Center of Gravity of the Line C B is placed at the Distance of $\frac{3}{4}$ of the Line A B, from the Point of Suspension A, therefore the Circumference of the Circle generated by the Center of Gravity of the Line C B, will be $\frac{3}{4}$ of c, or the Circumference of the Circle BDE Wherefore $\frac{1}{2}r \times \frac{3}{4}c = \frac{3}{8}rc$, will be the Area of the *Annulus* C B D E G F; but the Area of the whole Circle is $\frac{1}{2}$ or $\frac{4}{8}cr$; whence it follows, that the Area of the *Annulus* is to the Area of the whole Circle as $\frac{3}{8}$ to $\frac{4}{8}$, or as 3 to 4, consequently the *Annulus* is equal to $\frac{3}{4}$ of the Area of the whole Circle, whence the Circle generated by the Line A C will be $\frac{1}{4}$ of the whole Circle A B D E, and $\frac{1}{3}$ of the *Annulus* C B D E G F.

AGAIN, if we suppose the Semi-circle A D B to revolve about its Diameter A B as an Axis, the Semi-Circumference A D B will describe the Surface of a Sphere, as will at the same time the Center of Gravity C, of the same Semi-circumference A D B, describe the Periphery of the Circle C F Put therefore the Diameter A B $= 2r$, the Semi-circumference A D B $= \frac{1}{2}c$, then will the Distance of C, the Center of Gravity of the Semi-circumference A D B, from F the Center of the Circle, be $\frac{4rr}{c}$ Wherefore as r is to c so is $\frac{4rr}{c}$ to $4r$, the Circumference of the Circle described by the Center of Gravity C. This therefore being multiplied by the Semi circumference,

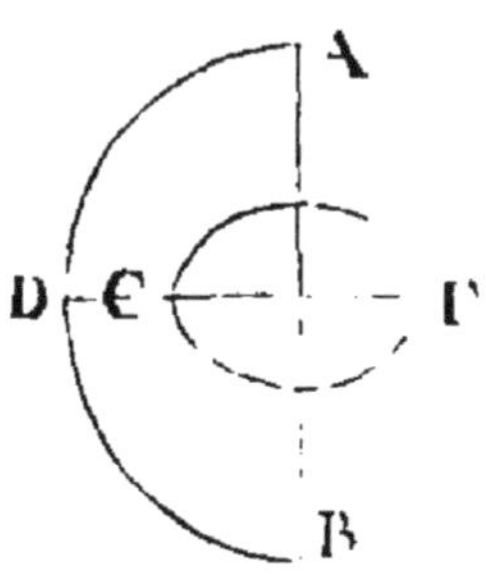

circumference, or generating Line, equal to $\frac{1}{2}$ c, will give $4\,r \times \frac{1}{2}\,c$ equal to $2\,r\,c$ for the Surface of the Sphere equal to $4 \times \frac{1}{2}\,c\,r$, or four times the Area of its greatest Circle.

AGAIN, if we imagine the Triangle A B P to revolve about the Line A P as an Axis, the Line A B, whose Center of Gravity is D, will describe the Surface of a Cone, as will at the same time the extreme Point B of the Line A B describe the Circumference B C, and the Center of Gravity D the Circumference D E.

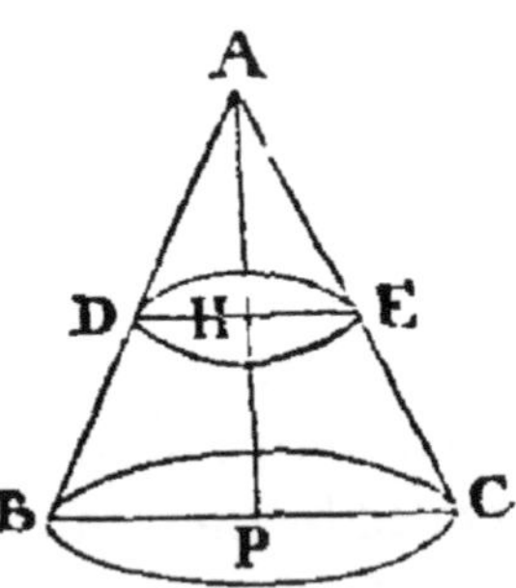

NOW put A B $= 2\,a$, the Circumference generated by the Point B $= c$, then will the Circumference generated by the Point D be $\frac{1}{2}\,c$; for as $2\,a$: a :: c : $\frac{1}{2}\,c$. This therefore being multiplied by $2\,a$, the generating Line, will give $2\,a \times \frac{1}{2}\,c = a\,c$, for the Surface of the Cone; whence if a be put for the Altitude of a Triangle, and c for the Base of the same Triangle, it will then follow, that the Area of this Triangle is equal to the Conic Surface, and consequently that the Surface of every Cone is equal to a Triangle, whose Base is equal to the Circumference of the Base of the Cone, and Altitude equal to the Side of the same Cone.

AGAIN, let A E B D C represent a Circle, A B its Diameter, and C its Center of Gravity. Now if we imagine the same Circle A E B D C to be carried with an uniform Motion along the right Line A F, in the Direction A F, it will describe or generate the Cylindric Solids A B I K and A F G B, while the Center of Gravity C describes or generates the Lines C P and C H, which are as the Cylindric Solids generated in the same Time (*by the* 11*th of Euclid* 12*th*), wherefore the Values of the Solids themselves (*by Example* I. *Sect.* IV. *Part* III)

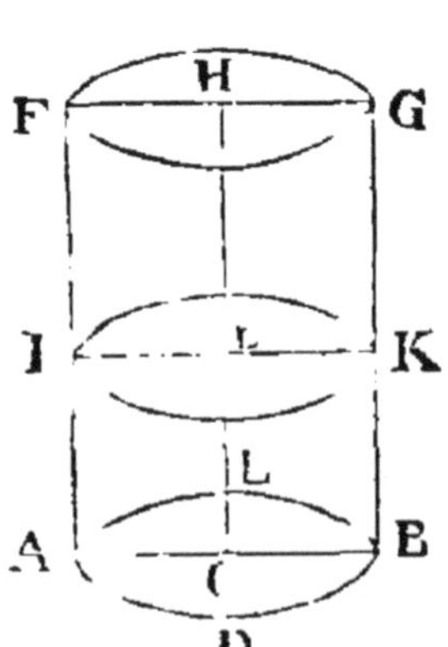

will be as the Products arising from the Area of the generating Circle A E B D C, and the Lines C P and C H, generated by the Center of Gravity C in the same time

BUT if the generating or describing Plane be of any other Form, suppose a Triangle, a Square, or Pentagon, *&c* the Value of the Prismatic Solid, generated by the Motion of this Plane, will always be a Result of the Product of the Value of the generating Plane, and the Line described by the Center of Gravity

LET us now consider the Cylinder as generated by the Rotation of the right angled Parallelogram H G B C, whose Center of Gravity is the Point P, about the right Line H C, as an Axis, 'till it return to the Place from whence it began to move Now it is evident, that in the same Time that the Extremity B, of the right Line G B, describes the Circumference of the Circle B D A E C, the Center of Gravity P, will describe the Periphery P Q Put therefore the Line G B $= a$, the Circumference B D E A C $= c$, then because the Center of Gravity P, of the Parallelogram, is found in the Middle of that right Line that divides the right-angled Parallelogram C H G B into two equal Parts, the Circumference of the Circle, described by the Center of Gravity P, will be equal to $\frac{1}{2}c$, and putting C B, the Radius of the Circular Base or Side of the generating Rectangle C H G B, equal to r, we shall have ar for the Area of the generating Parallelogram, consequently $\frac{1}{2} c \times ar = a \times \frac{1}{2} c \times r$, will give the Value of the Cylindric Solid A F G B, the same as was before investigated

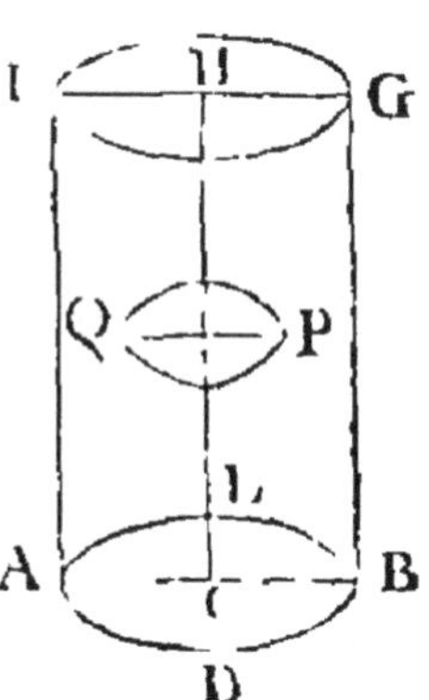

AGAIN, if we imagine the Semi circle A D B, (*See the following Figure*) whose Center of Gravity is E, to revolve about the Diameter A B, as an Axis, in the same time as the Semi-circle A D B shall generate a Sphere, the Center of Gravity E will describe the Circumference of a Circle F E Now putting

putting the Circumference of the generating Circle equal to c, its Radius C D $= r$, because the Distance of E, its Center of Gravity from C the Center of the Circle, has been found (*in Example* VII. *of Sect.* V *of Part* III) to be $\frac{8rr}{3c}$, it will be as r c : $\frac{8rr}{3c}$ $\frac{8r}{3}$ the Circumference of the Circle generated by the Center of Gravity E This therefore being multiplied by $\frac{1}{4}cr$, the Area of the generating Semi-circle A D B, will give $\frac{8crr}{12}$ equal to $\frac{2}{3}crr$, for the Solidity of the whole Sphere, the same as was investigated in *Example* III of *Section* IV. of *Part* III

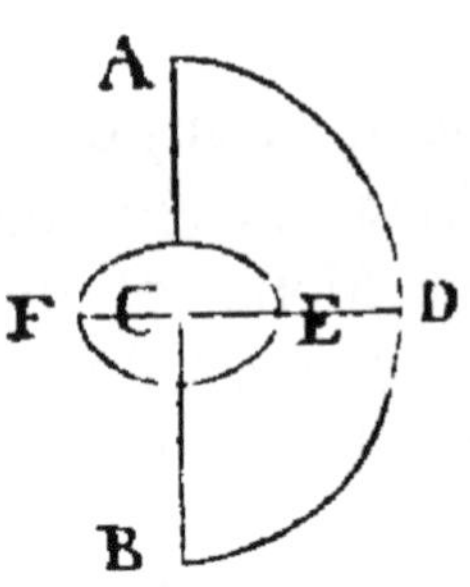

AGAIN, let us imagine the right-angled Triangle A P C, whose Center of Gravity is F, to revolve about its Perpendicular A P as an Axis. Now in the same time as the Triangle A P C, by this Revolution, shall generate the Cone B A C, the Center of Gravity E will describe the Circumference of the Circle F F, but (by *Example* II. of *Section* V. of *Part* III) the Distance of the Center of Gravity from A, the Point of Suspension, is $\frac{2}{3}$ of A H Wherefore putting A P $= a$, P C $= r$, and the Circumference generated by the Point C $= c$ we shall find the Circumference of the Circle F F, generated by the Center of Gravity F, to be $\frac{c}{3}$ This therefore being multiplied by $\frac{ar}{2}$, the Area of the generating Triangle A P C, will give $\frac{car}{6}$ for the Solidity of the whole Cone, the same as was investigated

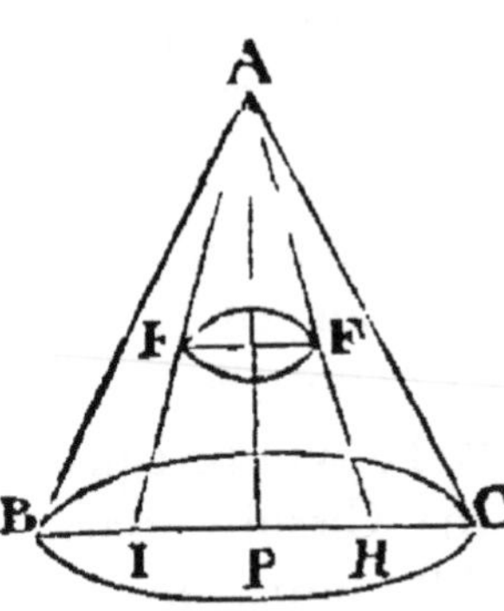

vestigated in *Section* IV of *Part* III. *Example* II and after the same manner may the Value of any Surface or Solid be determined.

LET A D K E B C represent the Section of a Prismatic Solid cut by a Plane thro' the Axis C K, and at right Angles to the Base ACB, then will the Line C P K represent the Line that is described by the Center of Gravity of the describing Plane, and let the same Solid be cut by another Plane N H S, which forms oblique Angles with the Plane of the same Base.

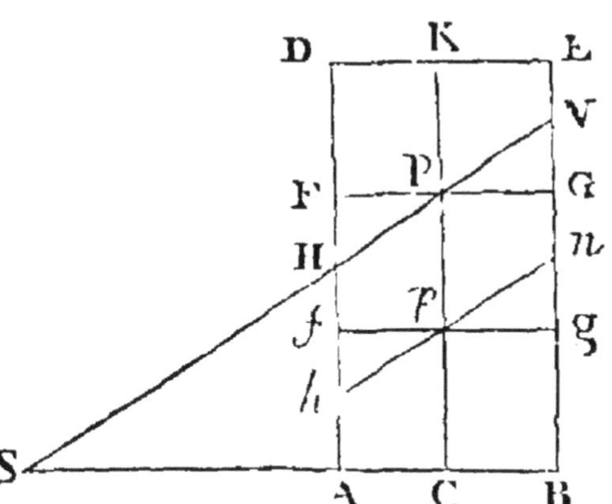

Now I say, that if through the Point P, where the Plane cuts the Line C K, described by the Center of Gravity, another Planebe imagined to cut the Prismatic Solid A D E B, so as to cut the Axis KC at right Angles, it will cut off a Segment A F P G B equal to the Segment A H P N B, cut off by the oblique Plane N H S

FOR if we consider the Point S as the Axis of Suspension, it is evident, that the *Momenta* of the Points A, C, B, are as their respective Distances S A, S C, S B, from the Point of Suspension S, but by the 4th of the 6th of *Euclid*, the Lines A H, C P, B N, are as the Distances S A, S C, S B, consequently the *Momenta* of the Points A, C, B, are as the Lines A H, C P, BN, and may therefore be expounded by them Now if we consider the Lines S A and A H in a flowing State, and imagine the Point A to move with an uniform Velocity along the Line A B, in the Direction A B, at the same time that the Point A arrives at, or coincides with the Point B, the Line A H will arrive at or coincide with the Line B N, and by its uniform Motion will describe the Space A H N B, as will the Line A F, equal to the Line C P, by which the *Momentum* of the Center of

Gravity C, is expounded, describe the Space A F P G B, and consequently the Spaces A H P N B and A F P G B will be equal the one to the other. Whence it follows:

First, THAT if the Prismatic Solid be cut by several Planes, howsoever inclined, yet if they pass through the same Point P, in the Line C K, described by the Center of Gravity, they will cut off Segments, or Ungulas, equal to each other, and to the Prismatic Solid A F G B.

Secondly, THAT if another Plane, as *n p h*, cut the same Prismatic Solid, and if through the Point *p*, where it cuts the Line C K, described by the Center of Gravity C, a Plane, as *f p g*, be imagined to pass, it will cut off a Segment A *h p n* B, equal to the Prismatic Solid A *f g* B, and consequently that the Solid *h* H N *n* comprehended between these two Planes, will be equal to the Solid *f* F G *g* comprehended between the two parallel Planes F G and *f g*, that is, to a Prismatic Solid, whose Base is equal to the Base A B of the given Prismatic Solid, and whose Altitude is equal to the right Line P *p*.

Thirdly, THAT the Surface of the Ungula A H N B, excepting its Bases, is equal to the Surface of the Prismatic Solid A F P G B, excepting its Bases also, for if C be consider'd as the Center of Gravity of the Perimeter of the Base A B of the Prismatic Solid A D E B, it is evident, that the *Momenta* of the several Points A, C, B will be as their respective Distances from S, the Axis of Suspension, and consequently may be expounded by the Lines A H, C P, B N. And consequently, by the former Method of reasoning, it will follow, that the Space A H N B, by which the Surface of the Ungula A H N B, excepting its Bases, is expounded, will be equal to the Space A F G B, by which the Surface of the Prismatic Solid, excepting its Bases, is expounded. And consequently,

Fourthly, THAT the Surfaces of all Ungulas cut off by Planes passing through the Point P or *p* in the Line C P, described by the Center of Gravity C, will be equal to each other, and to the Surface of the Prismatic Solid A F G B, or A *f g* B,

 the

the Bases excepted; and consequently, that the Surface of any Ungula, as H N *n h*, cut off by any two Planes H N and *h n*, howsoever inclined, will be equal to the Surface of the Prismatic Solid *f* F G *g*, the Bases excepted, cut off by two Planes F G and *f g*, parallel to each other, and to the Base A C B of the whole Prismatic Solid A D E B

LET us now imagine the Line A B, whose Center of Gravity is C, to revolve about the Point of Suspension S, as an Axis, then will the Points B C, A, describe the Arches B *b*, C *c*, A *a* in the same time, which Arches are to each other as their respective Radii SB, SC, SA, and inasmuch as the *Momenta* of the Points B, C, A, are as the same Radii S B, S C S A, it follows, that the *Momenta* of the Points B, C, A, are as B *b*, C *c*, A *a*, described by the same Points B, C, A, and may therefore be expounded by them. Let C P be made equal to the Arch C *c*, described by the Center of Gravity C, and draw the Line F P G parallel to the Base A B, also the Line S H P N Now because C P is equal to the Arch C *c*, and the Triangles S B N, S C P, S A H are similar, as also S B *b*, S C *c*, S A *a*, the Line B N will be equal to the Arch B *b*, the Line A H will be equal to the Arch A *a*, and the Space A H N B will be equal to the Circular Space A B *b a*, but the Space A H N B has been proved equal to the Space A E G B, wherefore the Surface A B *b a*, described by the Revolution of the Line A B about the Axis of Suspension S, is equal to a Parallelogram, whose Height is equal to the Periphery described by the Center of Gravity, and whose Base is equal to the generating Line.

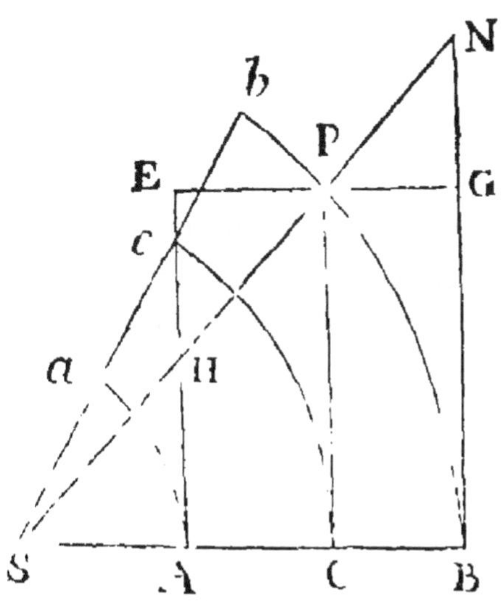

Now if we suppose the Line A B to represent a Surface of any Form whatsoever (for when Surfaces lie in the same Plane with the Eye they appear as streight Lines) and C the Center of Gravity of the same Surface, it will follow, from the same way of reasoning, that the Solid A B *b c a* A, generated by the Revolution of the Surface A C B about the Axis of Suspension S, will be equal to a Parallelopipedon, whose Height is equal to the Periphery described by the Center of Gravity, and whose Base is equal to the given revolving Surface Whence it follows,

First, That if the Distance of the Center of Gravity of any Line or Surface, from the Axis of Suspension, and the Magnitude of the Line or Surface be given, the Value of the Surface or Solid generated by a total or partial Revolution may be found, and consequently any two of the three being given, the third may be easily found

Secondly, That if the generating or revolving Lines or Surfaces are equal, but the Distances of their Centers of Gravity from the Axis of Motion be unequal, then the generated Surfaces or Solids will be as the Distances of their Centers of Gravity from the Axis of Motion directly.

Thirdly, That if the Distances of the Centers of Gravity of the generating or revolving Lines or Surfaces from the Axis of Motion be equal, but the generating Lines or Surfaces unequal, then the generated Surfaces and Solids will be as the generating Lines and Surfaces But,

Fourthly, If neither the generating or revolving Lines or Surfaces, nor the Distances of their Centers of Gravity from the Axis of Motion be equal, the generated Surfaces or Solids will be to each other, in a Ratio compounded of the Ratio of the generating Lines or Surfaces, and the Ratio of the Distances of their Centers of Gravity from the Axis of Motion

Thus, for Example, the Triangle is to its circumscribed Parallelogram as 1 to 2, and the Distance of the Center of Gravity of the Triangle from its Vertex is $\frac{2}{3}$ of the Axis; but the Distance of the Center of Gravity of the Parallelogram

2 from

from the same Point is $\frac{1}{2}$ of the Axis, therefore the Distance of the Center of Gravity of the Triangle from the Axis of Motion, is to the Distance of the Center of Gravity of the Parallelogram as 4 to 3 Now if both the Spaces are supposed to revolve about a Line touching the Vertex of the Triangle, and parallel to its Base, then the Solid generated by the Triangular Space, is to the Solid generated by the Parallelogramic Space as 4 to 6, or as 2 to 3

AGAIN, the common Parabola is to its circumscribing Parallelogram as 2 to 3, and the Distance of the Center of Gravity of the Parabola, is to the Distance of the Center of Gravity of the Parallelogram, from the same Point of Suspension, as 6 to 5, wherefore the Solid generated by the Parabolic Space, is to the Solid generated by the Parallelogramic Space, each revolving about the same common Axis passing through the Vertex of the Parabola, and parallel to its Base, as 12 to 15, or as 4 to 5, and consequently the Solid generated by the Triangular Space, is to the Solid generated by the Parabolic Space, in a Ratio compounded of the Ratios of 5 to 4, and of 4 to 6; that is, of 20 to 24, or of 5 to 6, and after the same manner may the Value of any Surface or Solid be found, and the Values of all sorts of Surfaces or Solids be compared together.

WHENCE it is abundantly manifest, that the Value of any Surface or Solid is always equal to the Product arising from the Value of the generating Quantity multiplied into the Line described by the Center of Gravity, in the same time that the Surface or Solid is generated, which is the celebrated Property of the Center of Gravity.

SECT.

SECT. VII.

Containing the Use of FLUXIONS *in finding the Centers of* Percussion *of Lines and Surfaces.*

DEFINITION.

THE Center of Percussion of a Body in Motion, is that Point wherein all the Forces of that Body are united in one, or, which is the same thing, wherein the whole Percussive Force is collected, so that the Force of Percussion in that Point is greater than any where else, and if the Body meets with any Obstacle in its way, it will strike it with a greater Force in that Point than in any other Part of the Body.

So that as the Center of Gravity is that Point in which all the *Momenta* of a Body are united in one, and by which, if it be suspended, it will remain at Rest in any Situation whatsoever, the Center of Percussion is that Point in which the whole Percussive Force is collected, and if it meet with any Obstacle in its way, it will strike it with the greatest Force. And as the Distance of the Center of Gravity from the Point of Suspension is found by dividing the *Momentum* of the Body by the Quantity of Matter contained therein, so the Distance of the Center of Percussion, from the same Point of Suspension, is found by dividing the whole percussive Force by the *Momentum* of the same Body. For if we suppose the Line S *c b* to be suspended at the Point S, it is manifest, by the preceding fifth *Section*, that the *Momentum* of the Point *b* is to the *Momentum* of any other Point, suppose *c*, as S *b*, the Distance of the Point *b* from S the Point of Suspension,

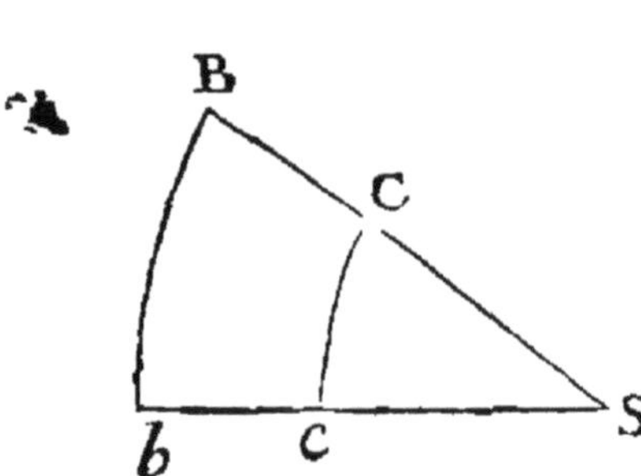

to

to Sc the Distance of the Point c, from the same Point of Suspension S. Now if we imagine the Line Scb to revolve about the Point of Suspension S, it is evident, that the Velocity of the Point b is to the Velocity of the Point c, as the Arch bB, generated by the Point b, is to the Arch cC, generated by the Point c in the same time; that is, as their respective Radii Sb, Sc; and consequently the *Momentum* of the Point B, acquired by this additional Velocity, which I call its percussive Force, is to the new acquired *Momentum* of the Point c, which I call its percussive Force, as $Sb \times SB$ to $Sc \times SC$, that is, as $\overline{SB}^2$ to $\overline{SC}^2$; and as the same Consequence will happen, wheresoever the Point c be taken, that is, in every conceiveable Point in the Line Sb, if SB, which we will suppose equal to x, expound the whole Velocity, then we shall have $xx\dot{x}$ for the Fluxion of the Forces, whose Fluent $\frac{xxx}{3}$ will be the whole percussive Force; which therefore being divided by $\frac{xx}{2}$, the *Momentum* of the same Line SB, will give $\frac{2}{3}x$ for the Distance of the Center of Percussion from S the Point of Suspension. For as the *Momentum* on each Side the Center of Gravity is equal, so the whole percussive Force on each Side the Center of Percussion is equal also. And if we consider the several percussive Forces on each Side the Center of Percussion at the Instant of Percussion, as the several *Momenta* on each the Center of Gravity, it is evident, that if the whole *Momentum*, in the present Case be divided by the total Gravity, the Quotient will give the Distance of a Point from the Point of Suspension, at which, if the Body be suspended, it will remain at Rest, and consequently the Center of Percussion is found in the same manner as the Center of Gravity is found, if we suppose the Gravity or Weight of the Body to be increased in Proportion to the Velocity at the Instant of Percussion; for since the Velocity of every Particle of a Surface or Solid revolving about an Axis is encreased in

Proportion

Proportion to its Distance from the Axis of Rotation, if the Fluxion of the *Momentum* be multiplied by this new acquired Velocity, the Product will give the Fluxion of the whole percussive Force, whose Fluent being divided by the *Momentum*, must give the Distance of the Center of Percussion from the Axis, from whence we may draw this general Rule for finding the Center of Percussion.

MULTIPLY the Fluxion of the *Momentum* of the whole Body by the Velocity, or multiply the Fluxion of the whole Mass by the Square of the same Velocity, and the Product in either Case will give the Fluxion of the whole percussive Force, whose Fluent being divided by the whole *Momentum*, will give the Distance of the Center of Percussion from the Point or Axis of Rotation, which will always be found in that Line in which is the Center of Gravity

EXAMPLE I.

Let it be required to find the Center of Percussion of a Line, as AB, *suspended by one of its Extremities* A, *about which it is supposed to revolve*

PUT $AB = a$, $AC = x$, then will $\dot{x}x$ be the Fluxion of the *Momentum*, which being multiplied by x, the new acquired Velocity, will give $\dot{x}xx$ for the Fluxion of the

A C B

Force, whose Fluent $\frac{xxx}{3}$, being divided by $\frac{xx}{2}$, the Fluent of $\dot{x}x$, the Fluxion of the *Momentum*, will give $\frac{2}{3}x$ for the Distance of the Center of Percussion of the Line AC from the Point of Suspension A, but when the Point C, by flowing, arrives at, or coincides with the Point B, the Line AC will become equal to AB, and x will become equal to a, whence

whence the Distance of the Center of Percussion of the whole Line will be $\frac{2}{3}a$ from the Point of Suspension A.

EXAMPLE II

Let it be required to find the Center of Percussion of a Parallelogram A H I D, *revolving about one of its Sides* A H.

It is evident that the Center of Percussion will be found somewhere in the Line S B E. Put S E $= a$, A H $=$ C C $= b$, and S B $= x$, then will $b\dot{x}$ be the Fluxion of the Mass, or whole Weight. This being multiplied by x, which represents the Velocity, will give $bx\dot{x}$, for the Fluxion of the *Momentum*, and this again being multiplied by the acquired Velocity x, will give $bxx\dot{x}$ for the Fluxion of the Force, whose Fluent $\frac{bxxx}{3}$, being divided by $\frac{bxx}{2}$, the Fluent of $bx\dot{x}$, the Fluxion of the *Momentum*, will give in the Quotient $\frac{2}{3}x$ for the Distance of the Center of Percussion from the Point S in the Axis of Rotation of the Space A C C H, but if we conceive the Line C C in a flowing State, and to move 'till it arrives at, or coincides with the Line D I, then the Point B will coincide with the Point E; whence x will become equal to a, and we shall have $\frac{2}{3}a = \frac{2}{3}$ S E for the Distance of the Center of Percussion of the Parallelogram A H I D, from the Axis of Suspension A S H

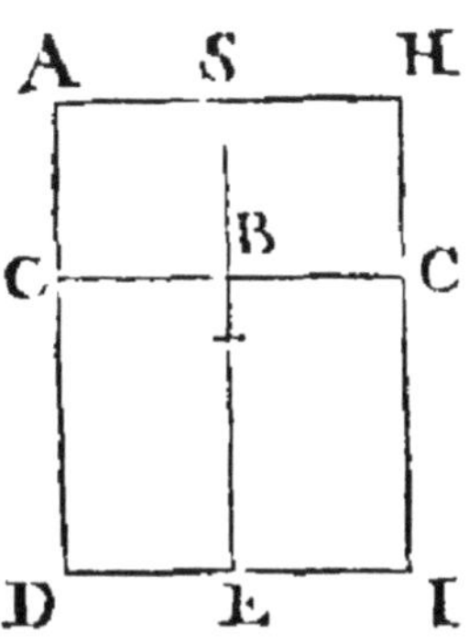

Let us now imagine the Parallelogram A H I D to oscillate or swing by the sole Force of its own Gravity about the Line A H, as an Axis, by which it is suspended, then the

Parallelogram may be conſidered as a compound Pendulum (that is, a Pendulum conſiſting of ſeveral Bodies, or Weights, fix'd together) which will perform an equal Number of Vibrations, in any given Space of Time, with a ſimple Pendulum conſiſting of one ſingle Body, or Weight, conſider'd as a Point, whoſe Length is equal to the Diſtance of the Center of Percuſſion from the Point of Suſpenſion, and which is impelled by a Force equal to that by which the Center of Percuſſion is impelled

For ſince all the Forces of the Parallelogram are united in the Center of Percuſſion, if we ſuppoſe the Parallelogram to be contracted into that Point, and the ſame Force to remain, it is manifeſt, that both Pendulums will be ſimple Pendulums, and becauſe they are agitated by equal Forces, their Vibrations muſt be Iſochronal. And as the Center of Oſcillation is a Point in the Axis of a Compound Pendulum, whoſe Diſtance from the Point of Suſpenſion is equal to the Length of a ſimple Pendulum iſochronal to the former, and as there is but one Point in the Parallelogram wherein all the Forces are united, there can be only one ſimple Pendulum, whoſe Vibrations, the Forces being equal, will be equal to that of the Parallelogram, and becauſe the Point in the Parallelogram, wherein all the Forces are united, determines the Length of the ſimple Iſochronal Pendulum, and is that Point wherein all the Forces are ſuppoſed to be united while it vibrates, and is therefore called the Center of Oſcillation, it follows, that the Center of Oſcillation and Percuſſion, in every Body, are the ſame; and conſequently the Method made uſe of for finding the one, will find the other alſo. Wherefore in

EXAM-

EXAMPLE III

Let it be required to find the Center of Percussion, or Oscillation, of an Isosceles Triangle A D E, *revolving, or oscillating about the Line* F H, *drawn parallel to the Base* D E, *and passing through the Vertex* A.

PUT A N $= a$, D E $= b$, A B $= x$, and C C $= y$, then will $y x$ be the Fluxion of the Mass, and because, from the the Property of the Triangle, as $x \; y \; a \; b$, therefore $y = \frac{x b}{a}$, and substituting this Value of y in the Expression $y x$, we shall have $\frac{b x x}{a}$ for the Fluxion of the Mass. This therefore being multiplied by the Velocity x, will give $\frac{b x x x}{a}$, for the Fluxion of the *Momentum*, and this being again multiplied by the same Velocity x, will give $\frac{b x x x x}{a}$ for the Fluxion of the Force, whose Fluent $\frac{b x^4}{4 a}$, being divided by $\frac{b x x x}{3 a}$, the Fluent of $\frac{b x x x}{a}$, the Fluxion of the *Momentum*, will give $\frac{3}{4} x$ for the Distance of the Center of Percussion, or Oscillation, of the Space C A C from the Axis of Rotation.

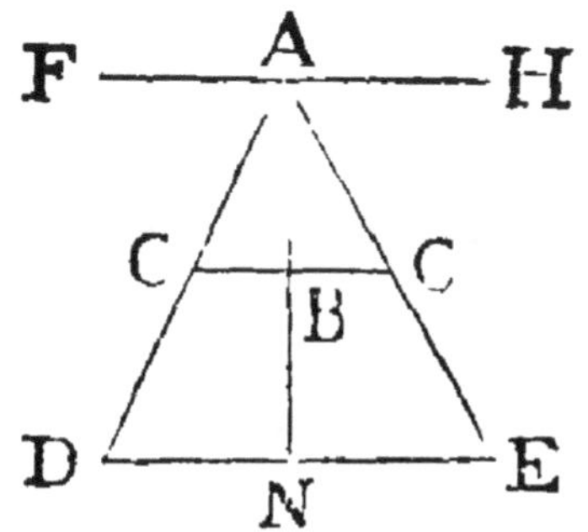

NOW if we conceive the Line C B C in a flowing State, and to move 'till it arrives at, or coincides with the Line D N E, then A B will become equal to A N, x will become equal to a, and we shall have $\frac{3}{4} a$ for the Distance of the Center of Percus-

 sion

ſion, or Oſcillation, of the Triangle A D E from the Point of Suſpenſion A, in the Axis of Rotation F A H.

AGAIN, let it be required to find the Center of Percuſſion, or Oſcillation, of the ſame Triangle A D E revolving about its Baſe D E.

PUT, as before, $AN = a$, $DE = b$, $CC = y$, $AB = x$, then will $BN = a - x$, becauſe $y\dot{x}$, the Fluxion of the Maſs, has been ſhewn in the former Part to be equal to $\frac{bx\dot{x}}{a}$. If this Expreſſion be multiplied by $a - x$, the Velocity in the preſent Caſe, we ſhall have $bx\dot{x} - \frac{bxx\dot{x}}{a}$ for the Fluxion of the *Momentum*, and multiplying this Fluxion again by the ſame Velocity $a - x$, we ſhall have $abx\dot{x} - 2bxx\dot{x} + \frac{bxxx\dot{x}}{a}$ for the Fluxion of the Force, whoſe Fluent $\frac{abxx}{2} - \frac{2bx^3}{3} + \frac{bx^4}{4a}$, being divided by $\frac{bxx}{2} - \frac{bx^3}{3a}$, the Fluent of $bx\dot{x} - \frac{bxx\dot{x}}{a}$, the Fluxion of the *Momentum* will give $\frac{6aa + 3xx - 8ax}{6a - 4x}$, for the Diſtance of the Center of Percuſſion, or Oſcillation, of the Trapezium D C C E from the Axis of Rotation D E, but if we conceive the Line C B C in a flowing State, and to move 'till it arrives at, or coincides with the Line D N E, then A B will become equal to A N, x will become equal to a, and we ſhall have (by putting a in the room of x, in the Expreſſion $\frac{6aa + 3xx - 8ax}{6a - 4x}$) $\frac{6aa + 3aa - 8aa}{6a - 4a} = \frac{9aa - 8aa}{2a} = \frac{1}{2}a$, or $\frac{1}{2}$ the Axis

A H,

A H, for the Distance of the Center of Percussion, or Oscillation, of the whole Triangle A D E.

EXAMPLE IV

Let it be required to find the Center of Percussion, or Oscillation, of a Parabolic Space E C A C E, *revolving or oscillating about the Line* H I, *parallel to its Base* E D E, *and passing through the* Vertex A *of the Figure.*

PUT A D $= a$, E E $= b$, A B $= x$, B C $= y$, then will $2\,y\,x$ be the Fluxion of the whole Mass but because from the Parabola $1\,x = y\,y$, therefore $y = x^{\frac{1}{2}}$, and $2\,y = 2\,x^{\frac{1}{2}}$ Substituting therefore this Value $2\,y$ in the Expression $2\,y\,x$, in the room of $2\,y$, and we shall have $2\,x^{\frac{1}{2}}\,x$, for the Fluxion of the Mass, which being multiplied by the Velocity x, will give $2\,x^{\frac{1}{2}+1}\,x$, for the Fluxion of the *Momentum*, and this again being multiplied by the same Velocity x, will $2\,x^{\frac{1}{2}+2}x$, for the Fluxion of the Force, whose Fluent $\frac{4}{7}\,x^{\frac{7}{2}}$, being divided by $\frac{4}{5}\,x^{\frac{5}{2}}$, the Fluent of $2\,x^{\frac{1}{2}+1}x$, the Fluxion of the *Momentum*, will give $\frac{5}{7}$ of x for the Distance of the Center of Percussion of the Space C A C B C from the Vertex A; but if we conceive the double Ordinate C B C in a flowing State, and to move 'till it arrives at, or coincides with the Base E D E, then A B will become equal to A D, x will become equal to a, and the Distance of the Center of Percussion, or Oscillation of the whole Parabolic Space E A E, from the Vertex A, will be $\frac{5}{7}\,a$, or $\frac{5}{7}$ A D, from the Point of Suspension A in the Axis of Rotation H A I.

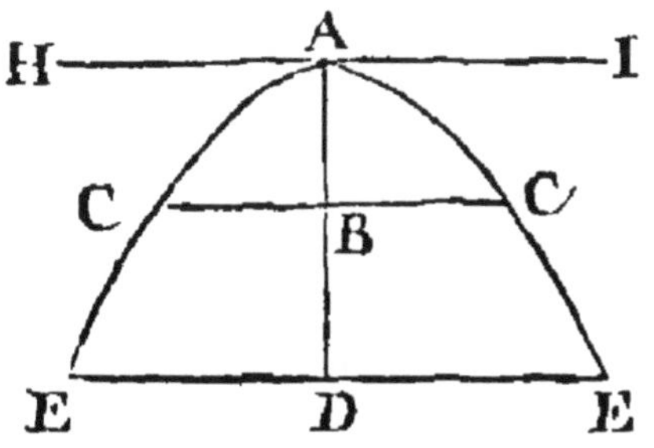

AND

AND universally if $x = y^m$, then $y = x^{\frac{1}{m}}$; whence we shall have $x^{\frac{1}{m}} \dot{x}$, for the Fluxion of the Mass. This being multiplied by x, the Velocity, will give $x^{\frac{1}{m}+1} \dot{x}$ for the Fluxion of the *Momentum*; this again being multiplied by the same Velocity x, will give $x^{\frac{1}{m}+2} \dot{x}$, for the Fluxion of the Force, whose Fluent $\frac{m}{3m+1} x^{\frac{1}{m}+3}$, being divided by $\frac{m}{2m+1} x^{\frac{1}{m}+2}$, the Fluent of $x^{\frac{1}{m}+1} \dot{x}$, the Fluxion of the *Momentum*, will give $\frac{2m+1}{3m+1} x$, for the Distance of the Center of Percussion, or Oscillation, of the Parabolic Space C A C B C from the Vertex A, but if we conceive the double Ordinate C B C in a flowing State, and to move 'till it arrives at, or coincides with the Base E D E, then A B will become equal to A D, x will become equal to a, and we shall have $\frac{2m+1}{3m+1} a$, for the Distance of the Center of Percussion, or Oscillation, of the whole Parabolic Space E A E, from the Point of Suspension A, in the Axis of Rotation H A I.

IF $m = 2$, as in the common Parabola, then $\frac{2m+1}{3m+1} a$, will be $\frac{4+1}{6+1} a = \frac{5}{7} a$.

IF $m = 3$, as in the Cubic Parabola, then $\frac{2m+1}{3m+1} a$, will be $\frac{6+1}{9+1} a = \frac{7}{10} a$.

IF $m = 4$, as in the Biquadratic Parabola, then $\frac{2m+1}{3m+1} a$, $= \frac{8+1}{12+1} a = \frac{9}{13} a$, &c.

LET

Let us now imagine the same Parabolic Space E C A C E to revolve about its Base E D E, then will D B $= a - x$, consequently $a x^{\frac{1}{2}} x - x^{\frac{1}{2}+1} x$, the Result of the Multiplication of $x^{\frac{1}{2}} x$ by $a - x$, the Velocity, will be the Fluxion of the *Momentum* This therefore being multiplied by $a - x$, the same Velocity, will give $a a x^{\frac{1}{2}} x - 2 a x^{\frac{1}{2}+1} x + x^{\frac{1}{2}+2} x$, for the Fluxion of the Force, the Fluent of which is $\frac{2}{3} a a x^{\frac{1}{2}+1}$

$$- \frac{4}{5} a x^{\frac{1}{2}+2} + \frac{2}{7} x^{\frac{1}{2}+3} = \frac{70 a a x^{\frac{1}{2}+1} - 84 a x^{\frac{1}{2}+2} + 30 x^{\frac{1}{2}+3}}{105}$$

which being divided by $\frac{10 a x^{\frac{1}{2}+1} - 6 x^{\frac{1}{2}+2}}{15}$, will give $\frac{35 a a - 42 a x + 15 x x}{35 a - 21 x}$ for the Distance of the Center of Percussion, or Oscillation, of the Parabolic Space E C C E from the Axis of Rotation E D E

But if we conceive the Line C B C in a flowing State, and to move 'till it arrives at, or coincides with the Line E D E, then A B will become equal to A D, x will become equal to a, and we shall have $\frac{35 a a - 42 a a + 15 a a}{35 a - 21 a} = \frac{8 a a}{14 a}$ $= \frac{4}{7} a$, for the Distance of the Center of Percussion, or Oscillation, of the whole Parabolic Space E A E from the Axis of Rotation.

Now if $y^m = x$, whence $y = x^{\frac{1}{m}}$, which is the general Equation for all kinds of Parabolas whatsoever, we shall have $x^{\frac{1}{m}} x$ for the Fluxion of the Mass, and this being multiplied by $a - x$, the Velocity, will give $a x^{\frac{1}{m}} x - x^{\frac{1}{m}+1} x$, for the Fluxion of the *Momentum* This being multiplied again by $a - x$, the same Velocity, will give $a a^{\frac{1}{m}} x - 2 a x^{\frac{1}{m}+1} x$ $+ x$

$+ x^{\frac{1}{m}+2}\dot{x}$, for the Fluxion of the Force, whose Fluent $\frac{m}{m+1}aax^{\frac{1}{m}+1} - \frac{2m}{2m+1}ax^{\frac{1}{m}+2} + \frac{m}{3m+1}x^{\frac{1}{m}+3}$, being divided by $\frac{m}{m+1}ax^{\frac{1}{m}+1} - \frac{m}{2m+1}x^{\frac{1}{m}+2}$, the Fluent of $ax^{\frac{1}{m}}x - x^{\frac{1}{m}+1}x$, the Fluxion of the *Momentum*, will give

$$\frac{\overline{6m^3+5mm+1m}\times aa - \overline{6m^3-5mm-2m}\times ax + \overline{2m^3-3mm+m}\times xx}{\overline{6m^3+5mm+1m}\times a - \overline{3m^3-4mm-m}\times x}$$

for the Distance of the Center of Percussion, or Oscillation, of the Parabolic Space E C C E revolving about the Base E D E as an Axis from the Point of Suspension, but when A B becomes equal to A D; that is, when the Line C B C, by flowing, arrives at, or coincides with the Line E D E, then x becomes equal to a, and we shall have $\frac{2m}{3m+1}a$, for the Distance of the Center of Percussion, or Oscillation, of the whole Parabolic Space E A E from the Axis of Rotation E D E.

If $m = 2$, as in the common Parabola, then $\frac{2m}{3m+1}a$, will give $\frac{4}{6+1}a = \frac{4}{7}a$, as in the former Example.

If $m = 3$, as in the Cubic Parabola, then $\frac{2m}{3m+1}a$, will give $\frac{6}{9+1}a = \frac{6}{10}a = \frac{3}{5}a$.

If $m = 4$, as in the Biquadratic Parabola, then $\frac{2m}{3m+1}a$, $= \frac{8}{12+1}a = \frac{8}{13}a$, &c.

EXAM-

EXAMPLE V.

Let it be required to find the Center of Percussion, or Oscillation, of the Space A D F, *inclosed between two equal Parabolic Curves* A C D, A C F, *touching one another in the Point* A, *and the right Line* D F, *parallel to the common Axis* E K, *about which it is supposed to revolve, or oscillate*

PUT A B $= y$, B C $= x$, A H $= a$, D H $= b$, then will $x\dot{y}$ be the Fluxion of the Space, but because, from the Property of the Curve, $x = yy$, if we substitute yy in the room of x, in the Expression $x\dot{y}$, we shall have $yy\dot{y}$ for the Fluxion of the Mass This therefore being multiplied by y, the Velocity, will give

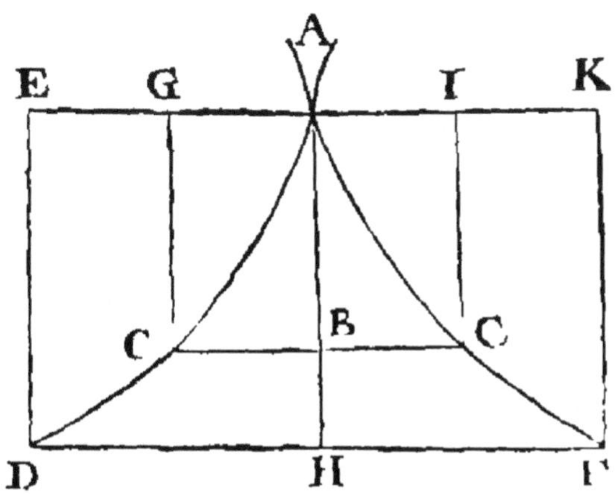

$y^3\dot{y}$ for the Fluxion of the *Momentum*, and being again multiplied by the same Velocity y, will give $y^4\dot{y}$ for the Fluxion of the Force, whose Fluent $\frac{1}{5}y^5$ being divided by $\frac{1}{4}y^4$, the Fluent of $y^3\dot{y}$, the Fluxion of the *Momentum*, will give $\frac{4}{5}y$ for the Distance of the Center of Percussion, or Oscillation, from the Point A of the Space C A C But if we conceive the Line C B C in a flowing State, and to move 'till it arrives at, or coincides with the Line D H F, then A B will become equal to A H, y will become equal to a, and we shall have $\frac{4}{5}a$ for the Distance of the Center of Percussion, or Oscillation, of the whole Space A D H F A, from E K the Axis of Rotation, or Oscillation

NOW if we suppose $x^n = y^m$, which is a general Equation for all Kinds of Parabolas, then $x = y^{\frac{m}{n}}$, whence $y^{\frac{m}{n}}\dot{y}$ will be the Fluxion of the Space, $y^{\frac{m}{n}+1}y$ the Fluxion of the *Momentum*, and $y^{\frac{m}{n}+2}y$, the Fluxion of the Force, whose Fluent $\frac{n}{m+3n}$ $y^{\frac{m}{n}+3}$, being divided by $\frac{n}{m+2n}y^{\frac{m}{n}+2}$, the Fluent of $y^{\frac{m}{n}+1}y$, the Fluxion of the *Momentum*, will give $\frac{m+2n}{m+3n}$ for the Distance of the Center of Percussion, or Oscillation, of the Space C A C from the Point A, but when C B C, by flowing, arrives at, or coincides with the Line D H F, then A B becomes equal to A H, y becomes equal to a, and we shall have $\frac{m+2n}{m+3n}a$, or A H, for the Distance of the Center of Percussion, or Oscillation, of the whole Space A D H F A, from the Axis of Rotation, or Oscillation, E A K

If $n=1$, and $m=2$, as in the common Parabola, then $\frac{m+2n}{m+3n}a=\frac{2+2}{2+3}a=\frac{4}{5}a$, will be the Distance of the Center of Percussion, or Oscillation, the same as was deduced from the preceding Investigation

If $n=2$, and $m=3$, as in the Cubic Parabola, then the Distance of the Center of Percussion, or Oscillation, from the Axis of Rotation, or Oscillation, will be $\frac{3+4}{3+6}a=\frac{7}{9}a$, &c.

SECT.

SECT. VIII.

Containing the Use of FLUXIONS *in finding the Centers of* Percussion, *or* Oscillation, *of* Solids.

THE Center of Percussion, or Oscillation, of a Solid in Motion will be always found in that Line in which the Center of Gravity is found. Wherefore in

EXAMPLE I.

Let it be required to find the Center of Percussion, or Oscillation, of a square Prism revolving, or oscillating, about one of its Extremities A.

PUT r for one Side of the Square of the Base, the Altitude $AD = a$, put $AB = x$, and $BC = y$, then will yyx be the Fluxion of the Mass, which being multiplied by the Velocity x, will give $yyxx$, for the Fluxion of the *Momentum*. This being multiplied again by the same Velocity x, will give $yyxxx$ for the Fluxion of the Force, whose Fluent $\frac{yyx^3}{3}$ being divided by $\frac{y^2xx}{2}$, the Fluent of y^2xx, the Fluxion of the *Momentum*, will give $\frac{2}{3}x$ for the Distance of the Center of Percussion, or Oscillation, from A the Point of Suspension of the Part ABC, but when the Point B, by flowing, arrives at, or coincides with the Point D, then x becomes equal to a, whence we shall have $\frac{2}{3}a$ for the Distance of the

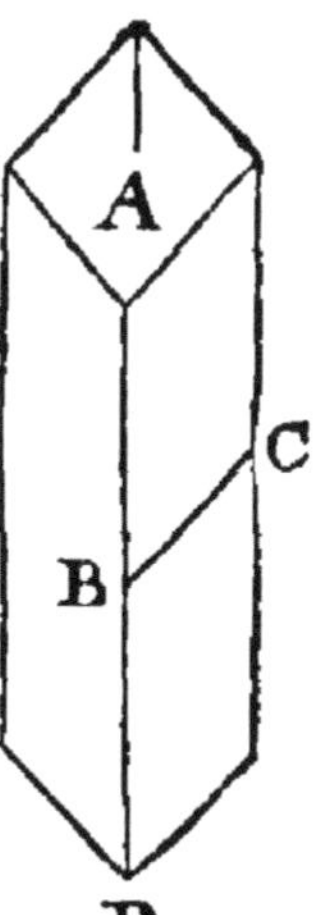

Center of Percussion, or Oscillation, of the whole Prism from the same Point A And the same Law will hold good in any other Prism, let the Base be of what Form soever, as will more evidently appear from the following Example

EXAMPLE II

Let it be required to find the Center of Percussion, or Oscillation, of a Cylinder suspended by one of its Extremities, about which it is supposed to revolve, or oscillate.

Let the Cylinder be suspended by the Extremity A of the Axis A B H, about which it is supposed to revolve, or oscillate Put A H $= a$, H E $=$ B C $= r$, and the Circumference of the Circle D H E $=$ C B C $= c$, then will $\frac{cr}{2}$ be the Area of the Circle generated by the Radius H E or B C. Put A B $= x$, then will $\frac{cr\dot{x}}{2}$ be the Fluxion of the Mass, or whole Weight, which being multiplied by x, the Velocity, will give $\frac{crx\dot{x}}{2}$ for the Fluxion of the *Momentum*, and this being again multiplied by the same Velocity x, will give $\frac{crxx\dot{x}}{2}$ for the Fluxion of the Force, whose Fluent will be $\frac{crxxx}{6}$. This being divided by $\frac{crxx}{4}$, the Fluent of $\frac{crx\dot{x}}{2}$, the Fluxion of the *Momentum,* will give $\frac{2}{3}x$ for the Distance of the Center of Percussion, or Oscillation, from A the Point of Suspension in the Axis

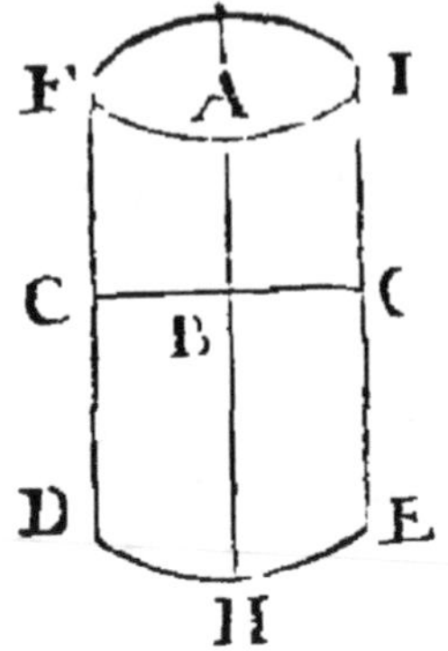

Axis A H of the Cylinder, which hath for its Altitude A B; but when the Point B, by flowing, arrives at, or is coincident with the Point H, then x becomes equal to a, and we shall have $\frac{2}{3}a$, or A H, for the Distance of the Center of Percussion, or Oscillation, of the whole Cylinder from the same Point of Suspension A.

EXAMPLE III.

Let it be required to find the Center of Percussion, or Oscillation, of a square Pyramid revolving, or oscillating, about an Axis H A F, *passing through the Vertex* A, *and parallel to the Base* D N E.

PUT A N $= a$, A B $= x$, C C $= y$, and D E $= r$, then will $y\dot{y}\dot{x}$ be the Fluxion of the Solid, but because, from the Nature of the Triangle D A E, it will be as $a : r :: x \; \frac{rx}{a} = y$; whence $yy = \frac{rrxx}{aa}$ Substituting this therefore in the Expression $yy\dot{x}$ in the room of yy, and we shall have

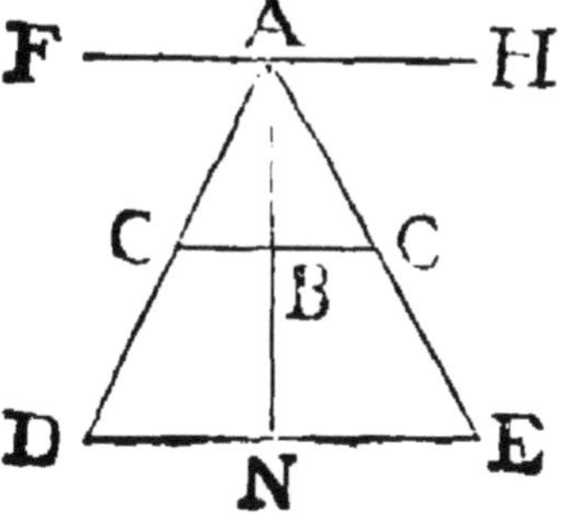

$\frac{rrxx\dot{x}}{aa}$ for the Fluxion of the Mass, which being multiplied by the Velocity x, will give $\frac{rrxxx\dot{x}}{aa}$ for the Fluxion of the *Momentum*, and this being again multiplied by x, will give $\frac{rrx^4\dot{x}}{aa}$ for the Fluxion of the Force, whose Fluent

rrx^5

$\frac{rrx^5}{5aa}$ being divided by $\frac{rrx^4}{4aa}$, the Fluent of $\frac{rrxxxx}{aa}$, the Fluxion of the *Momentum*, will give $\frac{4}{5}x$ for the Diſtance of the Center of Percuſſion of the Pyramid A C C from the Vertex A.

Now if we imagine the Line C B C in a State of flowing, and to move 'till it arrives at, or coincides with the Line D N E, then x will become equal to a, and we ſhall have $\frac{4}{5}a$ for the Diſtance of the Center of Percuſſion, or Oſcillation, of the whole Pyramid D A E from the Point of Rotation A. And the ſame Law will hold good, let the Baſe be of what Form ſoever, as will more evidently appear, if we ſuppoſe the Baſe to be a Circle, then will the Solid repreſent a Cone, as in the adjacent *Figure*, and let it be required to find the Center of Percuſſion, or Oſcillation, of this Solid revolving, or oſcillating, about an Axis H A I, paſſing through the Vertex A, and parallel to the Baſe E D E.

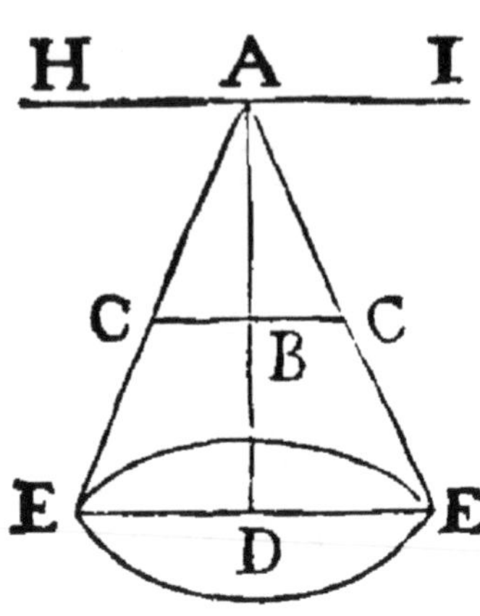

Put A D $= a$, D E $= r$, the Circumference of the Baſe E D E $= c$, A B $= x$, and B C $= y$; then will $\frac{cyy}{2r}$ be the Area of the Circle deſcribed by B C; and becauſe as $y : x :: r : a$, therefore $y = \frac{rx}{a}$, and $yy = \frac{rrxx}{aa}$. Subſtituting therefore $\frac{rrxx}{aa}$ in the Expreſſion $\frac{cyyx}{2r}$, in the room of yy, and we ſhall have $\frac{crxxx}{2aa}$ for the Fluxion of the Maſs. This therefore being multiplied by x, the Velocity, will give $\frac{crx^3x}{2aa}$ for the Fluxion

Fluxion of the *Momentum*, which being again multiplied by the same Velocity $\dot{x}$, will give $\frac{crx^4\dot{x}}{2aa}$ for the Fluxion of the Force, whose Fluent $\frac{crx^5}{10aa}$, being divided by $\frac{crx^4}{8aa}$, the Fluent of $\frac{crx^3\dot{x}}{2aa}$, the Fluxion of the *Momentum*, will give $\frac{4}{5}x$ for the Distance of the Center of Percussion, or Oscillation, from the Axis of Rotation of the Cone C A C.

Now if we conceive the Diameter C B C in a flowing State, and to move 'till it arrives at, or coincides with the Diameter E D E, then x will become equal to a, and we shall have $\frac{4}{5}a$ for the Distance of the Center of Percussion, or Oscillation, from A, the Vertex of the whole Cone, the same as in the Pyramid

EXAMPLE IV.

Let it be required to find the Center of Percussion, or Oscillation, of the same Cone A E F, *revolving, or oscillating, about its Base* E D L. (See the preceding Figure)

Put, as before, A D $= a$, DE $= r$, c for the Circumference of the Base, B C $= y$, and A B $= x$, then will B D $= a - x$, and as r c y $\frac{cy}{r}$, the Circumference described by the Point C, whence $\frac{cy}{2r} \times y = \frac{cyy}{2r}$ will be the Area of the same Circle, whence, because as a r x $\frac{rx}{a} = y$, whence $yy = \frac{rrxx}{aa}$, which being substituted in the Expression

pression $\frac{cyy}{2r}$, in the room of yy, will give $\frac{crxx}{2aa}$ for the Area of the same Circle, and this being multiplied by x, will give $\frac{crxx\dot{x}}{2aa}$, for the Fluxion of the Mass. This therefore being multiplied by $a-x$, will give $\frac{acrxx\dot{x}-crxxx\dot{x}}{2aa}$, for the Fluxion of the *Momentum*, and being again multiplied by the same Velocity $a-x$, will give $\frac{aacrxx\dot{x}-2acrx^3\dot{x}+2crx^4\dot{x}}{2aa}$, for the Fluxion of the Force, whose Fluent is $\frac{crx^3}{6}-\frac{crx^4}{4a}+\frac{crx^5}{10aa}$ $=\frac{10aacrx^3-15acrx^4+6crx^5}{60aa}$, which being divided by $\frac{4acrx^3-3crx^4}{24aa}$, the Fluent of $\frac{acrxx\dot{x}}{2aa}$ $-\frac{crxxx\dot{x}}{2aa}$, the Fluxion of the *Momentum*, will give $\frac{20aa-30ax+12xx}{20a-15x}$, for the Distance of the Center of Percussion, or Oscillation, from the Axis of Rotation H A I of the Frustum of the Cone E C C E, but if we imagine the Diameter C B C in a flowing State, and to move 'till it arrives at, or coincides with the Diameter E D E, then A B will become equal to A D, x will become equal to a, and we shall have $\frac{4}{5}a$ for the Distance of the Center of Percussion, or Oscillation, of the whole Cone E A E D E, from the Axis of Rotation E D E.

EXAM-

EXAMPLE V.

Let it be required to find the Center of Percussion, or Oscillation, of a Sphere revolving about, or oscillating, the Line P A M, *a Tangent, to the generating Circle* F A H *in the Point* A, *as an Axis*

IT is evident that the Center of Percussion, or Oscillation, will be found some where in the Diameter A D

PUT AB $= x$, BC $= y$, EF $= r$, and c for the Circumference of the great Circle of the Sphere,

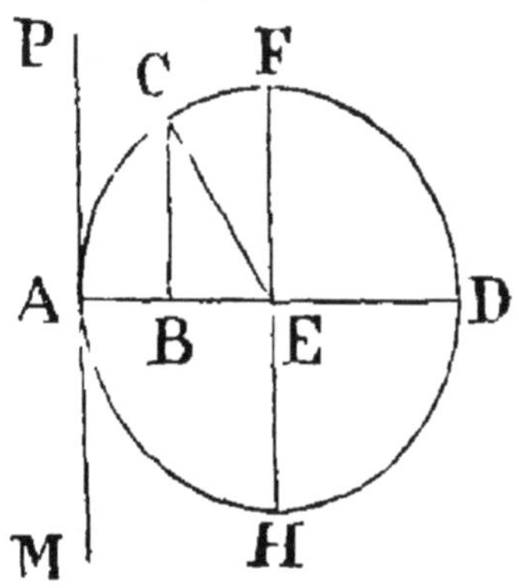

then will $\frac{cyy}{2r}$ be the Area of the Circle described by B C, equal to $\frac{2crx - cxx}{2r}$ (because yy is equal to $2rx - xx$), whence $\frac{2crx\dot{x} - cxx\dot{x}}{2r} = cx\dot{x} - \frac{cxx\dot{x}}{2r}$, will be the Fluxion of the Mass. This therefore being multiplied by the Velocity x, will give $cxx\dot{x} - \frac{cx^3\dot{x}}{2r}$, for the Fluxion of the *Momentum*, and this being again multiplied by the same Velocity x, will give $cx^3\dot{x} - \frac{cx^4\dot{x}}{2r}$, for the Fluxion of the Force, whose Fluent $\frac{cx^4}{4} - \frac{cx^5}{10r}$, being divided by $\frac{cxxx}{3} - \frac{cx^4}{8r}$, the Fluent of $cxx\dot{x} - \frac{cxxx\dot{x}}{2r}$, the Fluxion of the *Momentum,* will give $\frac{30rx - 12xx}{40r - 15x}$ for the Distance of the Center of Percussion, or Oscillation, of the Segment of the Sphere generated by the Semi-Segment of the Circle A B C, from the Axis of Rotation P A M

Now if we consider the Point B in a flowing State, and to move 'till it arrives at, or coincides with the Point D, then x will become $= 2r$, and $\frac{30rx - 12xx}{40r - 15r}$ will become $\frac{60rr - 48rr}{40r - 30r} = \frac{12rr}{10r} = \frac{6}{5}r$, for the Distance of the Center of Percussion, or Oscillation, of the whole Sphere from the Point of Rotation A, or $\frac{3}{5}$ of the whole Diameter A D

When the Point B, by flowing, arrives at E, the Center of the generating Circle, then x becomes equal to r, and $\frac{30rx - 12xx}{40r - 15x}$ will become equal to $\frac{18}{25}r$, which is the Distance of the Center of Percussion, or Oscillation, of the Hemisphere from the Point of Rotation A.

EXAMPLE VI.

Let it be required to find the Center of Percussion, or Oscillation, of a Parabolic Conoid revolving, or oscillating, about the Line AF *as an Axis, parallel to the Base* DE, *and passing through the Vertex* A.

It is manifest, that the Center of Percussion, or Oscillation, will be found somewhere in the Axis of the Solid A D

Put $AD = a$, $DE = b$, $AB = x$, $BC = y$, and c for the Circumference of the Base (*See the following Figure*), then will $\frac{cyy}{2r} = \frac{cx}{2r}$ (because $x = yy$) be the Area of the

Circle

Circle generated by B C, and $\frac{c x \dot{x}}{2r}$ be the Fluxion of the whole Mass; whence $\frac{c x x \dot{x}}{2r}$ will be the Fluxion of the *Momentum*, by multiplying $\frac{c x \dot{x}}{2a}$, by x the Velocity, and $\frac{c x^3 \dot{x}}{2r}$, the Fluxion of the Force, by multiplying $\frac{c x x \dot{x}}{2r}$ again by x the Velocity, whose Fluent $\frac{c x^4}{8r}$ being divided by $\frac{c x x x}{6r}$, the Fluent of $\frac{c x x \dot{x}}{2r}$, the Fluxion of the *Momentum*, will give $\frac{3}{4} x$ for the Distance of the Center of Percussion, or Oscillation, of the Solid generated by the Space A B C from the Axis of Rotation, but if we consider the Ordinate B C in a flowing State, and to move 'till it arrives at, or coincides with the Ordinate D E, then x will become equal to a, and we shall have $\frac{3}{4} a$ for the Distance of the Center of Percussion, or Oscillation, of the whole Solid from the Point of Rotation A.

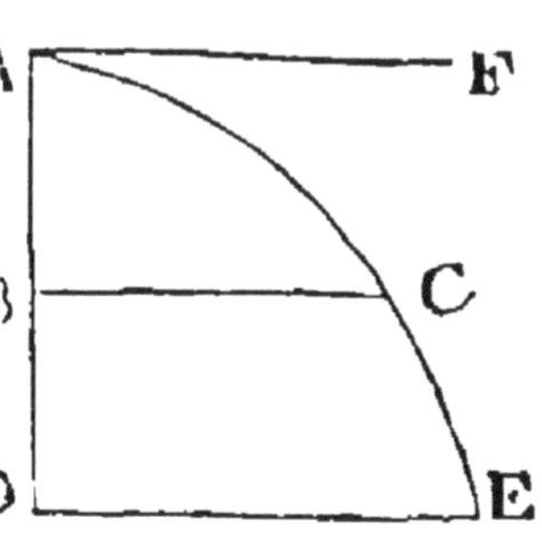

Now if $1 x = y^m$, whence $y = x^{\frac{1}{m}}$, which is the general Equation for all kinds of Parabolas, we shall have $y y = x^{\frac{2}{m}}$; and because $\frac{c y y}{2r}$ is equal to the Area of the Circle described by the Ordinate B C, if we substitute $x^{\frac{2}{m}}$ in the room of $y y$, in the Expression $\frac{c y y}{2r}$, we shall have $\frac{c x^{\frac{2}{m}}}{2r}$ for the Area of the same Circle, whence $\frac{c x^m \dot{x}}{2r}$, will be the Fluxion of the Mass

 This

This therefore being multiplied by the Velocity x, will give $\frac{c x^{\frac{2}{m}+1} x}{2 r}$ for the Fluxion of the *Momentum*, and being again multiplied by x, will give $\frac{c x^{\frac{2}{m}+2} x}{2 r}$, for the Fluxion of the Force, whose Fluent $\frac{m}{6 m + 4} \times \frac{c x^{\frac{2}{m}+3}}{r}$, being divided by $\frac{m}{4 m + 4} \times \frac{c x^{\frac{2}{m}+2}}{r}$, the Fluent of $\frac{c x^{\frac{2}{m}+1} x}{2 r}$, the Fluxion of the *Momentum*, will give $\frac{2 m + 2}{3 m + 2} x$ for the Distance of the Center of Percussion, or Oscillation, of the Solid formed by the Space A B C revolving about A B, from the Axis of Rotation A F; but when B C flows into, and becomes equal to D E, then x becomes equal to a, and we shall have $\frac{2 m + 2}{3 m + 2} a$, for the Distance of the Center of Percussion, or Oscillation, of the whole Solid from the Point of Rotation A.

If $m = 2$, as in the common Parabola, then $\frac{2 m + 1}{3 m + 1} a = \frac{5}{7} a$, will be the Distance required

If $m = 3$, as in the Cubic Parabola, then $\frac{2 m + 1}{3 m + 1} a, = \frac{7}{10} a$, will be the Distance required.

If $m = 4$, as in the Biquadrate Parabola, then $\frac{2 m + 1}{3 m + 1} a, = \frac{9}{13} a$, will be the Distance required, &c.

EXAM-

EXAMPLE VII.

Let it be required to find the Center of Percussion, or Oscillation, of a Spheroid (formed by the Rotation of a Semi-Ellipsis about its longer Axis) revolving, or oscillating, about A H *as the Axis of Motion, a Tangent to the Point* A.

It is evident the Center of Percussion, or Oscillation, will be found somewhere in the Axis of the Solid A D

Put FE $= r$, C B $= y$, A D $= 2a$, A B $= x$, then will $\frac{cyy}{2r}$ be the Area of the Circle described by the Ordinate B C, and $\frac{cyyx}{2r}$, the Fluxion of the Mass, equal to $\frac{2arcxx - crxxx}{2aa}$, because $yy = \frac{2arrx - rrxx}{aa}$, whence, by mul-

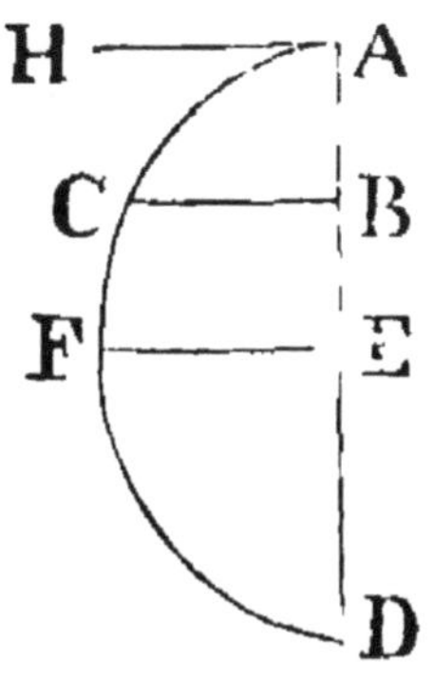

tiplying by the Velocity x, we shall have $\frac{2acrx^2x - crx^3x}{2aa}$ for the Fluxion of the *Momentum*, and multiplying this last Quantity again by the Velocity x, we shall have $\frac{2acrx^3x - crx^4x}{2aa}$ for the Fluxion of the Force, whose Fluent $\frac{crx^4}{4a} - \frac{crx^5}{10aa}$, being divided by $\frac{crx^3}{3a} - \frac{crx^4}{8aa}$, the Fluent of $\frac{2acrx^2x - crx^3x}{2aa}$, the Fluxion of the *Momentum*, will give $\frac{30ax - 12xx}{40a - 15x}$ for the Distance of the

† Center

Center of Percussion, or Oscillation, of the Segment of the Spheroid generated by the Semi-Segment of the Ellipsis ABC revolving about AB, but when the Point B, by flowing, arrives at D, then x becomes equal to $2a$; whence $\frac{30ax - 12xx}{40a - 15x}$, will become $\frac{60aa - 48aa}{40a - 30a} = \frac{12aa}{10a} = \frac{6}{5}a$ for the Distance of the Center of Percussion, or Oscillation, of the whole Spheroid from the Point of Rotation A

But because a is equal to the Semi-transverse Diameter, therefore $\frac{3}{5}$ of the whole Transverse Diameter AD will be the Distance of the Center of Percussion, or Oscillation, from the same Point of Rotation A.

When x becomes equal to a, that is, when the Point B arrives at the Center E, then $\frac{30aa - 12xx}{40a - 15x}$ will become $\frac{30aa - 12aa}{40a - 15a} = \frac{18aa}{25a} = \frac{18}{25}a$, whence we shall have $\frac{18}{25}$ of AE, the Semi-transverse Diameter, for the Distance of the Center of Percussion, or Oscillation, of the Semi Spheroid generated by the Space AEF revolving about AE, from the Point of Rotation A.

EXAMPLE VIII.

Let it be required to find the Center of Percussion, or Oscillation, of a Solid formed by the Rotation of the Semi-Hyperbolic Space ACFD, *about the Axis* AD, *the Solid being supposed to revolve or oscillate about the Line* AH *drawn through its* Vertex A, *parallel to the Base* DF.

Put $AD = a$, $AE = 2b$, $AB = x$, $BC = y$, $DF = r$, and c for the Circumference of the Circle described by the Point F (*See the following Figure*); then will $\frac{cyy}{2r}$ be the

Area

Area of the Circle describedby BC, whence $\frac{cy\dot{y}x}{2r}$ will be the Fluxion of the Solid But because, from the Nature of the Curve, $yy = \frac{rrxx + 2brrx}{aa + 2ab}$, if we substitute this Value of yy in the Expression $\frac{cyyx}{2r}$ in the room of yy, we shall have $\frac{crxxx + 2bcrxx}{2aa + 4ab}$ for the Fluxion of the Mass. This therefore being multiplied by x, will give $\frac{crx^3x + 2bcrx^2x}{2aa + 4ab}$ for the Fluxion of the *Momentum*; and this being again multiplied by the same Quantity x, will give $\frac{crx^4x + 2bcrx^3x}{2aa + 4ab}$ for the Fluxion of the Force, whose Fluent $\frac{crx^5}{10aa + 20ab} + \frac{bcrx^4}{4aa + 8ab} = \frac{2crx^5 + 5bcrx^4}{20aa + 40ab}$ being divided by $\frac{crx^4}{8aa + 16ab} + \frac{bcrx^3}{3aa + 6ab} = \frac{3crx^4 + 8bcrx^3}{24aa + 48ab}$, the Fluent of $\frac{crx^3\dot{x} + 2bcrx^2\dot{x}}{2aa + 4ab}$, the Fluxion of the *Momentum*, will give $\frac{12axx + 30bxa + 24bxx + 60bbx}{15ax + 30bx + 40ba + 80bb}$, for the Distance of the Center of Percussion, or Oscillation, of the Solid formed by the Revolution of the Space A B C, from the Axis of Rotation, or Oscillation, but if we

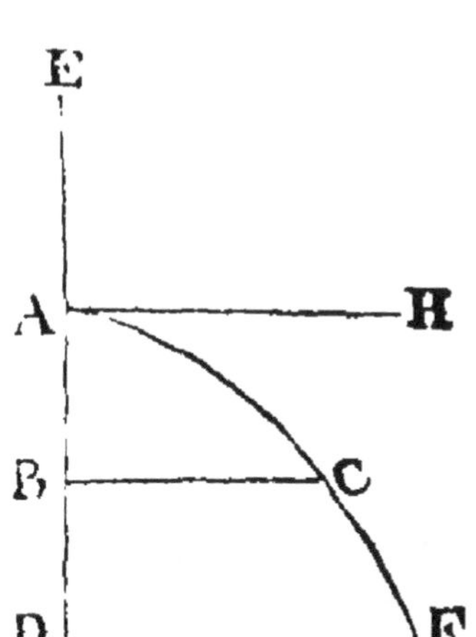

imagine

imagine the Ordinate B C in a flowing State, and to move 'till it arrives at, or coincides with the Ordinate D F, then A B will become equal to A D, and x will become equal to a, and we shall have $\frac{12aaa + 54aab + 60abb}{15aa + 70ab + 80bb}$, for the Distance of the Center of Percussion, or Oscillation, of the whole Solid from the Axis of Rotation, or Oscillation, *&c.*

EXAMPLE IX

Let it be required to find the Center of Percussion, or Oscillation, of a Cylinder oscillating or revolving about the Line N R N, *perpendicular to the Axis* A H *produced, and parallel to the Diameter* F I *and* D E *at the Top and Bottom.*

PUT R H $= a$, R A $= b$, and A B $= x$; then will R B $= b + x$, and A H $= a - b$ Now if we put c for the Circumference of the Circle C B C, and r for the Radius, we shall have $\frac{cr}{2}$ for the Area of the same Circle; whence $\frac{crx}{2}$ will be the Fluxion of the Mass. This being multiplied by $b + x =$ R B, the Velocity, will give $\frac{bcrx + crxx}{2}$ for the Fluxion of the *Momentum*, and this being again multiplied by the same Velocity $b + x$, will give $\frac{bbcrx + 2bcrxx + crxxx}{2}$ for the Fluxion of the Force, whose Fluent $\frac{bbcrx}{2} + \frac{bcrxx}{2} + \frac{crxxx}{6}$, being divided

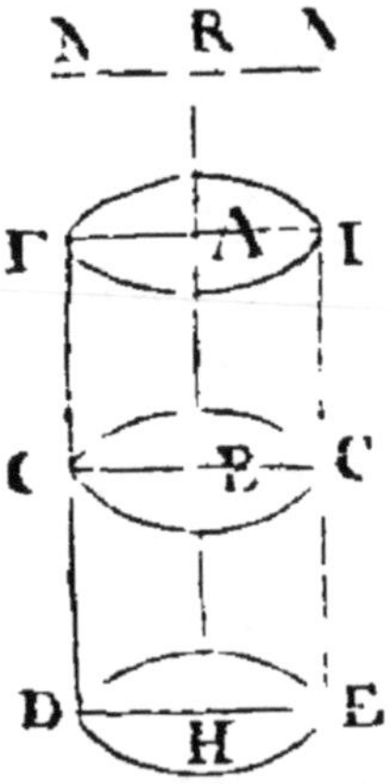

divided by $\frac{bcrx}{2} + \frac{crxx}{4}$, the Fluent of $\frac{bcr\dot{x} + crx\dot{x}}{2}$ the Fluxion of the *Momentum*, will give $\frac{6bb+6bx+2xx}{6b+3x}$ for the Distance of the Center of Percussion, or Oscillation, from the Axis of Rotation, or Oscillation, N R N, parallel to F I, or D E, of the Cylinder C I I C, which hath for its Altitude the Line A B; but if we imagine the Diameter C B C in a flowing State, and to move till it arrives at, or coincides with the Diameter D H E, then x will become equal to $a - b$, and we shall have $\frac{2aa+2ab+2bb}{3a+3b}$ for the Distance of the Center of Percussion, or Oscillation, of the whole Cylinder F I E D, and after the same manner may the Center of Percussion, or Oscillation, of any Surface, or Solid, be found, revolving, or oscillating about any Line, as N R N, drawn perpendicular to the Axis produced

THE celebrated Mr. *Huygens*, the first Man that adapted Pendulums to Clocks, in his *Horologium Oscillatorium*, published in the Year 1673, has shewn a Contrivance to make the Ball of a Pendulum, during its Vibration, to describe a Cycloid, and that is, by causing two Plates to be bent into the same Curvature, between which the Ball, being suspended by a Thread of a determined Length, will, by its oscillating Motion, describe a Curve of the same Kind For Example, if we suppose the two Plates P H A and P N C to be Semi-Cycloids, and the Pendulum to be suspended at the Point P, which while it oscillates, may apply itself to the Cycloidal Plates P H A and P N C, which it is supposed constantly to touch by the Application of the Thread to the Plates, the

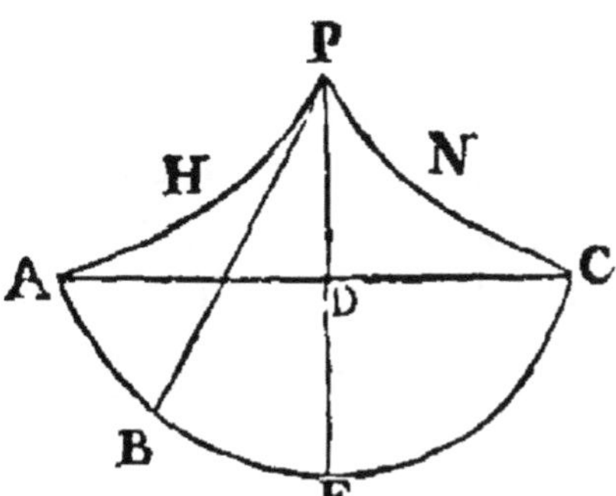

Motion of the Ball will be carried in the Curve A B E C, which Curve is described by the Evolution of the Cycloidal Curves P H A and P N C, and consequently will be a Cycloid, by *Example* VIII. *Sect* IV *Part* II. whose Axis is equal to E D, or P D, that is, to half the Length of the Pendulum; and that a Pendulum oscillating in this manner, whether it describes greater or less Arches, yet will perform its Vibrations in equal Times, may be demonstrated after the manner following.

LET H R B Q D represent a Semi-Cycloid inverted, and put H R, the Axis, or Height, equal to b, the Arch R B Q D of the Cycloid $= z$, and supposing Q the Point from whence the Pendulum begins to descend. Put P R, its Altitude, $= 2r$, also the Arch of the Semi-circle described about the Diameter P R $= c$; then putting P A $= x$, we shall have A R $= 2r - x$, and A N equal to $\overline{2rx - xx}|^{\frac{1}{2}}$, from the Nature of the Circle.

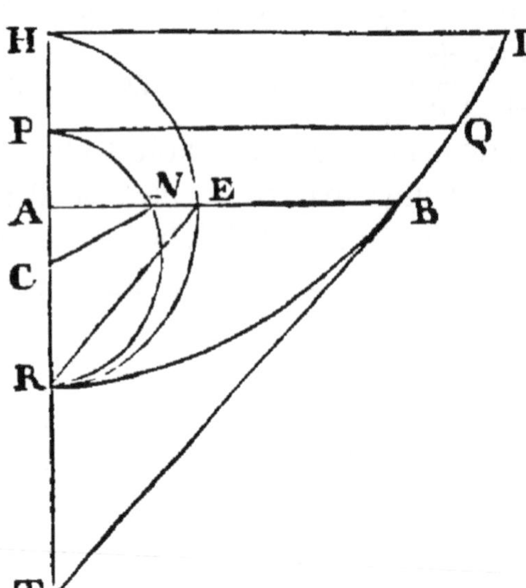

Now because the Velocity acquired by a falling Body, is as the Square Root of its perpendicular Descent, and as the same Body will acquire the same Velocity in descending through the Arch Q B, as it does in descending through its perpendicular Height P A, therefore the Velocity of the Pendulum in the Point B will be $x^{\frac{1}{2}}$; whence putting t for the time of the Descent through the Arch D Q B R, we shall have $\dot{t} = \frac{\dot{z}}{x^{\frac{1}{2}}}$. But from the Nature of the Cycloid, R E is parallel to T B, a Tangent to the Curve in the Point B, therefore the Triangles T B A

and

and R E A will be similar; consequently as T B · TA ∷ RE : RA, but (by *Proposition* II. *Section* I. *Part* III.) as $\dot{z} : \dot{x}$ ∷ TB : TA, therefore by Equality of Ratios, as $\dot{z} : \dot{x}$ ∷ RE : RA. Again, because the Lines HR, R E, and R A are continual Proportionals, therefore as R E : R A ∷ $\overline{HR}^{\frac{1}{2}} : \overline{AR}^{\frac{1}{2}}$; whence $\dot{z} : \dot{x} ∷ \overline{HR}^{\frac{1}{2}} : \overline{AR}^{\frac{1}{2}}$, or as $\overline{b}^{\frac{1}{2}} : \overline{2r-x}^{\frac{1}{2}}$, consequently $\dot{z} = \frac{\dot{x} \times \overline{b}^{\frac{1}{2}}}{\overline{2r-x}^{\frac{1}{2}}}$, and $\dot{t} = \frac{\dot{z}}{\overline{x}^{\frac{1}{2}}}$, will be equal to $\frac{\dot{x} \times \overline{b}^{\frac{1}{2}}}{\overline{2rx-xx}^{\frac{1}{2}}}$ $= \frac{2r\dot{x} \times \overline{b}^{\frac{1}{2}}}{2r \times \overline{2rx-xx}^{\frac{1}{2}}} = \frac{2 \times \overline{b}^{\frac{1}{2}}}{2r} \times \frac{r\dot{x}}{\overline{2rx-xx}^{\frac{1}{2}}}$; and because (by *Proposition* II. *Section* I. *Part* III.) as $\dot{c} : \dot{x}$ ∷ CN : N A, that is, as $r : \overline{2rx-xx}^{\frac{1}{2}}$, whence $\dot{c} = \frac{r\dot{x}}{\overline{2rx-xx}^{\frac{1}{2}}}$, if we substitute $\dot{c}$ in the room of $\frac{r\dot{x}}{\overline{2rx-xx}^{\frac{1}{2}}}$ in the Expression $\frac{2r\dot{x} \times \overline{b}^{\frac{1}{2}}}{2r \times \overline{2rx-xx}^{\frac{1}{2}}}$, we shall have $\dot{t} = \frac{2 \times \overline{b}^{\frac{1}{2}} \times \dot{c}}{2r}$, whence $t = \frac{2 \times b^{\frac{1}{2}} \times c}{2r}$, consequently $t \times 2r = 2b^{\frac{1}{2}} \times c$, whence as $t : b^{\frac{1}{2}} ∷ 2c : 2r$, but $\overline{b}^{\frac{1}{2}} = \frac{b}{b^{\frac{1}{2}}}$ = to the Time of the perpendicular Descent through the Axis H R, therefore the Time of an whole Oscillation through any Arch of a Cycloid is to the Time of the Descent through the Axis, as the Circumference of a Circle is to its Diameter, that is, in a constant Ratio, whence it follows, that the Vibrations of a Pendulum, whose Ball moves in the Curve of a Cycloid (whether it describes greater or less Arches) are Isochronal.

AND hence we see the Reason why the Times of Oscillation of a Pendulum performing small Vibrations in a Circle are equal, for since the Portion of the Cycloid near the Vertex E (*See the Figure in Pag* 449.) is described by the Motion of a Thread, whose Length is PE) revolving about the Point P, and since a Circle, whose Center is P, and Radius PE, almost coincides with the Portion of the Cycloid, near the Vertex, it follows, that a heavy Body will descend through small Arches of a Circle, whose Radius is equal to twice the Length of the Axis of the Cycloid, in the same Time nearly as it would do through small Arches of a Cycloid nearly coinciding with it.

WHEREFORE since the Time wherein a Pendulum performs a very small Oscillation in a Circle is equal to the Time wherein an Oscillation is performed through the Arch of a Cycloid, whose Axis is equal to half the Length of the Pendulum, and since the Time wherein an Oscillation is performed in a Cycloid, is to the Time of the perpendicular Fall through the Axis of the Cycloid equal to half the Length of the Pendulum, as the Circumference of a Circle is to its Diameter, it follows, that the Time of the smallest Oscillation is to the Time of the Fall through the Length of the Pendulum, as the Circumference of a Circle is to its Diameter, multiplied by the Square Root of the Number 2, since the Velocities acquired by falling Bodies, are in a Subduplicate Ratio of their perpendicular Descents, and hence it is manifest, that the smaller the Vibrations, the more Isochronal they will be

THE Copiousness of this Subject having swelled the Book more than I expected, the farther Use and Application of this *Doctrine* shall be published at a convenient Time

[ ]

THE

INDEX.

A

The INDEX.

—*In*

The INDEX.

—*In*

The INDEX.

2 *An*

The INDEX.

The INDEX.

Methods

The INDEX.

—*In*

The INDEX.

—*In*

The INDEX.

—*In*

The INDEX.

FINIS.

Lightning Source UK Ltd.
Milton Keynes UK
UKHW031958280219
338227UK00006B/361/P